Scientific and Technical Publication No. 582

Investment in Health

Social and
Economic Returns

Produced in collaboration with

 The Inter-American Development Bank and

 The World Bank

PAN AMERICAN HEALTH ORGANIZATION
Pan American Sanitary Bureau,
Regional Office of the
WORLD HEALTH ORGANIZATION
525 23rd Street, N.W.
Washington, D.C. 20037 U.S.A.

Also published in Spanish with the title:
Invertir en salud. Beneficios sociales y económicos
ISBN 92 75 31582 5

PAHO Cataloguing in Publication Data

Pan American Health Organization
    Investment in health: social and economic returns — Washington, D.C.: PAHO, © 2001.
viii, 284 p. — (Scientific and Technical Publication No. 582)

ISBN 92 75 11582 6

I.   Title   II.   Series
III.   Author
1.   HEALTH ECONOMICS
2.   HUMAN DEVELOPMENT
3.   EQUITY
4.   POVERTY
5.   SOCIAL CONDITIONS
6.   SUSTAINABLE DEVELOPMENT

NLM W74.P187i

CONTENTS

APPENDIX

PROLOGUE

The Pan American Health Organization (PAHO) as a whole, and myself in particular, have been concerned with the relationship between health and the economy for quite some time. When we first shared this concern with Enrique Iglesias, President, and Nancy Birdsall, then-Executive Vice-President of the Inter-American Development Bank (IDB), both concurred with us on the necessity to further analyze the different dimensions involved in this relationship. We then decided to implement two coordinated research projects: the first, sponsored by PAHO, dealt with the impact of health on economic growth; the second, promoted by IDB, focused on the impact of health on household productivity.

Encouraging reactions also emerged when we discussed this issue with the Economic Commission of Latin America and the Caribbean (ECLAC), the World Bank, and the United Nations Development Program (UNDP). As a result, a third research project—on investment in health, equity, and poverty reduction—was then launched as a joint initiative between PAHO, the World Bank and UNDP. This book summarizes the results of all three research projects.

In reiterating our gratitude to these organizations for their support, I hope that we will continue to work together and support the efforts of our member states towards bringing better health to their populations and, thus, contributing to their human development.

The researchers from Latin America and the Caribbean who carried out the studies reported here include economists interested in health issues, as well as health specialists interested in the broader consequences of good health. I thank them for their cooperation, and hope to continue to have them as our allies in the search for the explanations of the relationship between health and human development.

The results of these studies reaffirm what some of us in the health field have always believed to be true but could not always verify: the positive, still unquantified contribution of health to different dimensions of human development. They show that good health allows nations to accelerate their economic performance, and conversely that disease is an obstacle to development. They also show that household productivity benefits from health improvements and demonstrate how the reduction of health inequalities can contribute to poverty alleviation.

These findings open new possibilities for further exploring the role of health in human development, as well as opportunities for a better policy dialogue between health and development authorities. This dialogue will, I hope, benefit the people of the Americas.

George A. O. Alleyne
Director of the Pan American Sanitary Bureau

INTRODUCTION

This publication brings together the final reports from three research projects that explored how investments in health affected economic growth, household productivity, and poverty alleviation in Latin America and the Caribbean. The projects were carried out in 1998 and 1999, and came about through the coordinated efforts of the Pan American Health Organization (PAHO), the Inter-American Development Bank (IDB), the United Nations Development Program (UNDP), the United Nations Economic Commission for Latin America and the Caribbean (ECLAC), and the World Bank.

The first project was designed to explore the extent to which improvements in a population's health can help grow the national economy. PAHO's Research Grants Program called for research proposals on the topic based on terms of reference prepared by Harvard University Professor Robert Barro. Subsequently, a specially convened committee integrated by Dr. Barbara Stalling, ECLAC's Director of the Economic Development Division; Professor Maximo Vega Centeno, President, of the Latin American Econometric Society; and Professor José Luis Estrada, Autonomous University of Mexico, worked with PAHO to review the seventeen research proposals submitted by economic and health research centers from throughout the Region in response to this call. The selected proposal was submitted by a group constituted by two Mexican institutions—Centro de Investigación y Docencia Económicas (CIDE) and Fundación Mexicana para la Salud (FUNSALUD)—and one organization from Colombia—Fundación para la Educación Superior y el Desarrollo (FEDESARROLLO). The second project examined the effect of health improvements on household productivity. Sponsored by IDB, the project was based on terms of reference prepared by Professor T. Paul Schultz of Yale University and was carried out through IDB's Network of Research Centers. It involved six studies conducted in Colombia, Mexico, Nicaragua, and Peru.[1] The third project—"Investment in Health, Equity and Poverty" (IHEP/EquiLAC)—addressed issues of equity and poverty alleviation and was inspired on a similar study sponsored by the Organization for Economic Cooperation and Development (OECD) in the early 1990s.[2] Sponsored by PAHO, UNDP, and the World Bank the project conducted country studies in Brazil, Ecuador, Guatemala, Jamaica, Mexico, and Peru that were coordinated by José Vicente Zevallos from UNDP, Rubén Suarez from the World Bank, and Edward Greene from PAHO. In October 1999, experts in economics, social development, and health, as well as representatives from international and cooperation organizations, met at PAHO headquarters in Washington, D.C., to review the impact of investments in health on economic growth, household productivity, and poverty reduction. Reports from the

---

[1] A book with the all the reports from this project has been published by IDB: Savedoff W, Schultz T P. eds. *Wealth from Health: Linking Social Investments to Earnings in Latin America.*, Washington: IDB; 2000.

[2] Van Doorslaer, E., Wagstaff, A., and Rutten, F., eds., *Equity in the Finance and Delivery of Health Care: An International Perspective"*, Oxford Univwersity Press, NY, 1993.

three above-mentioned projects and their respective policy implications were presented and discussed at that time.

This book's structure mirrors the agenda for the October 1999 meeting. Part I presents the final report of the study "Investment in Health and Economic Growth," authored by the researchers who carried out the work. Part II includes the Colombia, Mexico, and Peru studies from the "Productivity of Household Investment in Health" project. And Part III presents the ten country case reports from the IHEP/EquiLAC project, plus a review paper, two works on methodological issues, and a review of experiences from other regions in the world regarding health inequalities and poverty alleviation. Finally, the book's annex includes the inaugural speech given by Dr. George A. O. Alleyne, Director of the Pan American Sanitary Bureau, at the opening of the October 1999 meeting; the meeting's agenda and list of participants; and a summary of discussions.

PAHO would like to acknowledge the efforts of the various groups and individuals that contributed to make this venture a success. We are especially grateful to our colleagues at IDB, ECLAC, UNDP, and the World Bank for working so closely with us to develop and review the studies published here. We also wish to commend the researchers' efforts to complete their reports under conditions that made a sometimes difficult task even more arduous. Third, we want to thank the participants at the October 1999 meeting, particularly for their recommendations regarding the future steps to be taken in this area. Finally, we want to acknowledge the work of the Organization's Public Policy and Health Program, Research Coordination Program, Publications Program, and Public Policy and Health Program for helping make this book a reality.

Health, Growth, and Income Distribution in Latin America and the Caribbean: A Study of Determinants and Regional and Local Behavior[1]

David Mayer,[2] Humberto Mora,[3] Rodolfo Cermeño,[4] Ana Beatriz Barona,[5] and Suzanne Duryeau[6]

INTRODUCTION

In recent years, Latin American and Caribbean countries have undergone an economic rationalization process in an attempt to achieve high levels of sustainable growth. Under these circumstances, important long-term policy decisions have arisen in the area of health investment. Although much attention is given to the problems of health-sector restructuring and efficiency, it is essential to determine how health affects economic growth, income distribution dynamics, and education. It also is necessary to determine the best health indicators and to identify possible policy proposals. We raise the following general questions:

- What is the importance of health in economic growth as an input for production?
- What is the importance of the distribution of health in terms of the distribution of income and economic growth?
- To what extent is health involved in the formation of educational capital resources in the different sectors of the population?
- What is the causal relationship between economic growth and health?
- What is the importance of the quality of health indicators in measuring the effects indicated above?

To answer these questions, we use several analytical frameworks developed in the field of economics. Our research ranges from studying the most aggregate relationships between socioeconomic and demographic variables at the country level to more disaggregated approaches to these relationships for specific population groups in a given country. We analyze the relationship between health and economic development as well as income distribution and the demographic transition in five studies with complementary analytical contexts.[7]

The quality of the data is fundamental to these studies. In particular, the health indicators were prepared specifi-

[1] Research report submitted by CIDE-FEDESARROLLO-FUNSALUD to the Pan American Health Organization. This project was the winner of the 1997 Regional Research Competition *Investment in Health and Economic Development*. The authors thank the following persons for their work in gathering health information on Mexico, Brazil, and Colombia, respectively: Rafael Lozano, Fundación Mexicana para la Salud (FUNSALUD, or Mexican Foundation for Health) and World Health Organization (WHO), Department of Epidemiology and Burden of Disease, Office 3070, CH-1211 Geneva 27, Switzerland; phone: (+41-22) 791-3623; fax: (+41-22) 791-4194, 791-4328; email: *lozanor@who.ch*. María Helena Prado de Mello Jorge, Professor at the University of São Paulo, School of Public Health, Department of Epidemiology, Avenida Dr. Arnaldo, 715, BRA-01246-904 São Paulo, SP, Brazil; phone: (+55-11) 282-3886; fax: (+55-11) 282-2920; email: *mphjorge@usp.br*. Henry Mauricio Gallardo, Specialist in Health Administration and Head of the Health Area, Corona Foundation, Calle 100 No. 8A-55, 9th floor, Tower C, Bogotá, Colombia; phone: (+57-1) 610-5555; fax: (+57-1) 610-7620; email: *hgallard@corona.com.co*.

[2] Researcher at the Centro de Investigación y Docencia Económicas, A.C. (CIDE, or Center for Research and Economic Studies), Economics Department, Carretera México-Toluca (Km. 16.5), No. 3655, Apartado Postal 10-883, Colonia Lomas de Santa Fé, Delegación Alvaro Obregón, MEX-01210 Mexico City, Mexico; phone: (+52-5) 727-9800; fax: (+52-5) 727-9878; email: *mayerfou@dis1.cide.mx*.

[3] Associate Researcher at FEDESARROLLO, Calle 78 No. 9-91, Santafé de Bogotá, Colombia; phone: (+57-1) 312-5300 or 530-3717, Ext. 310; fax: (+57-1) 212-6073; email: *hmora@fedesarrollo.org.co*.

[4] Researcher at the Centro de Investigación y Docencia Económicas, A.C. (CIDE, or Center for Research and Economic Sciences), Economics Department, Carretera México-Toluca (Km. 16.5), No. 3655, Apartado Postal 10-883, Colonia Lomas de Santa Fé, Delegación Alvaro Obregón, MEX-01210 Mexico City, Mexico; phone: (+52-5) 727-9800; fax: (+52-5) 727-9878; email: *rcermeno@ dis1.cide.mx*.

[5] Assistant Researcher at FEDESARROLLO, Calle 78 No. 9-91, Santafé de Bogotá, Colombia; phone (+57-1) 312-5300.

[6] Economist at the Inter-American Development Bank (IDB), 1300 New York Avenue, N.W., Stop W-0436, Office SW-404, Washington, D.C. 20577, USA; phone: (+202) 623-3589; fax: (+202) 623-2481; email: *suzanned@psc.lsa.umich.edu*.

[7] The full text of each of the studies summarized in this document is available from the Pan American Health Organization, Public Policy and Health Program, 525 Twenty-third Street, N.W., Washington, D.C. 20037, or visit http://www.paho.org.

cally for this project and are very high quality. We also assembled the detailed information required for the more disaggregate analysis of specific aspects of the relationship between economic growth and health. We constructed four databases of economic and health indicators—one by country for Latin America and the Caribbean and three by states (or department) for Mexico, Brazil, and Colombia.[8] In the case of Brazil, the economic database is organized by income deciles.

In the first study, the econometric framework uses functional specifications of the economic growth equations, such as those used by Barro (1996) and others,[9] which incorporate few constraints derived from economic theory. These functional specifications include health among an extensive list of other socioeconomic, demographic, and institutional variables that, in theory, may be associated with economic growth. We apply the methodology of Levine and Renelt (1992) to test for the robustness of these results. The second section of this paper contains the results of this analysis for the four databases.

In the second study (third section), the relationship between economic growth and human capital is evaluated in an analytical framework including far more restrictive constraints in the functional specification, which correspond to the augmented Solow model as developed by Mankiw et al. (1992) and applied by Islam (1995). In our specification, human capital is determined not only by education, as in the model used by these authors, but also by health. This analysis is applied to the four databases.

In the third study (fourth section) we analyze the long-term relationship between health and income for the case of Mexico, taking advantage of the length of the time period covered by the database. The analytical framework is similar to the one used by Barro (1996). However, it focuses on the causal relationship between health and income, using Granger's causality methodology to analyze the determinants of income growth and health improvement.

In the fourth study (fifth section), we study the role of health in the economic and demographic dynamics of Brazil. In this case, we take into account the different income levels, exploiting this aspect of the information contained in the Brazilian database. In particular, we examine the simultaneous relationship between economic growth, health, education, participation in the workforce, and fertility for the different income groups in Brazil.

In the fifth study (sixth section), which is similar to the study carried out for Mexico, we analyze the long-term effects of health on income growth for Latin America. This study also shares characteristics with the Brazilian study in terms of the health indicators used. The consistency of the results with those of the other two studies strengthens the hypothesis that the phenomena observed in Mexico and Brazil also occur for other Latin American countries.

Conclusions and policy recommendations are found in the last section.

HEALTH IN THE ECONOMIC GROWTH OF LATIN AMERICA

This component of the study conducts an empirical analysis of the impact of health capital on economic growth in the countries of Latin America and the Caribbean. Our point of departure is a verification of Barro's results (1996) for the worldwide sample of countries. We use three methodological approaches to address our objectives.

The first seeks to identify the existing correlation between alternative measures of health and economic growth, for which we empirically evaluate statistical models for growth similar to those formulated by Barro (1996). The measures of health used correspond to those available for a broad sample of Latin American countries. This is done to compare the results from Barro's global sample of countries (1996) with those obtained for Latin America.

To supplement the above information, the second approach seeks to analyze extreme limits of the type applied by Levine and Renelt (1992), in order to assess by econometric methods the strength of the results obtained from the Barro-type specifications. Specifically, the strength of the correlation between the variables of health capital and economic growth was analyzed.

Third, an effort was made to include in the analyses health measurements that are much more precise than those available for a broad sample of countries. These more precise measurements correspond to mortality by cause and/or years of life lost due to premature death (YLPD). To this end, the analysis described was carried out at two geographic levels. This was done first for a group of Latin American countries, in order to observe the performance of the Region in general and the impact of health capital on the economic performance of these countries in particular, using the available health indicators. Traditionally, intercountry analyses have used the variables of life expectancy at birth and infant mortality as health measures; these variables represent a highly aggregate measure. The second geographic level corresponds to a significantly more limited subset of coun-

---

[8] The information on health was prepared by Rafael Lozano, Fundación Mexicana para la Salud (FUNSALUD); Suzanne Duryeau, Inter-American Development Bank (IDB); María Helena Prado de Mello Jorge, Department of Epidemiology, University of São Paulo, Brazil; and Henry Mauricio Gallardo, Corona Foundation, Colombia.

[9] For an extensive list of works on economic growth that analyze the effect of different variables of interest, see, for example, Levine and Renelt (1992).

tries in the Region—specifically, Brazil, Colombia, and Mexico—where the most precise health indicators are available. In these cases, the analysis is performed by departments or states within each country.

Correlation between Economic Growth and Health

Health is a very important element in the formation of human capital. As Barro stated (1996), it is to be expected that its effect on economic growth is produced by the direct impact on human capital stock and a reduction in the rate of depreciation.

This section, using functional specifications similar to those of Barro (1996), summarizes the principal results obtained from evaluation of this relationship at the different geographic levels mentioned above.

When the geographic area changes, the available data change as well, particularly the data on health. Thus, it is not always possible to compare the effect of a single measurement of health on growth among different geographic areas. In addition, there are variables for which information cannot be obtained by department or state for a particular country.

Table 1 shows the main results of estimating growth models by three-stage least-squares analysis. As a point of departure in this research, an attempt was made to reproduce the results of Barro (1996), as recorded in the first column of Table 1. That study, using a sample of 138 countries worldwide, found that economic growth calculated for three periods (1965–1975, 1975–1985, and 1985–1990) correlates positively with schooling for males, the terms of trade, and variables that measure the level of democracy and the rule of law in countries. Moreover, health capital, represented by the variable of life expectancy at birth, shows a positive correlation with economic growth.

The second column shows the results of reestimating that model. Although Barro's results (1996) are not exactly reproducible, with the data used most of the variables included by Barro are indeed significant. However, there may be room to improve the quality of the sample and thus eliminate possible problems of bias in the estimations. Specifically, the rate of inflation did not turn out to be significant and the significance of the other variables proved to be less than in Barro's model.

The third column shows the results of estimating Barro's model for the sample of countries in Latin America and the Caribbean. Several of the correlations found in the sample of countries worldwide persist. Nonetheless, there are several variables, such as schooling, that traditionally have been identified as being closely linked to growth but that do not turn out to be significant. The indexes of democracy and inflation are also insignificant.

In addition, the fourth column shows the result of considering male life expectancy, with a lag of 15 years, for the Latin American and Caribbean countries. That variable is highly correlated with growth. The study sought to establish the lagged effect of health on growth over time. Unfortunately, information was not available for previous periods that would allow us to study this relationship to obtain more precise measurements of health. The sample of Latin American and Caribbean countries is the only sample in which that analysis could be carried out, although highly aggregate health indicators were used, as shown in the corresponding column of Table 1. These results are consistent with those on causality shown in the chapter on the reciprocal impact of health and growth in Mexico.

As mentioned previously, the most precise indicators of health are those available for the departments or states of a subgroup of Latin American countries (Brazil, Colombia, and Mexico). Unfortunately, the price of having greater precision in measuring health is not having information about other variables identified as being associated with growth at the country level. This is the main reason why several of the variables included in the growth equation for the sample of countries worldwide, or for Latin America and the Caribbean, are not included in the results in columns five through seven of Table 1.

In the case of Brazil and Colombia, information could be obtained on YLPD by cause of death. This variable, as well as the variable of schooling, is closely linked with growth. In the case of Mexico, information on mortality could be obtained only by cause; this is also highly correlated with growth, as shown in the last column of Table 1. The extended report shows the correlation between economic growth and other health variables by age groups and causes of death or causes of YLPD.

The above results indicate that, regardless of the sample of countries used, health and education are variables closely linked with the growth of national or local economies, at least in the functional specifications of Barro-type models. Policies aimed at achieving greater economic growth must necessarily affect the channels that influence the formation of greater human capital through health and education.

Analysis of Extremes

The analyses of extreme limits developed by Levine and Renelt (1992) evaluate the validity of the empirical results obtained from a given specification of the growth equation when the conditional set of data in that equation is modified.

TABLE 1. Contribution to economic growth, using growth of per capita gross domestic product (GDP) as a dependent variable and a three-stage least-squares analysis as a method of estimation.

Explanatory variable	Coefficients (t statistics)						
	Barro	Region 4	Region 5 Latin America and the Caribbean	Region 13 Latin America and the Caribbean	Region 2	Region 4	Region 8
	World	World			Brazil	Colombia	Mexico
Log (GDP)	−0.0254 (−8.193)	−0.032 (−7.778)	−0.0396 (−6.089)	−0.0434 (−6.08)	−0.043 (−7.09)	−0.032 (−4.62)	−0.076 (−7.85)
Male (secondary schooling and higher)	0.0118 (4.720)	0.0080 (2.747)				0.049 (4.99)	0.020 (5.89)
Log (life expectancy at birth)	0.0423 (3.087)	0.060 (3.285)	0.0554 (2.655)				
Log (GDP) male schooling	−0.0062 (−3.647)	−0.0033 (−1.702)	−0.0236 (−2.344)	−0.0384 (−3.44)			
Log (fertility rate)	−0.0161 (−3.037)	−0.0130 (−1.786)					
Government consumption ratio	−0.136 (−5.230)	−0.1657 (−5.734)	−0.0817 (−1.766)				
Rule-of-law index	0.0293 (5.425)	0.038 (5.520)	0.0459 (4.733)	0.04169 (4.67)			
Terms-of-trade change	0.137 (4.566)	0.2182 (4.062)	0.2415 (4.480)	0.1291 (2.26)			
Democracy index	0.090 (3.333)	0.0487 (1.702)					
Democracy index squared	−0.088 (−3.666)	−0.047 (−1.872)					
Inflation rate	−0.043 (−5.375)	−0.0427 (−1.220)					
Life expectancy 15-year lag (males)				0.0606 (3.40)			
Percentage of population with sewerage connection					0.028 (2.113)		
YLPD (male population)						−0.365 (−2.65)	
YLPD (total)					−0.289 (−3.44)		
Mortality from communicable disease (males)							−0.0123 (−5.43)
Participation of tertiary sector							0.042 (5.61)
Adjusted R² (Period 1, 1965–1975)	0.58	0.3795	0.1138	0.2418			
Adjusted R² (Period 2, 1975–1985)	0.52	0.3883	0.3793	0.3110			
Adjusted R² (Period 3, 1985–1990)	0.42	0.1562	0.2793	0.0934			

Levine and Renelt applied this analysis to evaluate the soundness of a large number of results obtained in various studies on the significance of the correlation between economic growth and different groups of explanatory variables. Many of those results showed a very close correlation between economic growth and a subgroup of explanatory variables selected in each study. However, when all the remaining variables that were predetermined in the equation were modified, the apparent soundness of the results broke down.

To carry out the analysis, Levine and Renelt begin by identifying a set of variables that are always or almost always included as explanatory variables in the different analyses and that generally show high statistical significance in the analyses. In Equation 1 these variables are included in Matrix I and they correspond to the initial level of per capita gross domestic product (GDP), to the rate of schooling, to the average annual level of population growth,[10] and to the intercept

---

[10] Levine and Renelt also consider the share of investment in GDP, a potential variable to be included in Matrix I. However, as explained by these authors, this variable is not included in the regressions primarily because of the ambiguity of the relationship: investment as a determinant of economic growth or economic growth as a determinant of investment. If investment is included, the only mechanism by which other variables affect growth is more efficient resource allocation.

$$Y = I\beta_I + \beta_M M + Z\beta_Z + u \qquad (1)$$

The other variables that enter Equation 1 are the M variable, whose soundness is being tested, and the Z variables, corresponding to the remaining explanatory variables included in the economic growth regression. Levine and Renelt include three type Z variables in each regression, taken from all the possible combinations of three variables. Thus, the total number of variables in each regression is seven.

This methodology was applied to confirm the soundness of each of the explanatory variables that proved to be significant in the analyses for the global sample of countries (for Latin America and the Caribbean and for Brazil, Colombia, and Mexico; see Table 1). Table 2 summarizes the results of the analysis of extremes.

Once the results were obtained for all the regressions for each M variable, the specification with the highest coefficient for the variable M was identified, with its respective t statistic. Table 2 records the t statistic for that specification that yielded the highest coefficient value and is denoted as the upper limit. Similarly, Table 2 records the t statistic for the specification that yielded the lowest coefficient, and it is denoted as the lower limit. Finally, for each M variable, the t statistic is reported in the case of the base regression. The base regression includes only the M variable and the I variables, as indicated above, and no Z variable.

It is said that a variable is solid in the growth equation if its statistical significance is high at the upper and lower limits as well as in the base regression and also if the sign of its coefficient does not change.

TABLE 2. Analysis of extreme limits (three-stage least-squares analysis).

				t statistics		
Variables	Limit	World	Latin America	Brazil	Colombia	Mexico
Democracy index	High	5.8671				
	Base	2.5028				
	Low	4.2793				
Democracy index squared	High	5.9793				
	Base	2.8543				
	Low	2.8001				
Government consumption	High	−0.7619	1.1543			
	Base	−4.6745	−1.1374			
	Low	−3.2659	−3.7064			
Inflation rate	High	4.5826				
	Base	3.8661				
	Low	2.1432				
Fertility rate	High	0.6791				
	Base	−1.2572				
	Low	−2.8967				
Life expectancy at birth	High	1.9275	1.3590			
	Base	2.4184	−1.7554			
	Low	−0.2495	−0.2826			
Rule of law	High	5.7535	3.5913			
	Base	1.7828	3.8391			
	Low	2.3475	1.4312			
Terms of trade	High	3.4482	3.7037			
	Base	3.5080	3.0044			
	Low	−0.3299	1.0989			
Exports/GDP	High	1.3201	0.6360		0.1017	
	Base	0.8349	−2.0063		−0.0366	
	Low	−0.8731	−2.3757		−0.1440	
Mortality (working-age population)	High		0.8733			
	Base		−3.5828			
	Low		−1.5684			
Initial GDP[a]	High		−0.3264			
	Base		−1.7570			
	Low		−2.1139			
YLPD per capita (total population aged 15–69)	High			−84.7880	4.8124	
	Base			−125.4382	−18.7039	
	Low			−186.3458	−9.5464	

(Continued)

TABLE 2. Continued.

Variables	Limit	t statistics				
		World	Latin America	Brazil	Colombia	Mexico
YLPD per capita (total population aged 0–4)	High			−6.8175	39.3687	
	Base			−8.0448	−14.1027	
	Low			−8.5256	−8.3922	
YLPD per capita (males)	High			−35.3517	32.3526	
	Base			−48.1392	−40.0092	
	Low			−50.0437	−21.4957	
YLPD per capita (total)	High			−38.5673	43.6136	
	Base			−51.1588	−23.8608	
	Low			−51.4556	−14.9298	
Log (mortality from noncommunicable diseases) $(\times 10^4)$	High			−0.9008	0.3772	0.8041
	Base			−1.0364	−0.3792	−0.8693
	Low			−1.2954	−0.1933	−0.9608
Log (mortality from communicable diseases) $(\times 10^4)$	High			−1.0681	0.9303	−1.0886
	Base			−1.3454	−2.7687	−1.6044
	Low			−1.6802	−2.9900	−1.4322
Log (mortality from injuries)	High			−0.7144	0.4246	0.1532
	Base			−0.8606	−1.1276	−1.5007
	Low			−1.0762	−1.1694	−2.6513
YLPD between the ages of 0 and 15 (males)	High				4.8124	
	Base				−18.7039	
	Low				−9.5464	
YLPD between the ages of 0 and 4 (males)	High				20.6086	
	Base				−6.6622	
	Low				−3.4322	
YLPD between the ages of 15 and 69 (males)	High				135.0077	
	Base				−367.8901	
	Low				−244.1799	
YLPD (females)	High				57.4533	
	Base				−5.4407	
	Low				−8.3278	
Log (mortality from noncommunicable diseases) (males)	High				2.0075	−0.9047
	Base				−1.3149	−0.9718
	Low				−1.8058	−1.0414
Log (mortality from noncommunicable diseases) (females)	High				2.5587	−1.0999
	Base				−1.8752	−1.1677
	Low				−1.9934	−1.2564
Log (mortality from communicable diseases) (males)	High				1.9225	−0.9726
	Base				−1.3565	−1.3259
	Low				−1.2269	−1.0607
Log (mortality from communicable diseases) (females)	High				1.9442	
	Base				−1.4287	
	Low				−1.0681	
Log (mortality from injuries) (males)	High				4.3987	−0.7545
	Base				−1.2479	−0.9553
	Low				−1.3237	−0.9719
Log (mortality from injuries) (females)	High				2.4126	−1.2167
	Base				−0.7455	−1.8477
	Low				−0.4179	−1.5486
Annual average number of governors	High				2.3372	
	Base				−1.5808	
	Low				−2.5003	
Number of votes in presidential elections as percentage of registered voters	High				−0.4788	
	Base				−3.6634	
	Low				−3.7870	
Standard deviation of average schooling by standard deviation of average per capita GDP	High				3.2466	1.6355
	Base				0.8159	0.7906
	Low				−4.7469	0.1390

TABLE 2. Continued.

Variables	Limit	World	Latin America	Brazil	Colombia	Mexico
					t statistics	
Gini coefficient at departmental level	High				−0.6550	
	Base				−8.9784	
	Low				−8.3073	
Total public spending per capita (departmental administration)	High				0.3822	
	Base				0.2676	
	Low				−0.0362	
Log (life expectancy) (males)	High					1.0091
	Base					−0.2119
	Low					−1.5721
Log (life expectancy) (females)	High					0.1532
	Base					−1.5007
	Low					−2.6513
Log (fertility rate with 20-year lag)	High					1.0823
	Base					−2.2920
	Low					−2.5069
Log (fertility rate with five-year lag)	High					1.9570
	Base					2.1743
	Low					−0.0762
Log (infant mortality rate with 20-year lag)	High					1.3067
	Base					0.3123
	Low					−0.6646
Log (infant mortality rate with five-year lag)	High					1.4166
	Base					1.4615
	Low					0.2151
Log (government spending/GDP ratio)	High					−0.4595
	Base					−2.3720
	Low					−2.1061

[a] Schooling.

For the worldwide sample, only the democracy index passes the extreme limits test. The rate of inflation is highly significant at the upper and lower limits as well as in the base regression. However, the sign of the coefficient is contrary to expectations from the standpoint of economic theory. Life expectancy at birth is highly significant at the upper limit and in the base regression, but it shows the opposite sign and low significance at the lower limit. Of the variables that are almost always associated with growth, only the population growth rate proved to be solid.

In the sample for Latin America and the Caribbean, none of the variables is robust from the standpoint of this methodology.

In the case of Brazil, YLPD for different causes and age groups are solid, with high statistical significance, as is initial GDP. This is not true for mortality by cause. Unfortunately, the results are less robust than in the other samples, because, owing to data constraints, the set of variables included in the regressions is much smaller.

In the case of Colombia, YLPD is highly significant in the base regression and at the lower limit. However, the sign of the coefficient changes at the upper limit. This is why it does not pass the extreme limits test. This also occurs with mortality by cause and by age group, although in this case the significance is less than for YLPD. The same situation occurs in the case of the Gini coefficient of income distribution.

In the case of Mexico, none of the explanatory variables is solid. Mortality by cause shows some significance.

In summary, the extreme limits test is rarely passed by any of the specifications in the growth equations and in the different samples. Variables passed the test in only two samples: the democracy index in the global country sample and YLPD in the case of Brazil.

It is not superfluous to point out that similar tests are rarely applied in other areas of economic research. Their use in the case of economic growth is justified because of the broad range of statistical models that obtain correlation results between the growth of countries and the many variables of interest to particular researchers. In areas where the functional specification of the equation to be empirically estimated is clearly derived from economic theory, application of this type of analysis is rare. Thus, from the standpoint of expanding knowledge of the correlation between economic growth and formation of human capital, it seems more relevant to delve further into the channels through which health and education of specific groups in society affect the population's sociodemographic dynamics and into the relationships between these variables and growth. This type of analysis is performed in other sections of the project. The next section presents the results of estimating functional specifications derived directly from the economic theory of growth, with health as one of the determinants of human capital.

EDUCATION, HEALTH, AND GROWTH: PANEL REGRESSIONS FOR LATIN AMERICA, BRAZIL, COLOMBIA, AND MEXICO

The objective of this work is to empirically evaluate the correlation between the level of production per person and education and health considered as components of human capital. This study was conducted for the Latin American countries (1960–1990) and the respective states or departments of Brazil (1980–1995), Colombia (1980–1990), and Mexico (1970–1995). We used panel information in five-year periods.

The analysis is based on a Solow-type growth model augmented by human capital, as formulated by Mankiw et al. (1992) and by Islam (1995). However, it should be pointed out, in reference to the aforementioned works, that this work considers health as a component of human capital. Thus, production per person depends on levels of education and health as well as on classic determinants such as savings rates and population growth rates.

According to the specified models, the level of production per person is expected to bear a positive relationship to the savings rate (investment) and level of education and a negative relationship to population growth rate. In the case of Colombia, the coefficient of the illiteracy rate is expected to be negative. With regard to the variable health, economic growth is expected to be positively correlated to life expectancy and the probability of survival in the next five years, and it is expected to be negatively correlated to mortality. All the estimated regressions include individual effects (to control for factors specific to each country, state, and department) and temporal effects (to control for factors common to all the economies that change over time). Both effects are modeled with fictitious or "dummy" variables.

Four different specifications of the model are considered in the study, depending on the treatment given to the dynamics of the product per person and to the Solow model restriction that the coefficients of the savings rate and of the sum of the growth rates of population and technology and depreciation be equal but of opposite sign (positive and negative, respectively). These specifications and their estimation are described in detail in the full report.

It is important to mention that, in the case of Latin America, information for Brazil and Colombia was available on health indicators by age and gender groups, which were included one by one in each regression, giving a large number of results. For this reason, the study concentrates on two important aspects: (i) evaluating to what point the expected relationships hold for the health indicators independently of the results obtained for the remaining variables in the model, and (ii) identifying the most consistent results of the model as a whole.

Table 3 reports the total number of estimated regressions and the number for which health variables gave significant results at the 1%, 5%, 10%, and 20% levels in

TABLE 3. Number of regressions estimated and significance of the health indicator coefficients.

	Positive effects				Negative effects				
	1%	5%	10%	20%	1%	5%	10%	20%	Total
Latin America									
Total LE[a]	20	31	7	7	0	0	0	0	136
Total PS[b]	14	10	6	7	0	3	0	5	128
Total Latin America	34	41	13	14	0	3	0	5	264
Brazil									
Total LE[a]	5	6	9	12	0	0	0	0	128
Total PS[b]	10	1	4	1	8	4	5	5	120
Total Brazil	15	7	13	13	8	4	5	5	248
Colombia									
Total LE[a]	0	14	8	16	2	0	1	8	128
Total PS[b]	16	4	9	14	0	0	0	1	128
Total Colombia	16	18	17	30	2	0	1	9	256

[a]LE = life expectancy.
[b]PS = probability of survival.

the cases of Latin America, Brazil, and Colombia. It must be stressed that the statistical significance of the individual parameters is evaluated by two-tailed t tests, which is quite demanding, and applying robust errors to problems of heteroskedasticity.

The proportion of regressions for which the health indicator coefficients are positive and significant at the 20% level or better is about one-third of all estimated regressions. Results have also been obtained in which, contrary to what was expected, the health indicator coefficients were negative and significant. However, these cases represent only 5% of the total. It must be noted that the greatest proportion of positive significant results is obtained in the case of Latin America.

The case of Mexico differs from the other three in that health indicators are not available by age groups. For this reason it is not included in Table 3. The results of models 3 and 4, which explore purely contemporary relationships between production and its factors, are better than those for the dynamic models 1 and 2 (see full report). The best results are obtained in the case of the unrestricted model. These results are very significant and have the expected signs when the education indicators are illiteracy, schooling, and complete primary education; they are somewhat less significant when "1 year of university" is used. In the other cases, the coefficients tend to have the expected sign and to be at least somewhat significant.

It is important to point out that the cases for which the expected relationships for the health indicators are most significant do not necessarily correspond to those cases for which the results for the remaining variables in the specified models are consistent. The full report presents some regressions selected according to their consistency with the expected results for the cases of Latin America, Brazil, and Colombia. In Table 4, we present those that correspond to the less restricted specification of the model (Model 1).

This specification includes the lagged dependent variable (lagged per capita product) in addition to the variables savings, population growth, health, and education. It is important to mention that in the case of Mexico the states of Campeche and Tabasco are excluded, because their petroleum production, which is registered as income, distorts the results. Similarly, in the case of Colombia the crime rate by department is included as an additional control variable.

The results presented in Table 4 show a high goodness of fit in every case, as measured by the adjusted R^2. Additionally, the F test supports the joint significance of the explanatory variables in the reported regressions. How-

TABLE 4. Growth regressions for Latin America, Brazil, Colombia, and Mexico (unrestricted model).

Sample (period)	Savings rate	Population growth	Health	Education	Adjusted R^2	F test	No. of objects
Latin America (1960–1990)							
(1)	0.157	−0.276	0.747	−0.217	0.992	1,485.8	85
	(3.431)°	(−3.511)°	(2.272)*	(−2.340)*			
(2)	0.219	−0.339	11.487	−0.157	0.993	1,127.8	62
	(3.787)°	(−3.032)°	(3.358)°	(−2.263)*			
Brazil (1980–1995)							
(3)	0.0108	0.168	0.163	0.812	0.995	3,013.8	74
	(0.049)	(4.071)°	(2.883)^	(4.214)°			
(4)	0.098	0.224	62.331	0.649	0.996	2,757.3	73
	(0.498)	(5.736)°	(5.171)°	(4.031)°			
Colombia (1980–1990)							
(5)	0.028	−0.113	0.469	−0.002	0.975	298.7	46
	(1.362)	(−1.488)	(1.830)^	(−1.084)			
(6)	0.037	−0.024	6.568	−0.000	0.979	307.2	46
	(1.636)	(−0.266)	(1.196)	(−0.023)			
Mexico (1970–1995)							
(7)	0.005	0.002	0.011	−0.011	0.950	401.0	150
	(2.735)°	(1.107)	(1.759)^	(−1.383)			
(8)	0.005	0.002	0.006	−0.009	0.950	400.2	150
	(2.710)°	(1.055)	(1.401)	(−1.254)			
(9)	0.006	0.002	−0.014	−0.014	0.950	402.8	150
	(2.674)°	(1.311)	(−1.519)	(−1.406)			

Note: The dependent variable is the level of production per person. All the regressions are panel regressions and include the lagged dependent variable and individual dummy and time variables. When the health indicator is the probability of surviving the next five years, the regression also includes the total rate of perinatal deaths. In the case of Colombia, the regressions also include the crime rate by department. Because of lack of space, the results for these additional variables are not reported. The health variables are not the same for all the regressions. Regressions (1), (3), and (5) use life expectancy for men at 5, 75, and 5 years of age, respectively. Regressions (2), (4), and (6) use the probability of surviving the next five years for men at the ages of 5, 5, and 15, respectively. Regressions (7), (8), and (9) use life expectancy at birth for men and women and the infant mortality rate, respectively. In the case of Brazil, the health indicators are lagged one period. Values in parentheses are t statistics, estimated with errors robust to problems of heteroskedasticity. °, *, and ^, significance levels of 1%, 5%, and 10%, respectively.

ever, it must be mentioned that these results are consistent with only some of the aspects of the model. In most cases, the expected signs are obtained for the coefficients of the explanatory variables, although in the case of Colombia, where there are few observations, acceptable levels of significance are not obtained. Possibly the weak consistency of the results occurs because, in the case of Brazil and partially in the case of Mexico and Latin America, the periods under study are periods of economic adjustment instead of growth, which weakens the application of the Solow model.

The traditional factors (rate of investment in physical capital and population growth) are related to the level of production per person as would be expected a priori. In particular, production per capita shows a positive correlation with the rate of investment (savings rate) and a negative correlation with the population growth rate. In the case of Brazil, both factors show a positive correlation, although the investment rate is not statistically significant. In the case of Mexico, the population growth rate has a positive but insignificant correlation with per capita production.

Education, here considered as a component of human capital, relates negatively to the level of production per person in the case of Latin America, which is inconsistent with a priori expectations. This also occurs in other studies, such as Barro's study (1996), with no clear explanation. In the case of Mexico, there is also a negative relationship, which is not significant. The presence of information limitations must be taken into account, as in the case of Colombia, for which the illiteracy rate is used as an education indicator. In this case, the expected (negative) sign is obtained, although it is not statistically significant. In the case of Brazil, there is evidence of a significant positive correlation between production per person and education.

Finally, it should also be mentioned that the study finds evidence that the per capita products of groups of countries or states (according to the database used) tend to grow at the same rate but maintain differences in their levels (conditional convergence). In practically every case, the parameter corresponding to lagged per capita income has a positive sign, is less than unity, and is statistically significant, consistent with this type of dynamics. Also, except for the case of Colombia, the technological tendency obtained, modeled as a temporal tendency, is negative. These results can be found in the complete report.

In general terms, some evidence is found in this study in favor of a positive relationship between health and per capita product. On the other hand, the results obtained are consistent with certain aspects of the model but not with the model as a whole. This could be because the samples include periods of economic adjustment instead of growth.

Regarding the relationship between health and per capita product, in the case of Latin America and also to an extent in the case of Colombia, a relatively important number of results (but not the majority) are positive and significant at the 10% level. However, these results are not necessarily accompanied by consistent results for the remaining variables of the growth model used for the analysis. Therefore, these results can be considered evidence in favor of a positive relationship between health and economic growth (not necessarily causal) but not in favor of the model as a whole.

On the other hand, for those results that are as consistent as possible with the model as a whole, the health indicators correspond in general to age and gender groups at the extremes and not necessarily the most statistically significant. These results constitute partial evidence in favor of the models used, although it must be recognized that these are obtained in few cases.

It is possible that the inconclusive results of this study follow from information limitations, possible omission of additional control variables, and statistical problems of simultaneity between the variables studied.

LONG-TERM RECIPROCAL IMPACT OF HEALTH AND GROWTH IN MEXICO

Fogel's study on the historical association between nutrition, longevity, and economic growth is a source of motivation for the contemporary study of the interaction between health and the economy. One the most interesting findings of Fogel's research is the persistence of improvements in health. When health improves during the initial years of life, it improves in all later stages and life expectancy increases, which leads to the hypothesis that increases in health can have a long-term effect on income. The database on the Mexican states offers an opportunity to examine whether this type of correlation exists between health and future income, because it includes the following five-year health indicators:

- Life expectancy for men and women, fertility, and infant mortality for the years 1955–1995.
- Mortality by age group and gender for the years 1950–1995.

It also contains five-year economic and educational indicators for the period 1970–1995. The time series of health indicators, which is much longer than that of the economic indicators, makes it possible to analyze the interaction between health and growth over a relatively long period within the context of growth studies for developing countries. We estimate economic growth regressions in which we examine the role of health indicators with lags of up to 15 and 20 years. We also examine the symmetrical equivalent—that is, regressions of growth (improvement) in health, specifically in life expectancy for men and women, which turned out to be the most significant health indicator in this database. The results yield evidence of long-term two-way causality. In particular, the magnitude of the coefficients indicates a significant channel of causality from health to income.

For economic growth regressions, we used the respective mortality indicators to disaggregate the results of long-term interaction by age group and sex. We found a pattern of lags similar to that for life expectancy associated with the more economically active age groups and with maternity.

Econometric Approach

The technique we used is similar to that of Barro in *Health and Economic Growth* (1996). We estimated economic growth as a function of a series of explanatory variables. We performed these estimations not only for the log of income y_t but also for life expectancy for men and women EV_t.[11] We estimated equations such as the following:[12]

$$(y_{t+T} - y_t)/T = \alpha_0 y_t + \alpha_p EV_{t-pT} \alpha_p EV_{t-pT} + \beta_1 X_1 + ... + \beta_r X_r + u_t \quad (1)$$

$$(EV_{t+T} - EV_t)/T = \gamma_0 EV_t + \gamma_q y_{t-qT} + \delta_1 Z_1 + ... + \delta_s Z_s + v_t \quad (2)$$

In these equations, T is the period of growth, t is the initial period, α_0 and γ_0 are coefficients with negative signs expected in the case of convergence, α_p is the coefficient of life expectancy with a lag of pT years, and γ_q is the coefficient of per capita income with a lag of qT years. Finally, $X_1, ..., X_r, Z_1, ..., $ and Z_s represent additional explanatory variables—dummy variables for each time period in the case of Equation 1 and the constant term for Equation 2.

Economic growth:

- The initial value of per capita income,
- Some health indicator (life expectancy, fertility, infant mortality, mortality by age group and gender),

- Percentage of the population speaking an indigenous language,
- Public spending (ln),
- Percentage of the population up to 4 years old,
- Fixed temporal effects, and
- Education indicators.

It would be desirable for the database to contain better indicators of savings as well as public and private investments in health. Those obtained were acquisition of banking resources, construction, public spending on education and health, and the population eligible to use public health services. However, these were not very significant, nor was an indicator for migration.

When the rate of improvement in life expectancy is estimated, the initial value is that of life expectancy itself, and a lagged GDP is used as an explanatory variable.

Equations 1 and 2 constitute a Granger causality test between y_t and EV_t, except for the presence of the additional explanatory variables, and the use of a pattern of lags constrained by the available information. Thus, it is a conditional Granger causality test that studies causality once the effects of the additional variables have been controlled.

A significant coefficient for a lagged variable indicates that the hypothesis that the correlation indicates causality cannot be rejected. The magnitude of the coefficients establishes the magnitude of the causal relationship suggested by the regression.

The results indicate that, in economic growth regressions, the coefficients of life expectancy and their significance reach their maximums for lags of 15 or 20 years. In the opposite direction, for which the horizon is shorter, the coefficients and their significance reach their maximums for lags of 10 years. The magnitude of the coefficients indicates that the first Granger causality relationship is considerable, whereas the second relationship is smaller. This second result leads us to believe that the income per capita of the Mexican states may not be a good indicator of actions, including channeling of resources, that improve health.

We also broke down the effect of life expectancy on economic growth by using indicators of mortality according to age and gender. This confirmed the results of lagged impact that we have mentioned, and we found that the results cluster around the health of the economically active population and possibly maternal health.

Results: Income Growth and Health

Here we summarize the results of the income growth regressions.

---

[11] For life expectancy we use the transformation $-\ln(80 - EV)$; for the other health indicators we use logarithms.

[12] We used least-squares estimates for Mexico's 31 states—i.e., all the states including the Federal District, with the exception of the state of Campeche, which we excluded because the oil boom it experienced is recorded as part of its income and it introduces considerable distortions in the regressions.

TABLE 5. Economic growth regressions: comparison of the impact of several health indicators[a] (main coefficients).

	Life expectancy for men	Life expectancy for men	Life expectancy for women	Life expectancy for women	Fertility	Infant mortality
Lag	0	15	0	15	0.	0.
Health indicator	**0.118** (3.569)	**0.153** (3.356)	**0.085** (3.631)	**0.114** (2.887)	−0.057 (−1.58)	***−0.046*** (−2.041)

[a] We write the results by their confidence intervals according to the following scheme. Better than 1% ($|t| \geq 2.61$), boldface; between 1% and 5% ($1.97 \leq |t| < 2.61$), boldface and italics; between 5% and 10% ($1.65 \leq |t| < 1.97$), italics.

Life Expectancy, Fertility, and Mortality

Life expectancy for men and women shows a significant positive correlation with growth of per capita income for time lags ranging from 0 to 15 years after the initial period, with the maximum at 15 years. The coefficients have the expected sign, are highly significant, and tend to increase as the lag increases from 0 to 15 years. The first four columns of Table 5 show these coefficients for 0 and 15 years. The results are not significant when fertility is used, whereas infant mortality has a significant coefficient with only 0 years of lag time.

Mortality by Age and Sex

We sought to identify the age groups and sex for which health has a lagged impact on income growth. In Tables 6 and 7, we show the coefficients of the regression that yield the most significant coefficient for each age group and sex for time lags of 15 and 20 years. Except for the group aged 30–49 years, the results are more significant for women, for whom significant coefficients in the group aged 5–14 and 15–29 years are obtained. The coefficients are even higher for men between 30 and 49 years of age. In the case of women, the age groups point to maternity and economic participation as relevant to causality, given the characteristics of women's participation in the workforce. In the case of men, the economically active ages are the most important. It is noteworthy that mater-

TABLE 7. Impact of female mortality by age on economic growth regressions: 15- or 20-year lag with the most significant coefficient for each age group[a] (main coefficients).

Age group	0–4	5–14	15–29	30–49	50–69	70+
Lag	15	15	15	15	15	15
Health indicator	−0.009 (−1.337)	*−0.011* (−1.909)	**−0.015** (−2.078)	−0.016 (−1.568)	−0.011 (−1.148)	−0.018 (−1.77)

[a] We write the results by their confidence intervals according to the following scheme. Better than 1% ($|t| \geq 2.61$), boldface; between 1% and 5% ($1.97 \leq |t| < 2.61$), boldface and italics; between 5% and 10% ($1.65 \leq |t| < 1.97$), italics.

nal mortality is an indicator of the availability of technologically feasible health services and thus shows the importance of broad coverage of health services.

Tables 8 and 9 are similar to the previous tables but deal with a lag of 0 years, where the causal relationship is less clear. These results are significant for women from the age of 15 on, but they are not significant for men. Several phenomena are present here. It is evident that older women are more vulnerable than men. For younger women, the increased vulnerability may be related to maternity and other health conditions that receive less care when economic resources decline.

In summary, there is strong evidence of causality from life expectancy of men and women to economic growth occurring in the five-year period beginning 0–15 years later; both the coefficients and the confidence levels grow during this time. When we use the mortality indicators by age group and sex, we find that this causal relationship has greater significance for men aged 30–49 and for women aged 5–14 and 15–29. Thus, the causal relationship detected is associated with the more economically active groups and with maternity.

TABLE 6. Impact of male mortality by age on economic growth regressions: 15- or 20-year lag with the most significant coefficient for each age group[a] (main coefficients).

Age group	0–4	5–14	15–29	30–49	50–69	70+
Lag	15	20	15	20	20	20
Health indicator	−0.002 (−0.21)	−0.007 (−1.124)	−0.005 (−0.603)	***−0.018*** (−2.095)	−0.019 (−1.214)	−0.008 (−0.59)

[a] We write the results by their confidence intervals according to the following scheme. Better than 1% ($|t| \geq 2.61$), boldface; between 1% and 5% ($1.97 \leq |t| < 2.61$), boldface and italics; between 5% and 10% ($1.65 \leq |t| < 1.97$), italics.

TABLE 8. Coefficient of male mortality by age in economic growth regression: 0-year lag[a] (main coefficients).

Age group	0–4	5–14	15–29	30–49	50–69	70+
Health indicator	0.001 (0.147)	0.001 (0.101)	−0.007 (−0.772)	−0.008 (−0.842)	−0.014 (−1.079)	−0.007 (−0.462)

[a] We write the results by their confidence intervals according to the following scheme. Better than 1% ($|t| \geq 2.61$), boldface; between 1% and 5% ($1.97 \leq |t| < 2.61$), boldface and italics; between 5% and 10% ($1.65 \leq |t| < 1.97$), italics.

TABLE 9. Coefficient of female mortality by age in economic growth regression: 0-year lag[a] (main coefficients).

Age group	0–4	5–14	15–29	30–49	50–69	70+
Health indicator	0 (–0.068)	0 (–0.002)	*–0.022* (*–2.655*)	*–0.019* (*–1.664*)	*–0.025* (*–2.094*)	*–0.043* (*–3.526*)

[a] We write the results by their confidence intervals according to the following scheme. Better than 1% (|t| ≥ 2.61), boldface; between 1% and 5% (1.97 ≤ |t| < 2.61), boldface and italics; between 5% and 10% (1.65 ≤ |t| < 1.97), italics.

In addition, the strongest correlations in the case of the 0-year lag, in which causality is less clear, are found only for women, with two peaks—one for the age groups in the childbearing years and the other for the elderly.

Education

The education variables show colinearity with the health indicators. Although they may be significant in the absence of the health variables, their confidence levels decline when the latter are included. This may indicate that part of the effect of health on future growth occurs through education, as is found in the study on Brazil. It also may be a reflection of poor quality of the indicators.

Results: Life Expectancy Growth Regressions

In the life-expectancy growth regressions, the dependent variable is the rate of growth in life expectancy for men or women (i.e., its rate of improvement).[13] Tables 10 and 11 show the main results.

For both sexes, the income variable is notably more significant when the lag is 10 years from the initial period and with the expected positive sign. However, in the case of women, the coefficient for 15 years is somewhat higher. Note that the number of available observations declines with the lags. For the 10- and 15-year lags, the coefficient of initial life expectancy is negative, which indicates convergence. This sign is lost for the lag of 0 years, which may be the result of not having enough explanatory variables.

Education

Using per capita income with a 10-year lag, we now introduce the education variables (Table 11). The results

---

[13] The variable is –ln(80 – EV), as above, and minus the rate of growth of (80 – EV) is estimated. The independent variables are life expectancy in the initial period (for the same sex); per capita income, either at the beginning of the period or with a lag of 5, 10, or 15 years; indigenous language; public spending by unit of income; and the percentage of the population under the age of 4.

are much more significant for females than for males. For males, literacy and primary education are significant, whereas for females all the education variables are significant. The most significant variable for men is primary education; for women it is literacy. The negative life expectancy coefficient represents convergence in life expectancy.

Magnitude of the Coefficients

We read the magnitude of the coefficients of the interplay between life expectancy and income in the best regressions for each causal direction. We find that, for every permanent one-year increase in life expectancy, there is a 0.8% increase in the growth rate of per capita income in the five-year period beginning 15 years later. In Mexico, during the period in question, the five-year increases in life expectancy have values of 2.34 years for men and 2.77 years for women. This means that the contribution to income growth is on the order of 2% per year. The increases in life expectancy continue to be about two years per five-year period in 1990.

In the opposite direction, the magnitude is the following. If income with a 10-year lag is doubled, life expectancy increases by about 70 days. However, the R^2 of the regressions is smaller, which indicates that the variables of the regression are not sufficiently explanatory with respect to improvements in health.

Conclusions

The results strongly indicate that health is correlated with future economic growth—that is, it causes economic growth in the long term in the conditional Granger sense. When we examine the impact of mortality by age group and sex, we see that this causality is associated with maternity and with the most economically active age groups. We also detect causality in the opposite direction but the magnitude is small. This may be because the per capita income of the Mexican states is not a good indicator of actions that improve health, including public spending on health. It also may be because a significant portion of health improvements occur for reasons other than income, such as technological and cultural change. Growth regressions, as Solow notes, do not take account of such changes, which appear in the residual. Particularly in the case of the life expectancy growth regression, we should consider that the residual, which is higher, includes not only technology but also preferences—especially when fertility is being considered, which in turn interacts strongly with other health indicators. This means that

TABLE 10. Life expectancy growth regression with several per capita income lags[a] (main coefficients).

Income lag	Men				Women			
	0 years	5 years	10 years	15 years	0 years	5 years	10 years	15 years
Initial life expectancy	**0.026**	0.008	−0.023	−0.02	**0.02**	−0.004	**−0.036**	**−0.042**
	(2.773)	(0.709)	(−1.673)	(−0.908)	**(3.117)**	(−0.508)	**(−4.413)**	**(−3.327)**
Per capita income (ln)	0.006	**0.011**	**0.019**	*0.016*	**0.016**	**0.021**	**0.03**	**0.033**
	(1.646)	**(2.771)**	**(3.919)**	*(1.771)*	**(3.849)**	**(4.614)**	**(6.308)**	**(4.202)**
Observations	155	124	93	62	155	124	93	62

[a] We write the results by their confidence intervals according to the following scheme. Better than 1% ($|t| \geq 2.61$), boldface; between 1% and 5% ($1.97 \leq |t| < 2.61$), boldface and italics; between 5% and 10% ($1.65 \leq |t| < 1.97$), italics.

changes in health are highly dependent on technology advances, public policy, and behavioral patterns.

The 15- or 20-year lags between health and growth surely result from the persistence of improvements in health and the intergenerational nature of the formation of educational and health capital. Investment in bringing up children involves lags of this length and depends on the wealth of the parents.

In this study, we found that improvements in health indicators are correlated with future economic growth over long periods of time that do not exhaust the horizon of available information. The magnitude of the correlation indicates the possibility that the contribution of improvements in health to growth during this period of Mexican development may be as significant as 2% annually.

HEALTH IN THE ECONOMIC AND DEMOGRAPHIC TRANSITION OF BRAZIL, 1980–1995

Among the main objectives of studies on the economic impact of health is identification of the main channels of interaction. In addition to its direct effect on productivity, health has other effects on both economic develop-

ment and the demographic transition. For example, Barro (1996) stated that health reduces the depreciation rate of human capital, making investments in education more attractive. In fact, good infant health and nutrition directly increase the benefits of education (World Health Organization, 1999; World Bank, 1993). Ehrlich and Lui (1991) examined the impact of longevity on economic growth through intergenerational economic exchange. Health can facilitate the economic participation of women. This in itself is important for economic development (Galor and Weil, 1993). Health is a factor in fertility, itself a pivotal phenomenon of the demographic transition, which in turn has been studied extensively from an economic standpoint. Finally, it is important to study the impact of each of these mechanisms on income distribution dynamics and on the different sectors of the population.

Together, these interactions paint a complex picture. Their simultaneous presence poses considerable difficulties to their study and to empirical detection of the diverse processes. In the case of Brazil, an excellent database was compiled from Brazil's National Household Sample Survey (PNAD household surveys) and from the classification of mortality by causes as obtained from death certificates. The quality of this database allows us

TABLE 11. Life expectancy growth regression with several educational indicators (main coefficients; 93 observations).[a]

Educational indicator	Men				Women			
	Literacy	Primary complete	Degree started	Schooling	Literacy	Primary complete	Degree started	Schooling
Initial life expectancy	*−0.029*	*−0.033*	*−0.024*	*−0.046*	**−0.041**	**−0.040**	**−0.039**	**−0.068**
	(−2.030)	*(−2.355)*	*(−1.749)*	*(−2.246)*	**(−5.451)**	**(−5.067)**	**(−4.908)**	**(−6.309)**
Per capita income with a lag of 10 years	**0.015**	**0.020**	**0.017**	**0.015**	**0.019**	**0.029**	**0.023**	**0.018**
	(2.848)	**(4.169)**	**(3.224)**	**(2.787)**	**(3.955)**	**(6.576)**	**(4.550)**	**(3.529)**
Education	*0.001*	**0.001**	0.008	0.007	**0.001**	**0.001**	**0.032**	**0.016**
	(1.713)	**(2.575)**	(0.819)	(1.503)	**(4.733)**	**(3.081)**	**(3.238)**	**(4.125)**

[a] We write the results by their confidence intervals according to the following scheme. Better than 1% ($|t| \geq 2.61$), boldface; between 1% and 5% ($1.97 \leq |t| < 2.61$), boldface and italics; between 5% and 10% ($1.65 \leq |t| < 1.97$), italics.

to pursue the detection of complex phenomena related to the role of health in changes in income, education, economic participation, employment, and fertility. From this analysis emerges a picture that consistently shows that health has important economic, demographic, and distributive interactions that can be influenced by public policy.

Database

We consolidated the information from the eight PNAD surveys (1977–1995), summarizing the data at 10 income levels (i.e., by deciles) for each Brazilian state.[14] Along with other types of data, these surveys include information on the size and composition of households, on schooling and school attendance, on the economic participation and employment of men and women, on household income, and on the percentage of urban population. Two advantages of using this part of the database are that all the information is tied to income distribution and the number of observations is large.

The health data obtained from death certificates include mortality and YLPD classified by cause and by age group, sex, and life expectancy for five-year periods between 1980 and 1995. All these data are included for each state in Brazil.[15]

To harmonize the two sources of information, it was necessary to extrapolate the years 1980 (based on 1979 and 1981) and 1985 (based on 1983 and 1986) from the PNAD survey.

From a descriptive standpoint, the indicators reveal a major economic and demographic transition. Low-income households have more children, constitute a population that is less active economically (especially in the case of women) and that has greater unemployment and less education. These households also are less urban. These differences decline considerably over time, although inequality in income distribution does not.

Used together, the databases allow us to examine how the health variables by age group and gender correlate with the growth or decline in income, fertility, education, and economic participation of each decile of the population.

Econometric Estimation

To examine the role of health in Brazil's economic and demographic transition, we estimate a series of growth

regressions, similar to those used by Barro (1991, 1996), for several important indicators. This means that we examine how health and certain other economic indicators intervene in the explanation of changes—that is, in the dynamics—of the principal indicators of Brazil's economic development and demographic transition. In other words, the variables to explain (left-hand side) are the growth rates of

- Per capita income;
- Percentage of the population under 1 year of age (a proxy for fertility);
- Schooling and the percentage of children aged 7, 10, and 15 who attend school; and
- Economic participation, unemployment, and wages for men and women.

These variables describe the major aspects of the economic and demographic transition. As explanatory variables, we use economic and demographic variables as well as health variables (right-hand side, logarithms).

1. Economic and demographic variables (logarithms):
- Initial level of the variable whose growth rate is being studied,
- Per capita household income and its square (to obtain a flexible functional form),
- Schooling of the household head and its square,
- Average schooling in the household,
- Economically active population (male and female),
- Percentage of urban population,
- Population growth rate, and
- Percentage of the population under 1 or 6 years of age.

These variables include the principal indicators that describe (in averages) the economic situation of the households of each decile in each state. They are income, schooling of the household head, average schooling of the household as a whole, economic participation, percentage of urban population, and percentage of newborns and young children in the household. The population growth rate is included to take into account the distributive effects implicit in using per capita indicators from the left-hand side. However, it was not very significant, because population growth is taken into account by the percentage of the population under 1 year of age. The initial level of the variable to explain makes it possible to take into account convergence-type effects in which the growth rate of a variable depends on its initial level. The squares of the income and schooling-of-the-household-head variables are included to give the estimator functional flexibility, which simultaneously adjusts to the behavior of

---

[14] This work was compiled by Suzanne Duryeau of IDB.

[15] This is the work of María Helena Prado de Mello Jorge, Department of Epidemiology, University of São Paulo, Brazil.

households with different levels of income. These squares are also included as explanatory variables.

2. Health variables for ages 0, 1, 5, 10, ..., 70, or 75 and for men and women (logarithms):

- Life expectancy;
- Probability of survival to next age group, $p_t t+a$; and
- Maternal mortality, mortality from communicable diseases, and mortality from noncommunicable diseases.

Of these, we used mainly the probability of survival. The other variables were used mostly for comparative purposes. The probability of survival, a concept that in itself is an excellent health indicator, was defined in a manner consistent with the mathematical concept of life expectancy; that is, in time t, the probability $p_t t+a$ of surviving a years satisfies the following equation:

$$EV_t = p_t^{t+a} EV_{t+a} + \tfrac{1}{2}(1 - p_t^{t+a})a \qquad (1)$$

where EV_t is life expectancy at age t (if the subject does not survive, life expectancy of half the period is assumed). Excellent results were obtained with this indicator.

Finally, we state the system of equations that describes the estimation carried out for each dependent variable. Because information on health is not available by deciles, we estimated panel-type growth equations such as the following:

$$\frac{y_{sd(t+5)} - y_{sdt}}{5} = \alpha y_{sdt} + \sum_i \beta_i X_{sdt}^i + \gamma_d S_{st} + c_d \chi_d$$
$$+ \theta_{85} \chi_{85} + \theta_{90} \chi_{90} + \varepsilon_{sdt}$$

In this equation, states, deciles, and years are represented by the indices $1 \leq s \leq 24$, $1 \leq d \leq 10$, and $t = 1980$, 1985, and 1990, respectively. Each of the variables to explain takes the place of y. The independent economic and demographic variables are Xi. The health variable is S. The right-hand side also includes dummy variables by decile χ_d and by date χ_{85}, χ_{90} in order to control for the respective fixed effects.

The estimates include 24 Brazilian states. The regressions were estimated by generalized least squares, correcting for heteroskedasticity and correlation in the errors between deciles and states.

Interpretation of results must take into account the fact that the health indicators are state level indicators. These differ from the remaining data, which refer to both states and income levels. Thus, the regressions answer the question, "What is the correlation between the state health indicators S (for a certain age group and sex) and the growth rate of the economic indicator y of each income decile, once the variables Xi and the initial level of y have been taken into account?"

We estimate these regressions by sets in which the health indicator covers the population's classification by age and sex. For each regression, coefficient γ_d is obtained for each income decile d, which estimates the correlation for each decile between the state health indicator and the growth rate of the variable to be explained. We graph these coefficients in three dimensions in order to observe the pattern they follow with respect to age group, sex, and income decile (nonsignificant coefficients are graphed at zero).

To complete our analysis, in a different estimate we also included as a variable to be explained the probability of survival for men and women. In this case, we use the equation

$$\frac{S_{s(t+5)} - S_{st}}{5} e_d = \alpha S_{st} e_d + \sum_i \beta_i X_{sdt}^i + c$$
$$+ \theta_{85} \chi_{85} + \theta_{90} \chi_{90} + \varepsilon_{sdt} \qquad (2)$$

where $e_d = 1$. Here, the relationship between the change in the health variable and the economic and demographic explanatory variables by deciles is estimated uniformly for the different income levels but with the functional flexibility provided by the squares of income and education.

Analysis and Results

A considerable number of the health indicator coefficients were significant in many of the regressions. In certain cases, the graphs of these coefficients of correlation between health indicators and the growth rates of the main variables of the economic and demographic transition show a high degree of regularity and consistency, which allows us to draw a series of conclusions. In other cases, the graphs show diverse behaviors that raise more questions than they answer. Although we discuss the overall results, here we show only the numerical results of some of the groups of regressions. These correspond to cases in which the dependent variables are the growth rates of the following variables: income, female economic participation, percentage of the population under 1 year of age, and schooling. In general, the female health indicators yield higher and more significant coefficients. Accordingly, here we show only the graphs of the coefficients obtained by female health indicators for this set of variables. Table 12 summarizes the coefficients obtained for economic and demographic explanatory variables in the regression

TABLE 12. Average coefficients in main groups of regressions,[a] 711 observations in the periods 1980, 1985, and 1990 (GLS, CSW, white).[b]

Dependent variable	Income growth	Growth of economic participation	Growth of percentage of population under 1 year of age	Growth of schooling
Number of regressions	32	17	32	32
Health indicators	Both sexes	Female	Both sexes	Both sexes
Average of fixed effects	**1.532**	**0.33**	**–0.575**	**0.289**
of deciles	**(16.06)**	**(3.36)**	**(–9.82)**	**(2.72)**
Income	–0.4544	–0.1377	0.096	–0.0455
	(–14.48)	(–4.75)	(3.04)	(–0.06)
Income squared	0.0263	0.00924	–0.0188	0.00122
Schooling	0.0065	**0.0266**	0.0115	**0.0852**
	(8.3)	(4.75)	(–4.41)	
Schooling	0.0065	**0.0266**	0.0115	**0.0852**
of household head	(0.5)	(3.36)	(1.23)	(5.76)
	(0.5)	(3.36)	(1.23)	(5.76)
Schooling of	–0.0012	–0.0061	**0.0199**	–0.0095
household head squared		(–1.27)	**(6.35)**	(–1.5)
Average schooling	—	—	–0.0237	**–0.1767**
			(–1.15)	**(–31.74)**
Economically active	–0.0002	**–0.1129**	0.0075	**0.0114**
female population		**(–28.96)**	(0.21)	**(4.57)**
Economically	0.0101	0.0016	–0.0674	**–0.0794**
active male population	(0.38)		(–1.62)	**(–3.67)**
Percentage urban	0.0023	**–0.0214**	–0.0022	0.004
population	(0.61)	**(–6.83)**	(–0.01)	
Population growth	-7.15×10^{-9}	-8.27×10^{-8}	4.17×10^{-8}	-9.12×10^{-8}
		(–5.25)	(0.6)	(–6.48)
Percentage of population	**–0.0018**	0.0034	**–0.1894**	**0.0055**
under 1 year of age	**(–3.96)**	(0.88)	**(–26.23)**	**(2.82)**
Percentage of population	0.0003	–0.0072	**0.082**	**–0.0213**
under 6 years of age		(–0.78)	**(7.97)**	**(–6.57)**
Dummy variable 1985	**–0.0277**	**0.0255**	**–0.0406**	**0.0306**
	(–9.87)	**(16.61)**	**(–8.87)**	**(16.46)**
Dummy variable 1990	**–0.052**	**0.0248**	**–0.0509**	**0.0203**
	(–71.78)	**(21.28)**	**(–12.66)**	**(15.23)**
R^2 (minimum)	0.96	0.706	0.605	0.885
(maximum)	0.988	0.803	0.731	0.929
Adjusted R^2 (minimum)	0.958	0.692	0.586	0.88
(maximum)	0.988	0.794	0.718	0.926
Durbin-Watson (minimum)	1.935	2.156	2.189	1.965
(maximum)	2.386	2.251	2.285	2.055
F statistic (minimum)	528.01	52.54	32	163.06
(maximum)	1,823.91	89.33	57	277.97

[a] Health variable: probability of survival.

[b] GLS = generalized least squares; CSW = cross section weights; white = White's method to correct for heteroskedasticity.

Minimum t statistic in parentheses, if the signs coincide in all regressions.

groups mentioned, whereas Figures 1–4 show the coefficients of the health variables. The coefficients are comparable, because they represent elasticities.[16]

---

[16] The elasticity of dependent variable y with respect to independent variable x is $[\partial \log(y)]/[\partial \log(x)]$. This represents the percentage change in y when x changes by 1%.

Relationship between Health and Growth of Per Capita Income

We begin by using two indicators of health to study the growth of income per capita: life expectancy and the probability of survival. With the second indicator, $p_t t+a$ (see Figure 1), we obtain much more precise results, because it correctly separates the effects by age group, whereas

FIGURE 1. Significant coefficients (2.5%) in the correlation of the probability of survival for women and income growth rate (GLS, CSW, and white).[a]

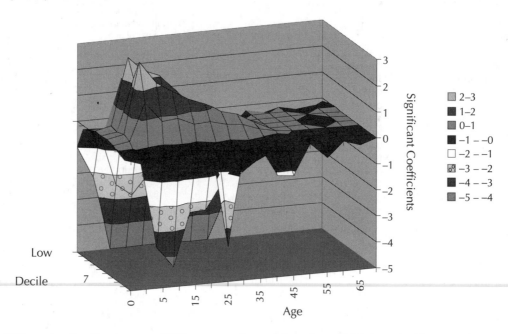

[a]GLS = generalized least squares; CSW = cross section weights; white = White's method for correcting for heteroskedasticity.

FIGURE 2. Significant coefficients (2.5%) in the correlation between the probability of survival for women and the growth rate of female economic participation (GLS, CSW, and white).[a]

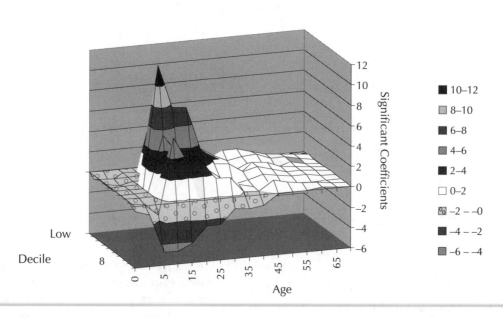

[a]GLS = generalized least squares; CSW = cross section weights; white = White's method for correcting for heteroskedasticity.

FIGURE 3. Significant coefficients (2.5%) in the correlation between the probability of survival for women and the growth rate of the percentage of the population under 1 year of age (GLS, CSW, and White).[a]

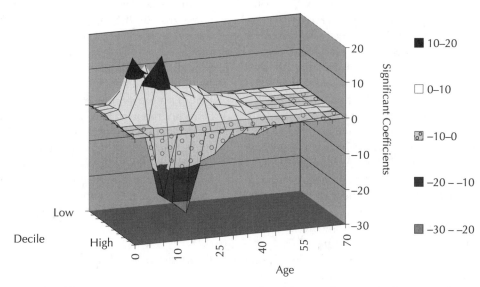

GLS = generalized least squares; CSW = cross section weights; White = White's method to correct for heteroskedasticity.

FIGURE 4. Significant coefficients (2.5%) in the correlation between the probability of survival for women and the growth rate of schooling (GLS, CSW, and White).[a]

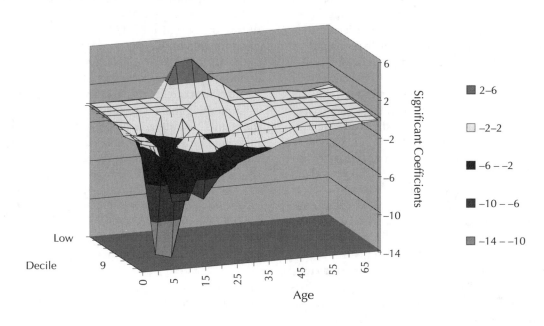

[a]GLS = generalized least squares; CSW = cross section weights; White = White's method to correct for heteroskedasticity.

life expectancy at age t is a weighted mean of health for age groups t and thereafter.

Figure 1 shows that the probability of survival for females aged 5–45 is positively correlated with income growth, except for the sectors of the population with very high or very low income levels. In these cases, the correlation is negative. In the case of high income, there appears to be a wealth effect on health in which women stop working and become involved in some other activity. The main such activity is motherhood, when women choose to remain at home. This hypothesis is strengthened by the results obtained when we take the growth rate of the economic participation of women, especially young women, as the variable to be explained (Figure 2). In upper-income levels, health correlates negatively with future female participation. This effect is corroborated when unemployment is used instead of participation. We deal with the results for the lower-income deciles in the section on participation and employment.

We consider it important to estimate the order of magnitude of the positive correlations between health and the growth of income and economic participation. For this, we used as a reference the average increases that occurred in the probability of survival $p_t t+a$ for women between 1985 and 1995. These estimates were hindered by the fact that there was a decline in the health indicators for some age groups in this period. Therefore, we estimated only the ranges in which the coefficients were observed. The maximum range for the direct effect on income of the average health increase from 1980 to 1995 is 0.19% per year. The average of the maximum range of the effect on female participation of $p_t t+a$ for women aged 15–35 is 0.39% per year. Because female participation is about 50% of male participation, and male participation is practically 100%, this increase in participation translates to an income growth of about 0.13% annually. It should be recalled that, because the increments in health are persistent, these effects are probably greater over longer periods of time, as indicated by the causality studies for Mexico and Latin America.

The results for the other explanatory variables for income growth are consistent with economic theory and are shown in Table 12. There is income convergence, which is somewhat greater for low incomes than for high incomes. Schooling of the household head contributes positively to growth, whereas schooling involving young people correlates negatively in that it represents an investment (in regressions not reported here). The appropriate indicator is an intermediate one. The percentage of the urban population contributes positively to growth. The percentage of the population under 1 year of age contributes negatively, and this is consistent with the impact on per capita income that arises from a larger population. On the other hand, a larger percentage of children under age 6 contributes positively, which may indicate that households with young children seek higher incomes.

With respect to the other explanatory variables for income growth, the results are consistent with economic theory (see Table 11). There is income convergence, a little more for low-income than for high-income groups. Schooling of the head of household contributes positively to growth, and average schooling, which refers more to that of young people, contributes negatively (in regressions not reported here), because it represents an investment. The ideal indicator is something in between. A higher percentage of the population living in urban areas contributes positively to growth. A higher percentage of the population under 1 year of age contributes negatively, which is consistent with the effect of a larger population on per capita income.

Relationship between Health and Fertility

To study the interaction between health and changes in fertility, we take as the dependent variable the growth rate in the percentage of children under 1 year of age in the household, a PNAD indicator determined by income levels.

The results show that health has a considerable impact on the demographic transition. Improvements in health are associated with higher rates of fertility in deciles 1–8 and with lower rates in deciles 9 and 10 (Figure 3). According to a Wald test, the difference among the coefficients is significant at the 0.0001 confidence level.

Average increases in the probability of female survival during the period 1985–1995 correlate with an increase of approximately 1% per year in the percentage of children under age 1 for low-income levels and with a reduction of the same order in the upper-income levels. These effects can be greater over longer periods of time.

Concerning the other explanatory variables (Table 12), the results indicate that, for the lower deciles, an increase in income correlates with an increase in fertility, whereas in decile 10 the relationship is reversed. This change in sign is consistent with economic theory. Schooling of the head of household contributes positively to fertility in all deciles and increases with wealth. However, average schooling contributes negatively—i.e., in new generations education reduces fertility. In addition, there is a declining trend in fertility over time.

Relationship between Health and Education

To study the interaction between health and changes in education we estimated regressions for the growth

FIGURE 5. Coefficients[a] of the lagged probability of survival in 204 economic growth regressions (GLS, CSW, White),[b] 18 Latin American countries.

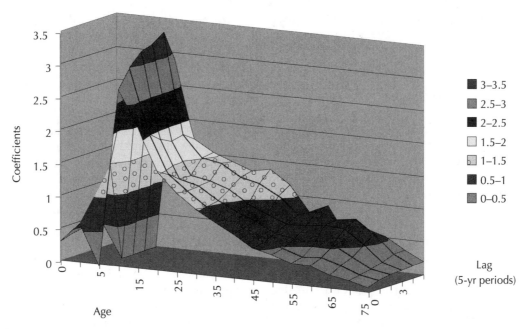

[a]Coefficients significant at the 1% level, women.

[b]GLS = generalized least squares; CSW = cross section weights; White = White's method to correct for heteroskedasticity.

rates of schooling and of school attendance at ages 7, 10, and 15.

In the case of schooling (Figure 5) as well as attendance, the results show effects of mixed signs. The following are some of our hypotheses about these results. Health, both for children (who study) and adults (who support them so they can attend school), has a positive impact on education indicators. However, with regard to negative effects, on observing the corresponding regions in the graphs on economic participation, it appears that healthier children join the workforce. This effect also may be correlated with higher fertility and female unemployment. Thus, it may be that a greater burden of young children in the home reduces the level of schooling of older children. Other explanations could be that there are conflicts in the allocation of public resources between health and education or that there is some association with phenomena of adolescence, including drug addiction, in which healthier adolescents drop out of school more frequently. Using the variable of violent deaths in males between the ages of 10 and 20 as a proxy for some juvenile problems, we obtain a decrease in the magnitude of the coefficients in the negative area but not their disappearance. This study cannot distinguish between these and other hypotheses. What the magnitude and

confidence levels of the coefficients do show is that the relationship between health and education is complex.

Again, using the increase in health from 1980 to 1995 as a reference, we estimate the magnitude of health's contribution to schooling, when this is positive. The maximum range is 0.29%. An estimate of the returns of education for the household head yields a coefficient of 0.90.[17] This implies, if the returns remain constant, that the contribution of health to economic growth through education has a maximum range of about 0.35% annually. As before, these effects may be greater over the longer term.

Concerning the other variables, in the case of schooling (Table 11), income levels lead to convergence, and schooling of the household head leads to divergence. Both processes are more intense at lower-income levels. The percentage of children aged 1–6 leads to growth in schooling. As for school attendance at 7, 10, and 15 years of age, the results yield a mosaic that is difficult to interpret. Some of the complexity may be due to stratification of the educational phenomena—for example, urban-rural or

---

[17] We control for participation and male and female employment, the population under ages 1 and 6, and temporal fixed effects. We use generalized least squares and correct for heteroskedasticity and correlation in the errors between deciles and states.

through the schooling of household heads. There is a positive correlation between female economic participation and increases in school attendance. The percentage of urban population has a positive effect on school attendance. Furthermore, there is a convergence effect on the initial level of each education variable analyzed.

Relationship between Health and Economic Participation, Unemployment, and Wages

The correlation between increases in health and female economic participation was mentioned in the section on income. In the case of males, there are increases in participation and decreases in unemployment.[18] These are especially sharp in the lowest decile and for the health indicators of young men and women. For corresponding regions of the graphs, we find a decrease in wages, with a very high implicit elasticity of approximately –6. These factors help to explain the reduction in income that occurs in the poorest decile when health indicators rise (Figure 1). Increases in health increase participation and employment in this decile (which is the one most vulnerable to unemployment, as indicated in the database) and the increased supply leads to a reduction in real wages and income.

With regard to the other explanatory variables (Table 12), the picture is consistent. Income correlates positively with an increase in male participation and negatively with female participation, consistently with increased fertility. Schooling of the household head correlates with an increase in female participation and with the wages of both sexes. This decreases a little with income. An increased percentage of the urban population reduces participation and increases unemployment and wages. An increased percentage of the population under 1 year of age increases female unemployment. An increased percentage of the population under 6 years of age increases male participation and the wages of both sexes. Furthermore, there is convergence on the initial levels of each variable analyzed.

Relationship between Health, Mortality, and Income Distribution

When we examine the correlation of income growth with the health variables maternal mortality, mortality from communicable diseases, and mortality from noncommunicable diseases, we find a surprisingly similar pattern. The correlation between increases in health (reduced mortality) and changes in income is positive for a broad segment of the intermediate deciles, following an inverted U shape. However, it is negative for the very high and very low deciles. We have shown that, in the high deciles, lower female participation reduces income, whereas in the lower deciles higher participation and employment reduce wages and income. Our previous explanations have assumed that state health indicators correlate with the health of every decile in every state and have been based mainly on the resulting sign. In fact, this assumption is confirmed by the existence of significant, differentiated, and consistent results for each decile. However, because the indicators are by state rather than by decile, the intensity of the correlation of the state indicator with the health of each decile may be different.

The inverted U shape of the correlation between health indicators and economic growth is evidence of such differences and is consistent with other work indicating that demographic segmentation of the health systems reinforces the existing inequities (Londoño and Frenk, 1997; González Block et al., 1997; Frenk, 1994). This implies the following: from its maximum on, which lies between deciles 4 and 6, state increases in health foster income convergence. In contrast, for the lower deciles, income divergence is fostered—i.e., less growth or even marginalization. The lower deciles receive fewer benefits from the health systems and must compete with deciles that receive better benefits. Additional evidence that health-related phenomena lead to divergence is that, when health indicators are included in the regressions, the coefficients indicating convergence become more significant.

In summary, we find evidence that increases in the state health indicators represent increases in health that are unevenly distributed among the population. Below decile 4, this inequality leads to divergence in income growth, and above decile 6 it leads to convergence. In contrast, we find little difference in the pattern of income change due to mortality from causes linked with maternity, communicable diseases, and noncommunicable diseases.[19]

Relationship between Income and Improvements in the Probability of Survival, p_t^{t+a}

The results of these regressions show a pattern in which health is increasingly sensitive to income with increasing

---

[18] The distinction between employment and participation is somewhat blurred in the results, probably because in surveys the questions and answers may be ambiguous on this point or may be understood differently by different population sectors.

[19] This finding in the relationship between causes of mortality and rates of income growth does not imply that the effect by income group of such causes of mortality is of a similar level.

age, especially for the older age groups, showing a larger correlation between income and survival for men, with a slightly smaller correlation for the lower income deciles.

Conclusions

Our results clearly indicate that health processes are part of Brazil's economic and demographic transition. The levels of health affect each of the principal aspects of the transition—namely, income, fertility, education, and economic participation.

According to our estimates, health increases income growth through three main channels: increases in educational levels, direct productivity effects, and increases in female participation. The period examined (1980–1995) is characterized by low or negative economic growth, which could mean that the economic potential of health might not have been fully realized. It is also a period of small increases in health status (see Figures 7 and 8 of the study on Latin America). In the case of Brazil, there are even some decreases in health status for some age and gender groups. This makes it difficult to measure the magnitude of the economic impact of health. The upper levels observed for the effects of improvements in health for the period are 0.35, 0.19, and 0.13 percentage points annually for the income growth rates due to increases in educational levels, direct productivity effects, and increases in female participation, respectively. Evidence from the long-term studies for Mexico and Latin America indicates that these effects are greater in the long run.

Health increases fertility (or limits its decline) at all income levels except for the highest, where it reduces fertility—a phenomenon consistent with the economic theory of endogenous fertility pioneered by Becker (see, for example, Becker et al., 1990; Dahan and Tsiddon, 1998). The 2% magnitude of these differences in fertility between upper and lower deciles could be even larger in the long term. However, education reduces fertility in the new generations, and fertility has a tendency to decline over time.

The health of both students and their parents increases the amount of schooling and school attendance. However, there are also negative correlations when minors apparently choose or are sent to work. This may be a secondary effect of greater fertility, in which homes with more children may provide less support from adults for school attendance. Both this effect and women's decisions to work or remain at home during motherhood are not adequately studied in economic theory. The reduction in schooling or in school attendance may also be the result of budgetary conflicts between health and education. In addition, there may be choices linked to adolescence that result in a reduction in human-capital formation.

When the effects of income on the probability of survival are studied, we confirm the conclusion arrived at in the study on the reciprocal impact of growth and health in Mexico (fourth section) in the sense that the causal relationship from health to income growth is much stronger than its inverse.

With regard to the distribution of income, increases in health can reduce inequality in principle, because their effects are greater when there is greater inequality. For example, increases in male and female participation occur especially in the low- and middle-income sectors. However, evidence shows that the distribution of health improvements is inequitable and, in fact, leads to divergence in incomes among the lowest 40% of the population. No really strong differences were detected in the patterns of the effects on income growth levels of mortality from causes related to maternity, communicable diseases, or noncommunicable diseases.

The results of the estimates show a high degree of consistency. The signs of the coefficients of income, education, proportion of urban population, and proportion of the population younger than 1 or younger than 6 years of age are the expected signs in almost every case. The Brazilian database we studied has enough indicators of the necessary quality to establish that health has complex interactions in the economic and demographic transition. Health manifests both positive and negative correlations with the trends of change of the main economic indicators. It increases income growth by fostering education, productivity, and economic participation. However, it also increases fertility at low and average incomes. This induces vicious circles in both income and schooling that revert only for high-income levels. Because of maternity, the economic participation of women in decile 10 decreases, which reduces income through what cannot be viewed as a negative effect because it is a result of the household's choice. Health also affects the distribution of income. Probably because of its poor distribution, it originates lower-income growth in the lower 40% of the population. Finally, the lowest 10%, who are most vulnerable to unemployment, see their income reduced because of increases in their economic participation that reduce their wages.

THE LONG-TERM IMPACT OF HEALTH ON ECONOMIC GROWTH IN LATIN AMERICA

In this study we analyze the long-term impact between health and economic growth in Latin America. Our motivation is the same as in the section on the long-term reciprocal impact of health and growth in Mexico, and we follow the conditional Granger causality methodology explained in that section. This analysis is possible because life tables have been available at five-year intervals since 1950 for many Latin American countries. Besides establishing a strong long-term relationship between health and economic growth, the results are interesting because they are directly comparable with both the above-mentioned study for Mexico and the study on the role of health on the economic and demographic transition in Brazil. The first of these studies uses life expectancy and mortality by age group and sex for several five-year periods but not the full life tables, whereas the second study uses only contemporary life tables.

The Study

We run the following economic growth regressions:

$$\frac{Y_{s(t+5)} - Y_{st}}{5} = \alpha y_{st} + \sum_i \beta_i X_{st}^i + \gamma S_{s(t-l)} + \sum_i c_i \chi_i + \varepsilon_{st}$$

Times t take the values 1975, 1980, and 1985. The variables are as follows: y_{st} is the logarithm of income per capita. Variable X_{st}^i is the logarithm of the average number of years of primary schooling of the population over 25 years of age, real investment as a proportion of product, and real "consumption" expenditure of the government as a proportion of product and total fertility (children per woman).[20] These variables include indicators for the basic explanatory variables of economic growth—namely, education, saving, and population growth. Variables χ_i are temporal dummies for the years 1975, 1980, and 1985, which take into account temporal effects common to the countries in the sample, such as macroeconomic and technological shocks. Subindex i runs through the following 18 countries: Argentina, Bolivia, Brazil, Costa Rica, Chile, Ecuador, El Salvador, Guatemala, Haiti, Honduras, Mexico, Nicaragua, Panama, Paraguay, Peru, the Dominican Republic, Uruguay, and Venezuela. During these years the average growth rates of these countries for the five-year periods 1960–1965 to 1985–1990 were 2.2%, 2.4%, 3%, 2.1%, –2.2%, and –0.6%, respectively.

The health variable S_{it} was the probability of survival to the next age group obtained from life expectancy by age groups and sex as described in the previous section. The age groups are 0–1, 1–5, 5–10, ..., and 75–80 years.

---

[20] The five variables are GDPSH5, PYR, INVSH5, GOVSH5, and FERT from the well-known Barro Lee database (available on the World Wide Web). The same database is used in this project for the Latin American economic indicators and is described in the second section of this paper.

The health variable was used with lags l of between 0 and 5 for the 5-year periods. This means that the number of regressions estimated was 17 age groups × 2 sexes × 6 lags = 204.

Results

The regressions were estimated by generalized least squares, correcting for heteroskedasticity and correlation in the errors between countries. The main statistics of these regressions are found in Tables 13 and 14. Initial income obtains a consistently negative sign (as expected by the hypothesis of conditional convergence) and is somewhat or very significant. "Average years of primary schooling for ages 25 and over" obtains a consistently significant negative sign [contrary to what is expected, as in Barro (1991)]. Investment obtains a consistently positive sign (as expected from economic theory), which is somewhat or very significant. The coefficients of the remaining variables change sign. Additionally, the R^2, F, and Durbin–Watson statistics are very good for all the regressions. Considering that each regression includes only 52 observations, the results are very good.

The coefficients of the female health variables are shown in Figure 5, with nonsignificant coefficients (less than 1% confidence) set to 0. The coefficients obtained by the male health indicators are somewhat smaller and less significant, as holds almost generally in the studies on Mexico and Brazil, but nevertheless follow the same pattern. The graph restricted to a zero lag is similar in shape and magnitude to the graph obtained for the Brazilian case (Figure 1). The highest coefficients are concentrated at the 10-year-old age group and diminish toward the younger and older age groups. What is important from the point of view of the long-term analysis is that the coefficients increase significantly toward the past for almost all the age groups. The coefficients of the adult age groups become larger (and, in the case of the male indicators, more significant). Such an increase would not take place, for example, if the lagged variable was income per capita.

These results are very similar to those obtained in the case of the study on Mexico. They confirm that there is a long-term relationship between health and economic growth and that adult health plays an important role in this relationship.

We analyze the magnitudes that these interactions between health and growth represent in real terms. To do this, we take into account the percentage increase in the probability of survival of men and women that actually occurred in the decades 1950–1960 and 1980–1990 and calculate the economic growth rates with which these health improvements would be associated. Figure 6

TABLE 13. Coefficients and their significance; results for 204 economic growth regressions for 18 Latin American countries (GLS, CSW, White).[a]

	Coefficient			Probability		
	Minimum	Average	Maximum	Minimum	Average	Maximum
Initial income	-9.17×10^{-6}	-7.26×10^{-6}	-1.82×10^{-6}	**6.20×10^{-12}**	**2.63×10^{-3}**	1.21×10^{-1}
Primary	-1.68×10^{-2}	-9.90×10^{-3}	-3.35×10^{-3}	**9.98×10^{-18}**	**1.22×10^{-4}**	**$9.13 \times 11,110^{-3}$**
Investment	1.67×10^{-2}	1.27×10^{-1}	1.66×10^{-1}	**2.19×10^{-11}**	**1.30×10^{-2}**	5.22×10^{-1}
Government consumption	-1.18×10^{-2}	1.96×10^{-2}	6.47×10^{-2}	8.29×10^{-2}	6.80×10^{-1}	9.98×10^{-1}
Fertility	-6.87×10^{-3}	-3.57×10^{-3}	3.10×10^{-3}	**3.40×10^{-6}**	3.30×10^{-1}	9.96×10^{-1}
Dummy 1975	$-3.30E+00$	-8.47×10^{-1}	8.65×10^{-2}	**8.93×10^{-6}**	**6.59×10^{-2}**	9.81×10^{-1}
Dummy 1980	$-3.34E+00$	-9.01×10^{-1}	4.22×10^{-2}	**1.18×10^{-6}**	**3.88×10^{-2}**	8.83×10^{-1}
Dummy 1985	$-3.33E+00$	-8.81×10^{-1}	6.17×10^{-2}	**2.98×10^{-6}**	**4.54×10^{-2}**	9.74×10^{-1}

Note: Boldface type indicates a confidence level better than 1%.

[a]GLS = generalized least squares; CSW = cross section weights; White = White's method to correct for heteroskedasticity.

TABLE 14. Global statistics.

	Minimum	Average	Maximum
R^2	0.86	0.92	0.97
Adjusted R^2	0.83	0.91	0.97
F statistic	32.19	71.15	179.25
Log probability	0.00000	0.00000	0.00000
Durbin–Watson	1.88	2.08	2.37
Number of observations	52	52	52

shows that these health increments are lower for the later decade, especially for women. Figures 7 and 8 show the economic growth associated with these decades' health increments obtained by using the coefficients of the regressions corresponding to the longest available lag (25 years to the initial period)—that is, the coefficients are multiplied by the health increments to obtain the associated economic growth.[21]

Because improvements in the probability of survival are relatively small between the ages of 5 and 15 (Figure 6), the shape of these graphs differs from the shape of the graph of the coefficients (Figure 5). The contribution of the different age groups is much more uniform, and the contribution to growth associated with the health increments of the old stands out. The male and female health increments of 1950–1960 are associated in the long term with income growth rates of about 0.8% and 1.1%, and the growth associated with the health increments of the older segment of the population would be even higher. The contribution that would be associated with the health increments of 1980–1990 is much smaller. In this case, men would contribute more than women, but the typical level would descend to 0.6% or more for adults, with the

female contribution running at 0.3%. Only in the case of 20-year-old men is the 1950–1960 level of contribution preserved. However, this seems to happen because of a notable negative perturbation in the health of this sector of the population that occurred in 1975 and 1980 (which extends to a lesser degree to 35 years of age).

The comparison shown in Figure 7 between the levels of economic growth associated with the health increments of two different decades has important implications. The changes in the quantity and distribution of health improvements can considerably affect long-term economic growth. The impact of each age group and sex on economic growth is very sensitive to the health improvement experienced by each sector of the population. Even when the coefficients of female health indicators are larger and more significant, male health improvements may contribute more to growth. The diminished health increments of the 1980–1990 decade (compared with those of the 1950–1960 decade), if not recuperated, may diminish income permanently between 4% and 8%.[22]

Overall, we can conclude that each health increment contributes permanently with an income increment, which takes time to fully take effect. The trajectory of the impact of health increments on income over time is shown in Figure 8, taking averages over female and male health indicators and also over all the indicators (vertical axis measures income in terms of percentage increments). Taking the form of this impact into account, as well as the different contributions for each five-year period, the approximate contribution of health increments to income in Latin America over the years 1950–1985 is shown in Figure 9 (vertical axis measures income in terms of percentage increments from 1950).

---

[21] We replaced the nonsignificant coefficients that occur for the 5-year-old age groups and for the 55-year-old female age group with the average of the neighboring coefficients.

[22] Examination of the health increments over the period 1950–1990 shows that the possibility that health improvements decrease in the long term plays a small role in the low performance of the 1980–1990 decade.

FIGURE 6. Percentage increase in the probability of survival, by age group and sex, 18 Latin American countries, 1950–1960 and 1980–1990.

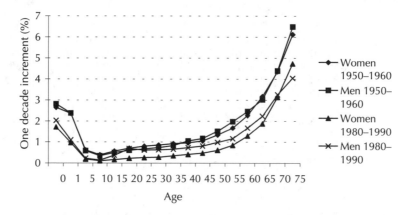

Conclusions

With regard to the long-term relationship between health and economic growth, this study confirms the results of the study on Mexico—namely, that there exists long-term conditional Granger causality from health to economic growth. The horizon of this phenomenon is not exhausted by the available information, which includes a lag of up to 25 years on the initial period—that is, a total of 30 years of lagged effects.

With regard to the coefficients of the impact on growth that the different age groups exert, there is a marked con-

sistency between the results for Brazil and Latin America, in which the largest coefficients correspond to young age groups and the most significant correspond to women. When the real changes in health are taken into account, the results coincide with those of the Mexican study in that adult health has a considerable long-term impact, which could be linked with intergenerational processes.

The impact of actual health increments at the longest lag of the period analyzed is found to be considerable, with an order of magnitude between 0.8% and 1.5% of annual economic growth. The impact of different age and sex groups depends on the health improvements each

FIGURE 7. Contribution by age group and sex of increments in the probability of survival to the annual income growth rate (five-year period beginning with a 25-year lag); health increments typical of the decades 1950–1960 and 1980–1990.

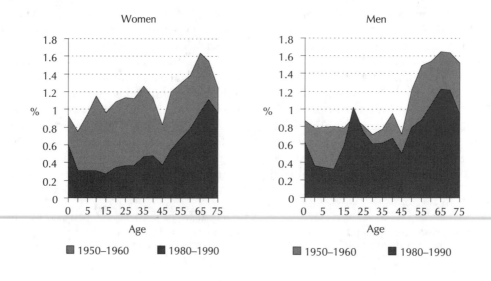

FIGURE 8. Temporal trajectory of the impact of health on income.

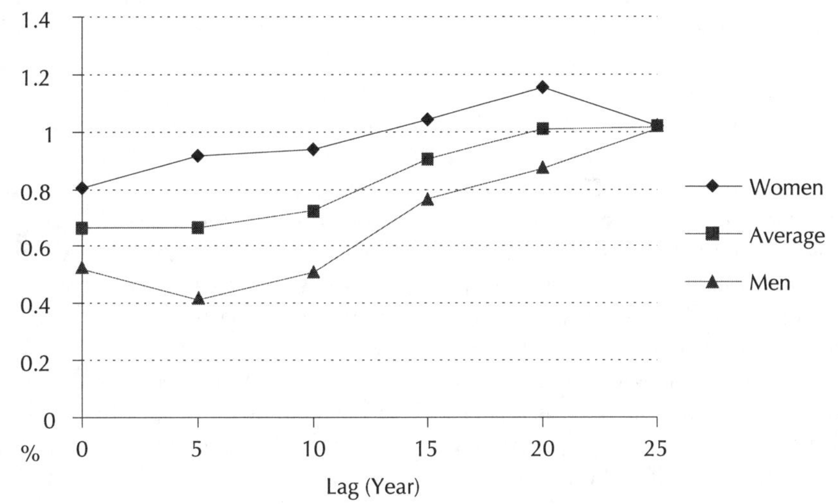

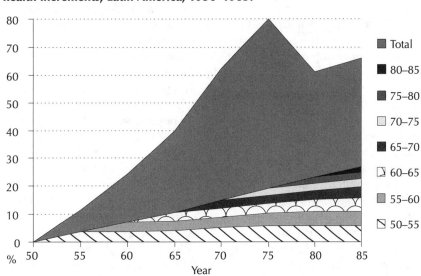

group may experience. In particular, it is notable that health improvements can contribute more in the elderly than in other age groups.

The results in the different studies show a high degree of consistency. Thus, the detailed and complex phenomena observed for Brazil, in which health affects income, education, economic participation, and fertility, as well as the causality results for Mexico probably take place not only in these countries but also in the Latin American region as a whole.

CONCLUSIONS AND POLICY RECOMMENDATIONS

The five research projects we have presented conclude that health plays an important role in economic growth. In the basic regressions of the Barro type (1991, 1996) on Latin America, as well as in the regressions for Brazil, Colombia, and Mexico, health plays a stronger role than education. The extreme limits test of Levine and Renelt (1992), which may be considered to be too strict, is confirmed in the case of Brazil for YLPD and in no case for

FIGURE 9. Approximate contribution to income growth of five-year-period health increments, Latin America, 1950–1985.

an educational indicator. From the point of view of economic theory, these analyses use relatively lax functional specifications, particularly compared with the augmented Solow model, which incorporates health as a determinant of human capital.

We include health in an application of the method of Islam (1995), who tests the augmented Solow model of economic growth of Mankiw et al. (1992). Given that significant results are obtained in the context of the economic constraints implied by a Solow-type growth model, the results may be considered as strong evidence of a reciprocal relationship between health and growth. In this same application, and contrary to expectations, the relationship between education and growth is generally negative, possibly because the indicators capture the level of education in age groups where it represents investment.

The panel regressions based on the method of Islam (1995) test an augmented Solow model in which health contributes to human capital. The results can be considered as evidence of a positive relationship between health and growth, because significant results are obtained in the restricted framework implied by the economics of the model.

The study on the long-term correlation between health and future income shows a very strong link for Mexico for the years 1955–1995, with lags of up to 15 and 20 years. These imply that there exists conditional Granger causality. The effects, which can be up to 2% of annual growth, cluster around the health of the economically strongest segment of the population and on maternity. The inverse causal relationship, from income to changes in health, also exists, although it is detected to be smaller. A larger residue is also present in these regressions. Improvements in health seem to depend more on public policies and on technological and behavioral changes as in the case of fertility.

The study of the role of health in the economic and demographic transition of Brazil (1980–1995) reveals complex relationships that induce both positive and negative correlations for all the indicators. This fact in itself explains the difficulties encountered in trying to find consistent and significant results in studies with a lower level of information, such as state-level studies or studies using samples of countries. With more information, a consistent picture emerges in which health plays a role that is not too different from what common sense would indicate.

Health increases income growth by fostering education, productivity, and economic participation, especially for women. The maximum positive ranges detected for these components, in a context of low growth and low and even negative health improvements, were 0.35%, 0.19%, and 0.13% percentage points of income, respectively. The channel with the largest contribution is edu-

cation. These effects can be larger in the long term, as established by the studies on Mexico and Latin America.

However, health increases fertility at low- and medium-income levels. This tends to reduce both income and schooling, except at high-income levels. The choice between working and staying at home, which occurs because of maternity, plays an important role as well.

Health also affects income distribution. In Brazil, the poor distribution leads to divergence processes in the income of the lowest 40% of the population. The lowest 10% even see their income reduced because of increases in economic participation that lead to reductions in real wages.

It is important to observe that the coefficients obtained by female health indicators tend to be larger and more significant. Health has economic impacts through maternity and female participation decisions, which also may have secondary effects on education. Thus, studies on the impact of health intersect with studies on women and the family.

The study of the long-term correlation between health and future income in the case of Latin America confirms the results of the study on Mexico, this time for a 25-year horizon. This study also reproduces the distribution of the regression coefficients by age groups and sex obtained for Brazil, and it shows that, once the real increments in health are taken into account, the contribution of adult and old age health improvements is the highest. The relative importance of male and female health depends on the health improvements that actually take place. Finally, the health improvements lost during the 1980–1990 decade may have a considerable impact on long-term economic growth.

Economic growth is linked to higher levels of health. Because of characteristics inherent to the health sector, an optimal allocation of investment resources in health necessarily involves the implementation of adequate public policies that not only make the health sector efficient but also take into account its effects on growth. These are long-term effects, an important portion of which occur through improvements in human capital in education.

Because this is another sector in which public policies are important, the efficiency problems are compounded. Except at the high-income levels, health may increase fertility and through this mechanism curb the increase in per capita income and education, which means that consistent policies must be maintained in health, education, and fertility. Policies that support women during motherhood and help make the choice between working and staying at home easier also may be successful. Health policies should also take distributive aspects into account. If the benefits do not reach the lower-income population, they contribute to a polarization of income and cease to have an effect on those sectors of the population for whom health investments produce the highest yield.

With regard to the magnitude of the aggregate impact of health on economic growth, the last three studies (on Mexico, Brazil, and Latin America) give a consistent picture once the different contexts are taken into account. The 2% estimate for the Mexican case corresponds to a high-growth environment with considerable health improvements. In the Latin American case, with an estimate of between 0.8% and 1.5%, the environment is one of medium growth with good health improvements. However, the parameters obtained for this case would yield a long-term contribution of only between 0.4% and 1% for the health improvements of the 1980–1990 decade. Finally, for the case of Brazil, which corresponds to this last period and for which the environment is of low or negative growth, the total short-term contribution obtained is a maximum of 0.67%, without taking into account some possible negative effects. In any case, these magnitudes must be considered as tentative, because the methodologies applied are not designed specifically for the purpose of estimating them and because of the deficiencies of the economic indicators in the databases.

Given the complexity of the interactions of health, and its relationship to education, the efficient implementation of public policies in a changing environment requires that information be sufficient to evaluate effects, costs, and benefits. The database we have worked with here represents a bare minimum that is nonetheless absent in practically every country in Latin America. We believe the systematic development of information sources of the breadth and depth necessary for these purposes should be promoted systematically both inside and outside the sphere of public services and health. This would yield enormous results. These sources should systematically cross-reference demographic (including maternity) and health indicators with information on education, economics, and the effect of public subsidies. Information should be obtained comprehensively from broader household surveys and from the institutions that furnish the various public services.

We now address the subject of efficiency in the allocation of resources among age groups. Recall first that economic growth is not an objective in itself. The theory of economic growth rests on the optimal allocation of consumption over time, in keeping with individual preferences. In this context, for example, better health may increase the number of women who choose to remain at home instead of working outside the home, which occurs in high-income households in Brazil because of a wealth effect, and a lower income may result. Far from being a negative effect, what we see here is a phenomenon whereby households are better able to pursue their

preferences. Analogously, the differentiated impact of health improvements by age and sex on increases in income, economic participation, and education only implies that an additional proportional weight should be given to the health of these groups, accounting for the intertemporal aspect of the allocation of health resources.

A topic for additional research could be the rigorous determination of these weights, which would also provide the economic basis for the weights involved in the formulation of life-year-type health indicators and would estimate the benefits to be obtained from using these to rationalize public spending. A related subject would be precise determination of the preferences that underlie the individual decisions that lead to the dynamics we have analyzed. This requires the development of theoretical and technical tools that include both the consideration of epidemiological risks and of household decisions on fertility, on whether mothers work outside the home or stay at home, and on education versus work at different stages in the family cycle. It is feasible to base this study on the information generated by this project.

Besides efficiency, technological absorption and development play an important role in the health sector, as they do in economic growth. It must be taken into account that facilitating the implementation of new health technologies, as well as updating existing health systems, has the potential of generating large benefits in terms of health and future economic growth at a cost that may be relatively low.

It is clear that, to carry out systematic analyses that incorporate the differences and socioeconomic and demographic characteristics of the various countries, it is necessary to count with enough comparable and periodic information. Such information must be obtained from household or life quality surveys, including questions on health, income, expenditure, availability of public services, economic participation, childcare, etc., for all members of the household. Based on this information, it would be possible to evaluate, in each period, the successes and limitations of those policies most closely related to economic growth, alleviation of poverty, and development. It is to be expected that the relationships between economic growth and health analyzed in this study may differ among countries and therefore that the emphasis on specific population groups, which public policies must have, could also be different.

Surveys incorporating measures of the state of health and of the use of health services by household members have been developed. Nevertheless, there exists an ample potential to obtain information that can be combined with other sources to periodically measure indicators such as YLPD or years of healthy life. In this study, it was possible to establish that such precise indicators can capture relationships with economic variables that are not significant when less accurate indicators are used.

This study analyzes the relationship between health and economic growth. However, it is necessary to investigate the processes that determine the conformation of a population's particular state of health, or, in other terms, how health capital is accumulated. This subject raises numerous questions. For example, it is necessary to analyze whether different subsidy schemes have different effects on the population's health; whether access to health services is differentiated across socioeconomic groups and service systems or is conditioned by employment; whether the insurance system induces the selection of risks among the population; etc.

From an economic point of view, health and education are both important components of human capital. However, the existing measures of one or the other variable do not incorporate the simultaneous determination of these two dimensions of human capital or their reciprocal interactions. The development of coherent and integral measures of these two dimensions of human capital as a factor of production is very important. However, besides productivity, health has other important channels of impact. One of them is education, in which important temporal lags exist. Another is female economic participation. Indicators complementary to health capital can be developed to account for the role of health as a factor of production of education and as a conditioning factor of female participation. Together, these different measures would highlight different aspects of a population's health. They could be used as observational variables to evaluate the effects of public policy in the areas of education and health as well as in the analysis of the relationship of health and other social, demographic, and economic variables. Measurement of the component of human capital that is determined by education has contributed valuable instruments for the analysis of such economic relationships and for policy design. However, a notable gap exists in relation to the economic effects of health.

REFERENCES

Barro R. Economic growth in a cross section of countries. *Quarterly Journal of Economics.* 1991; 196 (2/May):407–443.

Barro R. *Health and Economic Growth.* Annex I of *Convocatoria para propuestas de investigación sobre Inversión en Salud y Crecimiento Económico de la Organización Panamericana de la Salud.* Washington, D.C.: Pan American Health Organization (PAHO); 1996.

Becker GS, Murphy KM, Tamura R. Human capital, fertility, and economic growth. *Journal of Political Economy.* 1990; 98(5–2/Oct):S12–S37.

Dahan M, Tsiddon D. Demographic transition, income distribution, and economic growth. *Journal of Economic Growth.* 1998; 3(1/March):29–52.

Ehrlich I, Lui F. Intergenerational rade, longevity and economic growth. *Journal of Policital Economy.* 1991; 99 (5): 1029–1059.

Frenk J. Dimensions of health system reform. *Health Policy* 1994; 27.

Galor O, Weil DN. The gender gap, fertility, and growth. National Bureau of Economic Research Working Paper. 1993; (Nov.) No. 4550.

González Block *et al.* Experiencias de reforma en los sistemas de salud en el mundo. In: Frenk J., ed. *Observatorio de la salud: necesidades, servicios, politicas.* Mexico City: Fundación Mexicana para la Salud; 1997.

Islam N. Growth empirics: a panel data approach. *Quarterly Journal of Economics.* 1995; 110(4):1127–1170.

Levine R, Renelt D. A sensitivity analysis of cross-country growth regressions. *American Economic Review.* 1992; 82(4/Sept.):942–963.

Londoño JLL, Frenk J. Structured pluralism: towards an innovative model for health system reform in Latin America. *Health Policy.* 1997; 41 (1/July): 1–36.

Mankiw NG, Romer D, Weil D. A contribution to the empirics of economic growth. *Quarterly Journal of Economics.* 1992; May: 407–437.

World Bank. *World Development Report 1993. Investing in Health.* London/New York: Oxford University Press; 1993.

World Health Organization. *The World Health Report.* Geneva: World Health Organization; 1999.

Part II

Productivity of Household Investment in Health

PRODUCTIVITY OF HOUSEHOLD INVESTMENT IN HEALTH: THE CASE OF COLOMBIA

Rocio Ribero[1] and Jairo Nuñez[2]

INTRODUCTION

The purpose of this study is to understand how public and private investments in health in Colombia relate to the future earnings of individuals. The effects of being in good health as well as the determinants of health production functions are studied at the individual level. This chapter attempts to identify the magnitude of the returns of having good health status through the direct effect of health variables on the earnings of individuals. Regional (rural-urban)[3] and gender aspects are considered separately. The aim of this study is to use the information in the optimal design of policy interventions that may enhance health and increase labor productivity among low-income and disadvantaged groups.

This is the first study to analyze the links between primary indicators of health and individual labor productivity in Colombia and how additional public expenditures in health may improve individuals' health. Investments in health, as well as investments in schooling, affect an individual's productivity. Household resource allocation and consumption decisions determine nutritional status and the health of children and adults within the household. These decisions have an impact on adult anthropometric measures such as height or body mass index (BMI), acute and chronic morbidity, and patterns of illness and disability.

Human capital has many forms besides schooling. Migration, the capacity to avoid unwanted fertility, and health outcomes also are forms of reproducible human capital. The framework set up by Mincer (1974) is en-riched to allow for additional forms of human capital besides schooling. Schultz (1997) analyzed how state and family investments influence the formation of reproducible human capital and, also, how these affect labor earnings and growth. The main questions he studied are what determine the household demand for human capital and what are the wage returns of human capital stock in the labor market. Schultz (1997) found that adult height is an important determinant of adult productivity and that it emerges as inversely correlated to chronic health problems among the middle-aged and elderly. Moreover, results show that height is inversely related to mortality and, consequently, directly related to length of productive life. Fogel (1994) also found that height and BMI are related to male mortality at later ages and to chronic diseases between the ages of 20 and 50. This study confirms that height is positively related to individual earnings in Colombia.

According to Schultz and Tansel (1997), most studies that measure morbidity are related to high-income countries and focus on chronic disabilities among the elderly (degenerative diseases). Other studies have analyzed the productivity effects of nutrition in developing countries (Behrman, 1993; Deolalikar, 1988; Behrman and Deolalikar, 1988; Sahn and Alderman, 1988), and extensive literature has focused on child morbidity and malnutrition effects for children (Rosenzweig and Wolpin, 1988; Rosenzweig and Schultz, 1982a, 1983). Schultz (1984) has analyzed the relation between child mortality and public program interventions. Adult health status measures, such as height, reflect cumulative health, early childhood conditions, and nutrition investments undertaken by the parents of the individual (Strauss and Thomas, 1995; Martorell and Habicht, 1986). In addition, changes in height over time may be attributed to changes in reproducible human capital investments or in disease environments (Fogel, 1994). Strauss and Thomas (1997) used household urban Brazilian data containing height and BMI information and found that height has a large and

[1] Professor, Universidad de los Andes; Researcher, Centro de Estudios sobre Desarrollo Económico; Postdoctoral Fellow, Economic Growth Center, Yale University.
[2] Researcher, Departamento Nacional de Planeación.
[3] The patterns of illness in Colombia differ highly between rural and urban areas, and communicable diseases occur more frequently in rural areas. In 1993, approximately 30% of the Colombian population lived in rural areas (United Nations Development Program, 1998).

significant effect on wages for males and females. Based on this evidence, this study focuses on the relationship between height and other indicators of the current health of adults and their productivity. Exploring this relationship will help to identify policy tools to improve adult health outcomes and promote growth efficiently and equitably.

Strauss and Thomas (1995, 1997) used survey data from urban Brazil to show that, even after controlling for education, different dimensions of health such as height, BMI, calorie intake, and protein intake affect the wages of men and women positively. They found that, relative to the returns to education without controlling for health, the estimated returns to education with health controls were 45% smaller for literate men and 30% smaller for men with a secondary education or more. Schultz (1996) found that the estimated wage returns to schooling are reduced between 10% and 20% with the addition of three other human capital inputs in the regression: migration, BMI, and height. In this paper, however, it is found that the returns to education are almost invariant to the introduction of health in the earnings equations. They change from 9.7% without height to 9.1% with height for urban men and from 9.6% without height to 9.0% with height for urban women. They are identical when the dummy for disability or the number of days disabled is included in the instrument variable (IV) estimates of the earnings equation.

This study finds significant and positive effects of height on wages. Taller men receive hourly earnings 8% higher per centimeter and women receive hourly earnings 7% higher per centimeter. The size of the returns in Colombia are in line with the returns found in Ghana (Schultz, 1996), where a 1 cm increase is associated with a 5.7% wage gain for males and a 7.5% gain for females, holding constant for BMI and migration. In Côte d'Ivoire, the returns for male height are not significantly associated with a wage gain, holding constant for BMI and migration. These estimated returns to height in Colombia reveal that investments in nutrition may be important for future increases in productivity and growth.

Strauss and Thomas (1995) found that the effects of nutrition on height and adult productivity are subject to diminishing returns. The proportionate increase in height due to better nutrition may be greater for those who are especially malnourished. As a consequence, human capital returns are expected to be higher at lower levels of investments. In this way, nutritional programs targeted to the poor would help reduce income inequalities and promote efficient growth. Although information on nutritional programs to test this hypothesis was unavailable for this study, the models tried to capture nonlinear returns to adult health outcomes by introducing height

in linear and quadratic specifications in the earnings function. However, this study relies on the linear specification because the quadratic specification did not yield more precise estimates.

The approach used in this paper to evaluate health-related programs is an integrated human capital demand and wage framework presented by Schultz (1997) in which it is necessary to coordinate many types of data, some of which are not readily available. Two household labor market surveys were used to collect information on hourly earnings, labor force participation, and non-labor income and assets as well as measures of human capital stocks, such as height and disability.

The unit of analysis is the individual. The health indicators expected to be associated with current productivity of workers are a dummy for having been disabled[4] in the past month, the number of days disabled in the past month, and height. These are indicators of human capital because they can be affected by social investments, although they may vary across individuals because of genetic or environmental factors not controlled by the individual, family, or society. Based on an extended earnings function that includes health measures as human capital stocks in addition to schooling, productivity gains associated with these forms of human capital in Colombia are estimated. The possibility that health measures may be endogenous or measured with error is taken into account by the use of instrumental variable estimation.

This chapter's second section describes data sources and main characteristics of each survey as well as the health indicators. The third section presents descriptive statistics of the data. Empirical specification issues, estimation, and policy simulations are discussed further in the fourth section and the fifth section presents the main conclusions derived from the analysis.

THE DATA

This section describes the main sources of data and the variables used for the study. Apart from two major household surveys conducted by the Departamento Administrativo Nacional de Estadística (DANE), different sources were consulted to obtain regional data on environmental factors. That data were merged with the individual household survey data, so that each individual was linked to the characteristics of his or her community.

The socioeconomic characterization survey (CASEN) is a national survey conducted in 1993, which has specific modules on health, education, and child mortality. The survey interviewed 27,271 households: 22,257 in an

---

[4] Not able to attend work because of illness.

urban area and the remainder in rural areas. The size of the sample of individuals between 18 and 70 years old with positive wages or earnings was 35,395, of whom 64% were male and 74% lived in urban areas.

From this survey two indicators of health were used, which are the dependent variables of the health production functions:

1. Disability: a dummy variable equal to one if the individual reports that he or she was not able to work in the month before the survey because of his or her illness,[5] and

2. Number of days disabled: the actual number of days of work lost because of the specific illness[6] (as reported by the individual).

The variables to describe the individuals' characteristics are age, education, logarithm of hourly earnings, whether the person is a salaried worker, nonlabor income, and whether the individual lives in a house or an apartment.

To explain the health outcomes, a series of variables that describe the environmental factors was constructed from CASEN. By averaging the observations in rural and urban areas in each *departamento*,[7] the following community characteristics were linked to each individual:

1. Availability of credit (from either the public or the private sector) to buy a house in the *departamento* by rural and urban subareas;

2. Education level in the *departamento* by rural and urban subareas (illiteracy rates, primary and secondary coverage);

3. Percentage of persons affiliated with social security in the *departamento* by rural and urban subareas; and

4. Infrastructure conditions (water, electricity) in the *departamento* by rural and urban subareas.

The Instituto Geográfico Agustín Codazzi (1996) provided information about the following environmental factors used to account for health outcomes:

1. temperature, altitude, and rainfall in each municipality;

2. distance from each town to the capital of the *departamento*, where major hospitals are located;

3. average times to reach schools in the municipality;

4. average times to reach hospitals in the municipality;

5. availability of water in the municipality;

6. availability of electricity in the municipality;

7. availability of primary schools in the municipality;

8. availability of secondary schools in the municipality;

9. availability of hospitals in the municipality; and

10. availability of health centers in the municipality.

The Ministry of Health provided information about coverage of vaccination programs by municipality,[8] number of hospitals available in each municipality, and quality of those hospitals,[9] among others. From another external source[10] an index of the kilometers of paved roads per population and area in each *departamento* was obtained.

The urban part of the national household survey—stage 74 (ENH-91)[11] was collected in December 1991. This is a household survey that covers the 11 major cities of Colombia: Bogotá, Cali, Medellín, Barranquilla, Bucaramanga, Manizales, Pasto, Cúcuta, Pereira, Ibagué, and Montería. Surrounding metropolitan areas of the cities are included. These cities represent close to 40% of the total population of the country and about 70% of the urban population; the smallest of these cities at the time of the survey had at least 200,000 people.

The urban portion of ENH-91 is the only survey in Colombia that includes a person's height,[12] which is used here as the adult health outcome. This survey does not include the information about previous illness or lost days of work. The sample population was between 18 and 70 years old, but the age range is restricted in some estimations and figures (the wages and health equations are estimated for those between 18 and 60 years old). This cutoff is made because we believe that individuals may

---

[5] A preceding question included in the survey was: "During the last month did you have any illness, accident, and dental problem or health problem?" The question used here is: "During the last month did you not go to work or did not do your ordinary activities because of the illness or health problem mentioned above?" (in Spanish: "durante el último mes dejó usted de asistir al trabajo o realizar sus actividades ordinarias debido a la enfermedad o problema de salud señalado antes?"). The answers to these two questions were either "yes" or "no."

[6] The actual question used here says in Spanish "cuántos días estuvo incapacitado o en cama durante el último mes?" which can be translated as "for how many days during the last month did you not go to work or did you stay in bed?" In the questionnaire there is a space for the interviewer to write the number of days.

[7] Colombia is divided in 26 *departamentos*.

[8] This is measured as a percentage of coverage relative to the vaccination goal of the Ministry of Health for that municipality.

[9] A number between 1 and 6 to indicate the level of attention (from attending minor wounds to performing major medical interventions) in the institution.

[10] Económica Consultores (1996).

[11] We refer to this survey as ENH-91 to emphasize the year when it was conducted.

[12] The survey also includes a rural area, but it does not record the height of individuals for this rural area.

shrink after age 60 (not necessarily reflecting childhood nutritional status) and individuals may still be growing before age 18. From all persons who earn positive wages or earnings, those with unreasonable heights (less than 135 cm) were excluded,[13] leaving a working sample of 23,910 adults.

The variables used to describe individuals' characteristics are age, education, logarithm of hourly earnings, whether the person is a salaried worker, nonlabor income, and whether the house where the respondent lives is owned by him (her) or his (her) family (owner-occupied housing).[14]

To explain adult height, the following environmental health factors were derived from ENH-91:

1. percentage of households in the community with access to basic services (water, sewerage, and electricity);[15] and
2. percentage of households in the community with favorable population density according to poverty standards.[16]

The characterization of the community where the individual lives was made first by city and, within each city, by strata. In Colombia, the major cities are divided into six socioeconomic strata depending on the economic capabilities of the households, in order to charge differential rates for public services such as water, electricity, and telephone service.[17] Persons know how their houses are rated.[18]

It is assumed that a person's place of residence is exogenous, although people may have migrated to a specific area or community because of the variables treated here as exogenous, introducing potential bias in our estimates (Rosenzweig and Wolpin, 1988).[19]

---

[13] The number of observations dropped at this stage was approximately 7% of the total sample.

[14] In Spanish, "casa propia."

[15] The survey provides information of access to each service separately. The dummy variable used to construct the "percentage of households in the community with access to basic services" was 1 when the house had access to all three basic services and 0 otherwise.

[16] The percentage of households in the community without overcrowding in the houses based on DANE's definition of overcrowding.

[17] Because there are only 11 cities, a second characterization that gave more variability to the community variables for the sample was needed. Using strata, also provided by the survey, allowed having 66 different values for the community variables.

[18] Sometimes the interviewer is ordered to ask the respondent for receipts from the electricity, phone, and water companies to confirm that the information of strata is accurate.

[19] In this paper, we do not try to explain migration decisions, because the surveys do not provide sufficient information on migration histories or height information on rural populations.

DESCRIPTIVE STATISTICS OF THE COLOMBIAN DATA

Two samples were consulted. The first sample (CASEN) involves persons who lived in rural or urban areas in 1993, were earning a wage or had positive labor earnings, and were between 18 and 70 years old. This sample is 36% female and 64% male; only 9% have more than 13 years of schooling, 8% have 0 years of schooling, and 46% have partial or complete primary schooling; 74% live in urban areas. This sample is used to estimate the models with disability and the number of days disabled. The second sample (ENH-91) is urban only. It includes the health variable height. We used wage earners or individuals between 18 and 60 years old with positive labor earnings; 59% of this sample are males and 41% are females; 4% have 0 years of schooling and 13% have more than 13 years of education. The main characteristics of the samples and health indicators are reported in Tables 1–4.

In general, illness is more frequent among women than among men, and it increases with age. Illness is more common among less educated individuals than among the more educated (within rural and urban populations), and it occurs more frequently among rural than urban residents at all levels of education. The patterns for disability and number of days disabled shown in Tables 1 and 2 are similar to each other. However, the number of days disabled diminishes with education until 12 years of schooling; oddly, it increases at 13 or more years of schooling in urban areas. Note that this happens only for days disabled and not for disability. As shown in Table 1, the percentage of more educated individuals who have a disability is lower than among the less educated at all levels of education. This result is contrary to what was found by Schultz and Tansel (1997) in Ghana and Côte d'Ivoire, where the propensity of adults to report illness was positively related to education. The average number of days disabled may increase for urban residents with more than 13 years of schooling because they may have higher expectations about their health, be more able to perceive illness, or be more willing to seek professional advice (Johansson, 1991). In addition, more educated individuals may have more resources to indulge their illnesses and consume more days disabled when they are ill.

Figure 1 shows the histogram of the number of days disabled for the population with a positive number of days disabled. The bulk of this sample (78%) has fewer than 10 days of disability, 10% have 15 days of disability, and 7% of the sample have been disabled for the entire past month (they may be chronically disabled).

The patterns of height summarized in Table 3 refer to the whole sample between 18 and 70 years old and not

TABLE 1. Weighted share with disability by education, area, and sex.

Education	Area			Education	Sex		
	Rural	Urban	Total		Male	Female	Total
0 years	52,184	24,606	76,790	**0 years**	53,164	23,626	76,790
% population	9.60%	6.46%	8.31%	% population	7.99%	9.13%	8.31%
1–6 years	139,580	222,164	361,744	**1–6 years**	237,664	124,080	361,744
% population	6.78%	6.80%	6.79%	% population	6.46%	7.55%	6.79%
7–12 years	18,315	237,096	255,411	**7–12 years**	150,262	105,149	255,411
% population	4.83%	6.29%	6.16%	% population	6.11%	6.23%	6.16%
+13 years	1,298	42,179	43,477	**+13 years**	13,723	29,754	43,477
% population	3.61%	4.31%	4.28%	% population	2.44%	6.57%	4.28%
Total	211,377	526,045	737,422	**Total**	454,813	282,609	737,422
% population	7.01%	6.27%	6.46%	% population	6.17%	6.99%	6.46%

Age	Education					Age	Sex		
		1–6 years	7–12 years	>13 years	Total		Male	Female	Total
18–24	2,466	49,186	64,010	3,139	118,801	**18–24**	70,496	48,305	118,801
% pop.	3.84%	5.44%	5.77%	3.15%	5.45%	% pop.	5.03%	6.23%	5.45%
25–34	7,597	85,494	87,591	18,020	198,702	**25–34**	118,245	80,457	198,702
% pop.	5.88%	6.19%	5.33%	4.10%	5.53%	% pop.	5.22%	6.05%	5.53%
35–44	12,764	81,775	68,222	15,559	178,320	**35–44**	98,094	80,226	178,320
% pop.	6.29%	6.36%	7.44%	4.78%	6.53%	% pop.	5.85%	7.61%	6.53%
45–59	26,716	98,301	28,814	6,544	160,375	**45–59**	104,983	55,392	160,375
% pop.	8.23%	7.33%	7.21%	4.88%	7.29%	% pop.	6.99%	7.93%	7.29%
60–70	27,247	46,988	6,774	215	81,224	**60–70**	62,995	18,229	81,224
% pop.	13.40%	11.48%	8.75%	1.26%	11.49%	% pop.	12.11%	9.76%	11.49%
Total	76,790	361,744	255,411	43,477	737,422	**Total**	454,813	282,609	737,422
% pop.	8.31%	6.79%	6.16%	4.28%	6.46%	% pop.	6.17%	6.99%	6.46%

Source: CASEN.

% of total population below numbers. Sample including all persons in the labor force between 18 and 70 years of age.

only to participants in the labor market. They indicate that between young (18–24) and old (60–70) age groups, women have gained 2.88 cm and men have gained 2.91 cm. Most of the gain occurs between age groups 45–59 and 60–70, which suggests that gains to height from nutrition may be subject to sharply diminishing returns. However, part of the gain observed between these two age ranges may be because old people shrink for biological reasons and, therefore, the gain may be overstated. The best educated have an 8.36-cm advantage over the 0-year educated, although this result mixes age and class. There is less than 1 cm of gain within all the education groups and across ages (between the youngest and oldest age groups), except for the group with 0 years of schooling, where there was a 2 cm gain. Across education groups (between 0 and >13 years of schooling) and

within age groups, the gap has declined from 9 cm for the oldest to 5 cm for the youngest. However, for the 25- to 34-year-olds, the gap remains 9 cm.

Figure 2 shows the trends in height for the entire population aged 25–55 in 1991 in relation to their dates of birth. Figure 3 shows the same but only for participants in the labor force. There is a secular increase in height similar in shape and size to the one observed by Strauss and Thomas (1998) in Brazil. As shown in Table 3, the slope in the trend line is steeper for females than for males. Additionally, comparing the slopes in Figure 2 and Figure 3 shows that the slopes for labor force participants are higher than those for the entire population. This may indicate that the urban labor market has been selecting individuals who have higher child nutritional levels. Figure 2 implies an estimate that in Colombia the height

TABLE 2. Mean number of days disabled by age, sex, education, and area.

Age	Sex			Education	Area		
	Male	Female	Total		Rural	Urban	Total
18–24	6.87 (6.25)	4.28 (4.23)	5.82 (5.66)	**0 years**	8.54 (8.24)	10.55 (9.52)	9.18 (8.72)
25–34	6.38 (6.44)	6.36 (6.26)	6.37 (6.37)	**1–6 years**	8.77 (8.34)	7.37 (7.49)	7.91 (7.86)
35–44	7.53 (8.35)	7.05 (8.37)	7.31 (8.36)	**7–12 years**	6.62 (5.15)	6.22 (6.7)	6.24 (6.6)
45–59	10.17 (9.47)	7.12 (6.8)	9.12 (8.76)	**+13 years**	3.67 (0.95)	9.66 (10.29)	9.48 (10.19)
60–70	10.30 (8.57)	10.95 (9.61)	10.44 (8.82)	**Total**	8.49 (8.09)	7.18 (7.62)	7.56 (7.78)
Total	8.12 (8.09)	6.65 (7.17)	7.56 (7.78)				

Age	Education					Education	Sex		
	0 years	1–6 years	7–12 years	>13 years	Total		Male	Female	Total
18–24	6.153 (4.66)	5.862 (5.9)	5.51 (5.02)	11.244 (10.25)	5.82 (5.66)	**0 years**	9.38 (8.93)	8.74 (8.21)	9.18 (8.72)
25–34	7.821 (6.5)	6.943 (6.54)	5.866 (6.14)	5.521 (6.24)	6.37 (6.37)	**1–6 years**	8.45 (8.32)	6.87 (6.77)	7.91 (7.86)
35–44	8.026 (8.81)	6.936 (6.77)	6.213 (8.03)	13.551 (12.99)	7.314 (8.36)	**7–12 years**	7.07 (7.07)	5.06 (5.66)	6.24 (6.60)
45–59	8.922 (8.83)	9.549 (9.35)	7.672 (6.66)	9.737 (6.41)	9.115 (8.76)	**+13 years**	9.15 (9.67)	9.63 (10.41)	9.48 (10.19)
60–70	10.627 (9.14)	10.057 (8.97)	12.304 (5.26)	13.046 (13.08)	10.443 (8.82)	**Total**	8.12 (8.09)	6.65 (7.17)	7.56 (7.78)
Total	9.18 (8.72)	7.907 (7.86)	6.244 (6.6)	9.479 (10.19)	7.556 (7.78)				

Source: CASEN.
Standard deviations are in parentheses. Sample including all persons between 18 and 70 years of age in the labor force.

FIGURE 1. Histogram of number of days disabled.

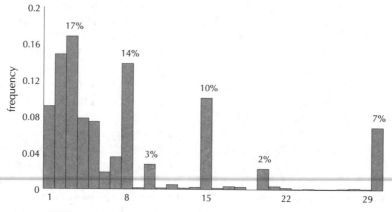

Source: CASEN

TABLE 3. Mean height in centimeters by age, sex, and education.

Age	Sex			Education	Sex		
	Male	Female	Total		Male	Female	Total
18–24	169.32 (11.43)	160.40 (9.98)	164.23 (11.49)	**0 years**	164.66 (9.52)	155.25 (12.79)	158.58 (12.46)
25–34	169.50 (10.10)	160.38 (9.93)	164.55 (10.96)	**1–6 years**	167.01 (9.10)	158.30 (10.28)	162.04 (10.68)
35–44	169.13 (9.57)	160.21 (9.75)	164.30 (10.57)	**7–12 years**	169.44 (10.63)	160.72 (9.80)	164.63 (11.05)
45–59	168.05 (8.51)	158.63 (10.86)	162.94 (10.91)	**>13 years**	171.64 (10.25)	162.01 (9.05)	166.94 (10.74)
60–70	166.41 (10.67)	157.52 (10.62)	161.32 (11.47)	**Total**	168.89 (10.14)	159.81 (10.17)	163.89 (11.08)
Total	168.89 (10.14)	159.81 (10.17)	163.89 (11.08)				

Age	Education				
	0 years	1–6 years	7–12 years	>13 years	Total
18–24	160.37 (14.81)	162.11 (11.06)	164.72 (10.97)	165.76 (14.03)	164.23 (11.49)
25–34	158.27 (15.98)	162.69 (10.82)	164.75 (10.97)	166.84 (9.97)	164.55 (10.96)
35–44	160.28 (8.27)	162.50 (10.53)	164.73 (11.20)	167.61 (8.15)	164.30 (10.57)
45–59	158.28 (13.19)	161.62 (10.53)	164.47 (10.86)	168.08 (8.56)	162.94 (10.91)
60–70	157.59 (10.74)	160.92 (10.41)	162.85 (12.44)	166.10 (19.11)	161.32 (11.47)
Total	158.58 (12.46)	162.04 (10.68)	164.63 (11.05)	166.94 (10.74)	163.89 (11.08)

Source: ENH-91.
Standard deviations are in parentheses. Sample includes all persons between the ages of 18 and 70 in and out of the labor force.

FIGURE 2. Mean height by year of birth, all sample ages 25–55.

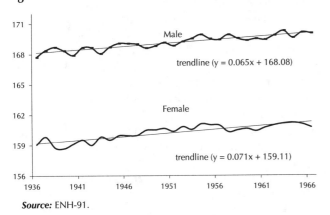

Source: ENH-91.

FIGURE 3. Mean height by year of birth, labor force ages 25–55.

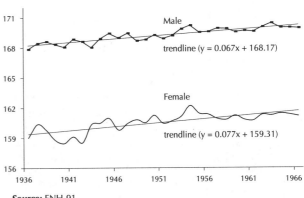

Source: ENH-91.

gains per decade are approximately 0.65 cm for urban men and 0.71 cm for urban women.[20]

To our knowledge, this is the first time secular height gains have been quantified in Latin America, except for in Brazil. This type of information is available for some European countries, some African countries, and Brazil. Strauss and Thomas (1998) showed that in the United States the mean male stature increased 1.25 cm. per decade between 1910 and 1950. The relative figure in Vietnam was 1.05 cm per decade and in Brazil it was 0.77 cm per decade. Fogel (1994) used historical European data on stature and weight and reported that, in Sweden, between the third quarter of the nineteenth century and the third quarter of the twentieth century, mean height in males increased 0.81 cm per decade and in France it increased 0.64 cm per decade. For the same period, the increase per decade in male stature was 0.57 cm in Norway and 1.07 cm in Denmark. Schultz (1996) reported that the gain in height per decade has been almost 1.33 cm for men and 1 cm for women in Côte d'Ivoire and 0.66 cm. for men and 0.33 cm for women in Ghana. Although the figures across countries are not strictly comparable because they were taken at different times and at different historical and economic moments of each country, they help to show that the order of magnitude of height changes in Colombia are similar to evidence from other countries in the world.

The main question of this study is whether health and productivity are related at the level of an individual. Table 4 shows the mean values of the natural logarithm of hourly earnings for males and females by education ranges and by different values of the health indicators. On average, labor earnings of persons who were disabled in the preceding month are lower than earnings of those who were healthy, although this is not true for females with more than 13 years of schooling. For both males and females, those who earn higher wages on average are those who had between 15 and 29 days of disability and more than 13 years of schooling. A very small percentage of the population lies in this category. These tables show that taller individuals (men and women) earn more at all education levels.

ESTIMATION OF PRODUCTIVITY OF HEALTH INVESTMENTS

To assess the returns to health investments, a Mincerian earnings function is estimated that depends on human capital. This section is divided into five subsections. In the first subsection, Mincerian log earnings equations are estimated considering the health indicators as hourly earnings determinants. In the second subsection, the selection bias introduced by considering only individuals with positive labor earnings is corrected. The third subsection analyzes the connection between local health policy instruments and adult health outcomes, similar to the one analyzed by Strauss and Thomas (1995). Once these health equations are estimated, the results are used to construct instrumental variable estimators of health that are inserted in the original hourly earnings equation. This procedure generates estimators of health that are free of noise and that better indicate the relationship between health status and productivity of adults. The instrumental variable estimation of earnings is shown in the fourth subsection, and the fifth subsection simulates the way changes in policy variables are likely to affect lifetime earnings. The sample means and standard deviations of the variables used in this section are shown in Tables A1 and A2 in the Annex.

Earnings Equations

An earnings function of the following type is estimated:

$$\log(w_i) = a + \sum b_j X_{ji} + \sum c_k C_{ki} + \sum d_h H_{hi} + f_i \qquad (1)$$

where w_i is the productivity measure (hourly earnings), X_{ji} contains only exogenous endowments that are not modified by the individual or the family, C_{ki} are reproducible forms of human capital, and H_{hi} are the health status indicators. In this section, the health status indicators are assumed to be exogenous to the hourly earnings function and not correlated with the errors f in Equation 1. The parameters a, b, c, and d are estimated; the error term f is assumed to be 0 mean independently distributed; i refers to individuals; and j, k, and h refer to the specific variables in the sets denoted X, C, and H, respectively. The sample includes wage earners as well as nonwage workers with positive earnings.

Among the exogenous endowments X, age, and age squared are included. The variable in C_{ki} is the number of years of schooling. Although a dummy variable for migration (equal to 1 if the person lives in a different place from where he or she did five years before the survey and 0 otherwise) was initially included in set C, this did not substantially affect the coefficients of health or education in any manner; therefore, these results are not reported.

As health status indicators H_{hi}, three variables are considered in separate regressions:

---

[20] The age ranges in these figures are restricted to avoid bias at the ends of age ranges. Younger people may still be growing and therefore have a lower height than their actual adult height, and older people may be shrinking. The growth reported here is free of biological growth or shrinkage.

TABLE 4. Ln (hourly earnings) by education and health indicators.

Health indicators		Males					Females				
		Years of schooling					Years of schooling				
		0	1–6	7–12	>13	Total	0	1–6	7–12	>13	Total
Disability	No	5.64	5.95	6.37	7.20	6.16	5.41	5.68	6.22	6.99	6.05
		(0.88)	(0.85)	(0.82)	(0.78)	(0.92)	(1.14)	(1.02)	(0.86)	(0.73)	(1.03)
	Yes	5.55	5.99	6.42	7.10	6.11	5.37	5.65	6.24	7.13	5.99
		(1.12)	(0.90)	(0.74)	(0.81)	(0.96)	(1.08)	(1.01)	(0.78)	(0.64)	(1.03)
	Total	5.63	5.96	6.37	7.20	6.16	5.41	5.68	6.22	7.00	6.05
		(0.90)	(0.85)	(0.81)	(0.78)	(0.92)	(1.14)	(1.02)	(0.86)	(0.72)	(1.03)
Days disabled	0	5.64	5.95	6.37	7.20	6.16	5.41	5.68	6.22	6.99	6.05
		(0.88)	(0.85)	(0.82)	(0.78)	(0.92)	(1.14)	(1.02)	(0.86)	(0.73)	(1.03)
	1–7	5.41	5.97	6.41	6.96	6.11	5.36	5.57	6.24	7.12	5.99
		(1.21)	(0.86)	(0.71)	(0.80)	(0.94)	(1.27)	(1.04)	(0.79)	(0.65)	(1.06)
	8–14	5.77	6.04	6.49	7.42	6.16	5.49	5.80	6.26	6.97	6.01
		(0.90)	(0.96)	(0.72)	(0.46)	(0.93)	(0.77)	(0.95)	(0.68)	(0.60)	(0.89)
	15–29	5.72	5.95	6.38	7.78	6.09	5.30	5.62	6.11	7.44	5.83
		(1.05)	(0.91)	(0.90)	(1.01)	(1.00)	(0.96)	(1.01)	(0.74)	(0.77)	(1.04)
	30	5.58	6.04	6.56	7.02	6.10	5.28	6.18	6.35	7.18	6.33
		(1.15)	(1.04)	(0.80)	(0.55)	(1.06)	(1.13)	(0.73)	(1.00)	(0.56)	(0.92)
	Total	5.63	5.96	6.37	7.20	6.16	5.41	5.68	6.22	7.00	6.05
		(0.90)	(0.85)	(0.81)	(0.78)	(0.92)	(1.14)	(1.02)	(0.86)	(0.72)	(1.03)
Height (cm)	135–154	6.90	7.14	7.43	7.94	7.24	6.59	6.73	7.15	7.93	7.02
		(0.61)	(0.71)	(0.78)	(0.47)	(0.74)	(0.72)	(0.72)	(0.72)	(0.60)	(0.81)
	155–159	6.78	7.14	7.41	8.20	7.29	6.58	6.83	7.27	8.02	7.19
		(1.00)	(0.65)	(0.66)	(0.73)	(0.72)	(0.63)	(0.73)	(0.72)	(0.66)	(0.82)
	160–164	6.94	7.16	7.38	8.19	7.33	6.65	6.88	7.31	8.01	7.28
		(0.65)	(0.63)	(0.70)	(0.67)	(0.72)	(0.59)	(0.65)	(0.65)	(0.69)	(0.77)
	165–169	6.96	7.16	7.47	8.26	7.43	6.90	6.86	7.34	8.03	7.36
		(0.60)	(0.66)	(0.62)	(0.75)	(0.74)	(0.69)	(0.73)	(0.64)	(0.68)	(0.79)
	>169	6.98	7.21	7.51	8.34	7.58	6.56	6.84	7.34	8.07	7.39
		(0.62)	(0.59)	(0.63)	(0.78)	(0.77)	(0.94)	(0.70)	(0.63)	(0.65)	(0.79)
	Total	6.95	7.18	7.48	8.31	7.50	6.65	6.83	7.29	8.02	7.26
		(0.64)	(0.62)	(0.64)	(0.76)	(0.76)	(0.68)	(0.71)	(0.67)	(0.67)	(0.80)

Sources: CASEN (excluding domestic servants) for disability and number of days disabled. ENH-91 for height
Standard deviations are in parentheses.

1. A dummy variable that is 1 when the person did not go to work at least 1 day in the previous month because of illness (incidence of disability);
2. The number of days the person was disabled in the previous month[21] (duration of disability); and
3. Height of individual (measured in centimeters).

The "number of days disabled" uses the threshold of inability to work to make the sickness less subjective and adds the information on how long the individual is incapacitated, although much of the information is contained in the first binary variable "disability." However, as the empirical results show, both variables explain more or less the same facts. On the other hand, height for adults is used as an indicator of child nutritional status, expo-

sure to diseases, and variation in other environmental factors (Schultz, 1997).

The equation was estimated with and without domestic servants but the parameters did not differ.[22] Similarly, the model was estimated separately for wage earners and self-employed persons without uncovering many interesting differences. These factors are summarized in terms of two dummy variables: one for domestic service and one for wage earners. The working assumption is that they are exogenously determined. Similarly, although in estimating Equation 1 the human capital variables may be correlated with the error, education is treated as an exogenous variable. The earnings function was estimated separately for men and women, taking into account that some of the health status and control variables may dif-

---

[21] Persons who were not disabled in the previous month had a value of 0 in this variable.

[22] The coefficients of all the other variables except for the intercept are the same when domestic servants are included and excluded from the sample.

TABLE 5. Hourly earnings equations: dependent variable log(hourly earnings).[a]

	Male										
	Urban							Rural			
Individual variables[b]	(1)	(2)	(3)	(4)	(5)	(6)	(7)	(8)	(9)	(10)	(11)
[1] Age	0.069* (25)	0.069* (25)	0.069* (25)	0.069* (25)	0.057* (16)	0.056* (16)	0.057* (16)	0.036* (6.9)	0.036* (7)	0.036* (7)	0.036* (6.9)
[2] Age squared/1000	−0.674* (20)	−0.675* (20)	−0.675* (20)	−0.675* (20)	−0.507* (11)	−0.502* (11)	−0.504* (11)	−0.349* (5.6)	−0.352* (5.7)	−0.352* (5.7)	−0.350* (5.6)
[3] Years of schooling	0.087* (61)	0.087* (61)	0.087* (61)	0.087* (61)	0.098* (76)	0.095* (71)	0.095* (71)	0.078* (19)	0.078* (19)	0.078* (19)	0.078* (19)
[4] Dummy salaried worker (person earns a wage = 1)	0.003 (0.23)	0.003 (0.24)	0.003 (0.24)	0.003 (0.23)	−0.070* (6)	−0.068* (6)	−0.067* (6)	0.210* (8)	0.210* (8)	0.210* (8)	0.210* (8)
[5] Dummy domestic servant = 1	(3)	(2.9)	(2.9)		−0.326*	−0.311*	−0.312*				
[6] Number of days disabled/100		0.200 (0.89)	0.865 (1.38)						0.400 (0.99)	−0.221 (0.21)	
[7] (Number of days disabled)^2/10^3			−0.292 (1.14)							0.278 (0.63)	
[8] Dummy disabled = 1				0.028 (1.07)							0.021 (0.45)
[9] Height/100						0.782 (8.7)	−9.02* (3.7)				
[10] Height^2/10^4							2.88* (4)				
[11] Intercept	4.160	4.159	4.158	4.159	5.397	4.201	12.430	4.496	4.492	4.493	4.495
Test joint significance [1]–[2]	607*	607*	607*	607*	698*	715*	712*	49*	49*	49*	49*
Test joint significance [6]–[7]			1.88							0.05	
Test joint significance [9]–[10]							46*				
Maximum ln(w) attained at age	51.09	50.95	50.95	51.06	55.79	56.21	56.07	52.19	51.52	51.52	52.13
Critical ln(w) attained at days disabled			14.83							3.97	
Critical ln(w) attained at height							156.75				
Adjusted R^2	0.20	0.20	0.20	0.20	0.33	0.33	0.33	0.08	0.08	0.08	0.08
Number of observations	18,666	18,666	18,666	18,666	13,721	13,721	13,721	4,966	4,966	4,966	4,966

Sources: ENH -91 for columns 5, 6, 7, 16, 17, and 18. CASEN (excluding domestic servants) for all others.

[a] Hourly labor income measured in pesos of the year of the survey. A 1991 peso is equivalent to 1.53 pesos of 1993.

fer by sex, especially height. The earnings function was also estimated separately for rural and urban areas, although they are linked by the choice of migration.

The hourly earnings regressions are shown in Table 5. A surprisingly weak correlation is observed between wages, the number of days disabled, and disability. The variables are not significant and do not even have the expected signs. Otherwise, the basic logarithms of earnings regressions are plausible. Because the health vari-

ables may be simultaneously determined and measured with error, a next step of instrumenting for health status is undertaken. The model is also estimated excluding the health variables from the right-hand side of Equation 1. Note that inclusion of health variables in the regressions does not alter the returns to education.

The regressions with height show that this variable is significant and has the correct sign. Height benefits men's earnings more than women's earnings (comparing the

| | Female | | | | | | | | | | |
| | Urban | | | | | | | Rural | | | |
Individual variables[b]	(12)	(13)	(14)	(15)	(16)	(17)	(18)	(19)	(20)	(21)	(22)
[1] Age	0.074* (16)	0.074* (16)	0.074* (16)	0.074* (16)	0.047* (10)	0.047* (10)	0.047* (10)	0.047* (3)	0.047* (3)	0.047* (3)	0.047* (3)
[2] Age²/10³	−0.705* (13)	−0.705* (13)	−0.704* (13)	−0.705* (13)	−0.429* (6.8)	−0.424* (7)	−0.420* (7)	−0.421* (2.5)	−0.421* (3)	−0.420* (2.5)	−0.417* (2.5)
[3] Years of schooling	0.106* (47)	0.106* (47)	0.106* (47)	0.106* (47)	0.096* (55)	0.095* (53)	0.095* (53)	0.102* (11)	0.102* (11)	0.102* (11)	0.102* (11)
[4] Dummy salaried worker (person earns a wage = 1)	0.211* (11)	0.211* (11)	0.211* (11)	0.211* (11)	0.141* (8)	0.139* (8)	0.139* (8)	0.276* (4)	0.276* (4)	0.274* (4)	0.274* (4)
[5] Dummy domestic servant = 1					−0.322* (14)	−0.317* (13)	−0.303* (13)				
Health variables											
[6] Number of days disabled/100		0.297 (0.92)	−0.601 (0.73)						0.004 (0.0)	−1.532 (0.63)	
[7] (Number of days disabled)²/10³			0.411 (1.18)							0.738 (0.69)	
[8] Dummy disabled = 1				0.010 (0.30)							−0.055 (0.5)
[9] Height/100						0.48* (4.7)	10.08* (3.1)				
[10] Height²/10⁴							−2.99* (2.9)				
[11] Intercept	3.488	3.487	3.490	3.487	5.294	4.542	−3.143	3.890	3.889	3.896	3.899
Test joint significance [1]–[2]	607*	607*	607*	328*	262*	265*	267*	17*	17*	17*	17*
Test joint significance [6]–[7]			1.88							0.50	
Test joint significance [9]–[10]							15*				
Maximum ln(w) attained at age	52.21	52.39	52.28	52.36	54.82	55.17	55.43	56.44	56.43	56.41	56.66
Critical ln(w) attained at days disabled		7.32							10.39		
Critical ln(w) attained at height							168.43				
Adjusted R²	0.25	0.25	0.25	0.25	0.35	0.35	0.35	0.12	0.12	0.12	0.13
Number of observations	10,464	10,464	10,464	10,464	9,332	9,332	9,332	1,299	1,299	1,299	1,299

Sources: ENH -91 for columns 5, 6, 7, 16, 17, and 18. CASEN (excluding domestic servants) for all others.

[a]Hourly labor income measured in pesos of the year of the survey. A 1991 peso is equivalent to 1.53 pesos of 1993.

[b]t statistics are in parentheses.

*Statistically significant.

coefficient of the linear term for males and females). Quadratic terms in height and in number of days disabled are included to check for nonlinearities, and only height and height squared are significant. Along the relevant interval of height (1.35 to 2 m), the productivity effects of height were always increasing and convex. In additional regressions (not included), it was found that height and education are positively correlated in Colombia, so that, when controlling for education, the coefficient of height

drops markedly.[23] Estimations of the model for the whole sample with a gender dummy indicated that being female is negatively related to productivity, a result that had already been found in other studies (Ribero and Meza, 1997). Similarly, rural areas have lower produc-

[23] In similar earnings equations, the coefficients of height/100 without education were 2.1 and 1.5 for men and women, respectively. When education is included, they drop to 0.71 and 0.47, respectively. These coefficients are significant.

tivity, a result also previously documented by Leibovich et al. (1997). The age variables are significant and have the expected signs.[24]

Being a salaried worker exerts different effects in the two data sources. With the survey of 1993, which includes urban and rural sectors (CASEN), a salaried worker has higher wages. The variable is positive and significant for rural males and females and for urban females, but it is not significant for urban males. In the urban survey of 1991 (ENH-91), the effect of being a salaried worker is negative for males and positive for females. Domestic servants have systematically lower earnings.[25]

Hourly Earnings Equations with Selection Bias Correction

When an earnings equation is estimated to calculate the returns to human capital in the population based on only a sample of individuals who are participating in the market, the estimated returns may be biased (Heckman, 1979). The selection bias may be particularly serious in estimations of female earnings, because relatively fewer women decide to enter the labor force. If other variables that determine the decision of participation and are unrelated to the market wage offers are observed, it is possible to obtain corrected estimates of the returns to human capital by joint estimation of the probability of receiving positive earnings and Equation 1.

The econometric model to estimate has the following two parts:[26]

1. Probit for labor force participation (selection mechanism):

$$z_i^* = \gamma' p_i + u_i \qquad z_i = 1 \text{ if } z_i^* > 0$$
$$z_i = 0 \text{ if } z_i^* \leq 0$$

$$\text{Prob}(z_i = 1) = \Phi(\gamma' p_i)$$
$$\text{Prob}(z_i = 0) = 1 - \Phi(\gamma' p_i) \qquad (2)$$

where $z_i = 1$ when individual i participates in the labor market, and $z_i = 0$ when individual i does not participate in the labor market. Φ is the standard normal cumulative distribution function, the error term u is assumed to be

distributed with mean 0 and variance 1, i refers to individuals, and γ' are the parameters estimated in the probit model. The variables p_i determine the decision of participation and are exogenous to the market wage offer. In theory, the individual will enter the market if the wage offer he or she receives is higher than his or her reservation wage. It is theoretically appealing to consider variables such as nonlabor income as determinants of the probability of working, because those variables determine the reservation wages of individuals and may affect their entrance into the labor market.

2. Hourly earnings equation:

$$\log(w_i) = a + \sum b_j X_{ji} + \sum c_k C_{ki}$$
$$+ \sum d_h H_{hi} + f_i, \text{ observed if } z_i = 1$$

$$(u_i, f_i) \sim \text{bivariate normal}(0, 0, 1, \sigma_f^2, \rho) \qquad (3)$$

The hourly earnings in Equation 3 are equal to that in Equation 1, but it is observed only when the individual is a participant in the market. σ_f is the standard deviation of the error term f, and ρ is the correlation coefficient between the error terms u and f. The variables z_i and p_i are observed for a random sample of individuals, but $\log(w_i)$ is observed only when $z_i = 1$. The model to estimate is as follows:

$$E[\log(w_i) \mid z_i = 1] = a + \sum b_j X_{ji} + \sum c_k C_{ki}$$
$$+ \sum d_h H_{hi} + \rho \sigma_f \lambda(\gamma' p_i) \qquad (4)$$

where $\lambda(\gamma' p_i) = \varphi(\gamma' p_i)/\Phi(\gamma' p_i)$ and φ is the standard normal probability density function.

Besides age and education, the additional variables used to explain participation in the labor force p_i were nonlabor income,[27] the dummy for living in a house or apartment,[28] a dummy variable for having adequate floors[29] in the house, and a dummy for owning the house where the individual lives.[30] These variables proxy the

---

[24] When the regressions involve quadratic terms in the explanatory variables and the coefficients are significant, the critical values are reported at the bottom of the tables. These are calculated by differentiating totally the fitted equation of the model with respect to the variable of interest, equating the derivative to 0, and solving for the optimal value.

[25] When the model was estimated with the domestic servants in the CASEN sample and the dummy for domestic servants (these regressions are not reported), the same pattern was found, but the variable is not significant for rural males.

[26] The model is based on Greene (1997).

[27] Nonlabor income is defined as the sum of four variables in the survey. The actual question in the survey is: did you receive money in the last month from any of the following sources: a) interest (yes, no, amount), b) rent (yes, no, amount), c) pensions or retirement benefits (yes, no, amount), and d) monetary assistance (yes, no, amount). Because nonlabor income was not a very powerful instrument for explanation of participation in the labor force, other housing variables were used as proxies for wealth. Note that nonlabor income is measured at the level of the individual and not for the family.

[28] The survey question for "tipo de vivienda" (type of housing) has four options: a) "casa" (house), b) "apartamento" (condominium or apartment), c) "cuarto o cuartos" (room or rooms), and d) "otro: vivienda móvil, refugio natural, carpa, etc." (other: trailer, natural shelter, tent, etc.). The dummy built here takes the value 1 when the answer is a or b and 0 when the answer is c or d.

[29] Adequate floors are defined as those made of tile, brick, carpet, marble, or hardwood. The alternatives were cement and dirt ("tierra").

[30] This variable, called "owner-occupied housing," is a dummy variable equal to 1 if the individual lives in a house that is owned by him (her) or his (her) family, and 0 if he (she) lives in a rented or other place.

individual's nonhuman wealth and are expected to reduce his or her likelihood of participating in the labor force. When the coefficient of the λ value is positive and significant, the unobservables that contribute to the probability of participation are positively associated with receiving higher market earnings for reasons not accounted for in the earnings equation. When the coefficient for λ is negative and significant, the opposite happens. It is not obvious a priori what sign to expect for λ.

The results of this estimation for females are shown in Table 6. The variables explaining participation in the labor force are significant and have the expected signs. The nonlabor income and the other proxies for wealth diminish the probability of participation for the rural and urban samples, except for adequate floors in the rural sample.

The returns to schooling in Table 6 are basically equal to those shown in Table 5 for the urban areas,[31] but they are smaller (less than one-third) for the rural areas. The significance of the coefficient for λ indicates that the returns to schooling estimated without the Heckman correction are not biased for the urban sample, but they are biased for the rural sample. According to the sign of λ, rural women who work, holding the observables in Equations 2 and 3 constant, are those who are paid less.

The productivity effects of disability remain nonsignificant after the correction. The coefficients of height and height squared change when selection bias is corrected, but the derivatives of earnings with respect to height evaluated at the sample mean remain equal with and without the correction. The parameter λ is significant in the specifications of columns 5, 7, and 8 but remains insignificant for the others.[32]

The model was also estimated for males, but these results are not reported. The negative effect of the wealth proxies on participation that was found for females holds for males. However, for males the parameter λ was insignificant, which implies no sample selection bias. In the absence of selection bias, the uncorrected estimates are more efficient as well as consistent (Heckman, 1979).

Health Equations

In this subsection the determinants of the observed health outcomes are explored. Using information on an individual's education and wealth, local prices (O), and the community health infrastructure prices and policies (P), the model tries to account for the individual indicators of health status (H). The estimated equation is as follows:

$$H_i = g + \Sigma c_l X_{li} + \Sigma h_j O_{ji} + \Sigma r_k P_k + t_i \qquad (5)$$

where g, c, h, and r are estimable parameters; t is the error term; l, j, and k index the sets of exogenous endowments to the individual (X), private opportunities (O), and public policies (P), respectively; and i indexes the individual. Equation 5 was estimated with probit models when the health variable was the dichotomous variable for disability. The model was estimated with ordinary least squares (OLS) when the health variables were "number of days disabled in the last month"[33] and "height."

When the health variables are "disability" and "number of days disabled in the last month," the data are rural and urban for the year 1993. Age of the individual is specified as an exogenous endowment.[34] Considering that wealth might shift health outcomes positively (given that wealthier individuals have more resources to spend on health), nonlabor income and a dummy to indicate the type of housing[35] were specified as individual private opportunities (O). With data from CASEN and from other sources,[36] a list of variables to describe the community-specific environment (P) was matched to sample clusters. The variables P are defined for 52 regions (approximately twice the number of *departamentos*, because most of the regions have rural and urban areas).[37] At the municipality level, characteristics that were expected to be related to the health outcomes were climate,[38] availability of health centers, enrollment in social security,[39] transportation infrastructure, transportation time to reach hospitals, transportation time to reach schools, and availability of water and electricity. Among those, few result in significant correlations and some have a counterintuitive sign. At the *departamento* level, the only significant variable was the num-

---

[31] Note that in these cases the coefficient for λ is not significant.

[32] Although the correction for selection bias was found relevant in some cases, in the rest of the paper it is ignored because it is particularly difficult to implement instrumental variables together with selection bias correction.

[33] Because the variable is truncated at 0 and 30, Tobit models were also, but the results do not differ substantially from the OLS.

[34] Because older individuals tend to have lower levels of health, age and age squared were taken into account to capture possible diminishing returns.

[35] The same variable "lives in house or apartment" defined in the second subsection.

[36] The Ministry of Health and the Instituto Geográfico Agustín Codazzi.

[37] Some regions are urban only and others are rural only.

[38] Altitude, temperature, and average yearly rainfall for each municipality.

[39] In 1993, approximately 25% of urban residents and 8% of rural residents were affiliated with or beneficiaries of the Social Security Institute for health services, 10% of the Colombian population used private health care, and 5% were covered by other services.

TABLE 6. Heckman selection model, female.

	Urban					Rural		
	Probit[1] (1)	Earnings[2] (2)	Earnings (3)	Probit (4)	Earnings (5)	Probit (6)	Earnings (7)	Earnings (8)
Individual variables[3]								
1–Age	0.127*	0.083*	0.083*	0.286*	0.099*	0.066*	–0.016	–0.016
	(35.63)	(12.80)	(12.82)	(41.37)	(24.97)	(8.20)	(1.04)	(1.05)
2–Age squared/1,000	–1.558*	–0.826*	–0.826*	–3.551*	–1.040	–0.693*	0.244	0.248
	(35.26)	(10.17)	(10.18)	(38.60)	(20.10)	(7.22)	(1.35)	(1.37)
3–Years of education	0.051*	0.106*	0.106*	–0.014*	0.090*	0.062*	0.032*	0.032*
	(22.64)	(37.90)	(37.93)	(4.24)	(66.64)	(9.43)	(2.78)	(2.79)
4–Dummy salaried worker (person earns a wage = 1)		0.224*	0.224*		–0.032*		0.155*	0.155*
		(11.72)	(11.70)		(2.79)		(2.25)	(2.25)
5–Dummy domestic servant = 1		–0.700*	–0.700*		–0.029		–0.580*	–0.579*
		(25.49)	(25.46)		(0.26)		(6.33)	(6.31)
6–Non-labor income/10⁶	–0.946*			–1.160*		0.161		
	(6.69)			(11.37)		(0.28)		
7–Dummy lives in house or apartment = 1 (a)	–0.135*					–0.366*		
	(3.63)					(4.11)		
8–Dummy adequate floor (b)	–0.009					0.103*		
	(0.49)					(2.02)		
9–Dummy owner ocuppied house (c)	0.021							
	(1.24)							
Health variables								
10–Number of days disabled/100		–0.480					–1.543	
		(0.61)					(0.71)	
11–Number of days disabled squared/1,000		0.302					0.821	
		(0.92)					(0.87)	
12–Dummy (disabled = 1)			0.004					–0.032
			(0.14)					(0.33)
13–Height/100					–0.986*			
					(5.89)			
14–Height squared/10⁴					0.515*			
					(7.98)			
15–Intercept	–2.653	3.225	3.222	–3.970	4.764	–1.865	7.099	7.102
16–Lambda[d]		0.113	0.114		0.404		–1.291	–1.292
		(0.06)	(0.06)		(0.02)		(0.08)	(0.08)
Critical values								
Max. dependent variable attained at age	40.87	50.46	50.45	40.26	47.64	47.74	32.85	32.75
Min. ln(w) attained at height					95.68			
Rho		0.131	0.132		0.628		–0.851	–0.851
Sigma		0.865	0.865		0.643		1.518	1.519
Log. likelihood		–32807	–32807		–19395		–5200	–5200
Number of observations	27,292	11,956	11,956	16,974	9,824	5,390	1,472	1,472

Sources: ENH-91 for columns (4) and (5); CASEN for all others.
[1]Dependent variable: participation in labor force.
[2]Dependent variable: log (hourly earnings)
[3]Z-statistic in brackets
*Statistically significant
(a) Type of housing: rents or owns house or apartment = 1; rents room or other = 0
(b) Floors made of tile, brick, marble, hardwood, or carpeted = 1; otherwise = 0
(c) Figure in brackets for lambda is standard error

ber of yearly transfers from the central government to the *departamento* for health.[40]

Regional differences are very important in Colombia. Levels of earnings, formality of labor markets, and levels of education and health are generally worse in coastal regions than in the interior. The Pacific Coast in particular is known to be the poorest region in the country. Although the variable altitude may capture some of these regional differences,[41] cultural, racial, and institutional differences that persist among these regions go beyond

---

[40] Other variables that were available but not included in this final model were the number of primary and secondary schools, the number of hospital beds, average times to reach schools, and average hours spent in schools daily.

[41] Coastal regions are closer to sea level

the climate. To capture some differences due to these elements, two regional dummy variables were introduced: one for living in a Pacific Coast *departamento* and one for living in an Atlantic Coast *departamento*.[42]

When height is used as a health indicator, data are only for the urban population in 1991.[43] At the individual level the model controls for age,[44] nonlabor income, and a dummy to indicate owner-occupied housing.[45] The variables that capture environmental health risks (P) are two indicators constructed at the city level from ENH-91. The first one measures availability of basic services in the households of the community where the person lives.[46] The second one measures percentage of houses in the community that are not overcrowded. City and strata define the communities or sample clusters for urban areas.

The estimation results are presented Table 7. Age is an important factor that explains the three health indicators, with older individuals tending to have worse health. The coefficients of age and age squared are individually significant for the number of days disabled and jointly significant for the probability of having a disability.[47] The negative effects of age on health are greater in rural than in urban areas and among females than males. Nonlabor income is not significant, but the wealth proxy "living in a house or apartment" is negatively related to the number of days disabled and to the incidence of disability, and it is significant in the urban samples. Home ownership is positively related to height. These results coincide with the intuition that wealthier individuals tend to have better health, controlling for the individual and community characteristics listed in Table 7.

The number of hospitals or clinics per capita is not significant, except for the explanation of the number of days disabled for the male urban sample. In this case, however, this variable has a counterintuitive sign that implies that more hospitals or clinics per capita lead to more days disabled in this subsample.

In rural areas, the model shows the expected negative sign for the variable "percentage of people directly en-

rolled in or beneficiaries of social security," and it is significant when the health outcome is the number of days disabled. The econometric model reveals that a 10% increase in the percentage enrolled reduces the mean disability for a man in rural areas by more than 0.2 day. With that same increase, the incidence of disability for rural females is reduced by 2 percentage points. In urban areas, however, the "percentage of people directly enrolled or beneficiaries of social security" has a positive coefficient on disability, although theoretically access to social insurance is expected to improve health. This may be because in urban regions more individuals are affiliated with social security;[48] they may tend to report more disabilities because they can more readily access diagnostic services and not necessarily because they are more frequently ill.

The coverage of electricity was expected to affect health outcomes, because almost all households in rural areas have access to potable water,[49] but the coverage of electricity remains low.[50] However, electrification did not show any significance. Climate variables such as altitude[51] were significant in the rural samples for the number of days disabled, with a negative sign, which implies that health tends to be better in places with higher altitude. The negative sign of the coefficient for altitude was expected, given that regions closer to sea level are more humid and the prevalence of communicable diseases is more common. This coincides with a general perception that people who live in the lowlands in Colombia are less healthy (Rosenzweig and Schultz, 1982b).[52] Estimations with altitude and altitude squared (these regressions are not reported) suggested that nonlinearities in the effect of altitude on our health indicators are not strong.

The distance in kilometers between the municipality and the capital of the *departamento*[53] is an approximation of commuting time or the price of metropolitan health services. This variable was significant only for the explanation of the number of days of disability in the rural

---

[42] The reference category was living in the interior.

[43] It was impossible to find for 1991 the same information found for 1993 at the municipality level.

[44] Age is more important for height than for the other health outcomes.

[45] The same variable "owner-occupied housing" defined in the second subsection.

[46] The availability in the community of each basic service separately was insignificant. The variable used here, which aggregates the availability of the three basic services (electricity, water, and sewerage) in the households, provided significant estimates.

[47] Estimation of this model only with a linear term for age showed that one additional year of age increases the probability of having disability by 0.6% and 0.8% for urban males and females, respectively, and by 1.1% and 1.3% for rural males and females, respectively. These regressions are not reported.

[48] Only 8% of the rural labor force is covered by social insurance compared with 25% of the urban labor force.

[49] Usually the houses are built in places close to potable water sources (rivers, creeks, or irrigation systems).

[50] Because electricity allows households to have a refrigerator and keep food in safer conditions and also helps to make public health programs more widely known through television, it may be a more powerful explanatory variable than potable water in rural areas.

[51] When the model is estimated with temperature instead of altitude the results are very similar. The reader has to take into account that Colombia's proximity to the equator implies a strong correlation between temperature and altitude.

[52] They find that altitude and altitude squared are significant in the determination of child mortality and that child mortality is lower in regions with higher altitudes.

[53] It would have been more useful to have the commuting time to the nearest hospital or medical center, but unfortunately this information was not available.

TABLE 7. Individual Health Production Functions(a).

Dependent health variable:	Dummy disabled(b)				Number of days disabled				Height	
Region:	Urban		Rural		Urban		Rural		Urban	
Gender:	Male	Female	Male	Female	Male	Female	Male	Female	Male	Female
	(1)	(2)	(3)	(4)	(5)	(6)	(7)	(8)	(9)	(10)
Individual variables										
1–Age	-0.004 (0.62)	0.013 (1.32)	0.005 (0.42)	-0.004((0.16)	-0.013 (1.46)	0.013 (0.97)	-0.029 (1.59)	-0.070 (1.74)	0.088* (2.31)	0.119* (2.47)
2–Age squared/1,000	0.136 (1.58)	-0.058 (0.49)	0.075 (0.55)	0.204 (0.74)	0.311* (2.84)	-0.009 (0.05)	0.608* (2.80)	1.205* (2.56)	-1.989* (4.04)	-2.514* (3.90)
3–Dummy type of housing (rents or owns house or apartment = 1; rents room or rooms or other, e.g., squatter = 0)	-0.215* (3.58)	-0.280* (3.54)	-0.182 (1.14)	-0.166 (0.58)	-0.131 (1.62)	-0.355* (2.89)	-0.270 (1.04)	-0.060 (0.13)		
4–Dummy owner occupied housing (house or apartment is own = 1; rented or other = 0)									0.29* (2.41)	0.32* (2.11)
5–Non-labor income/10^6 [c]	0.012 (0.09)	0.308 (1.19)	0.447 (0.59)	1.049 (0.69)	0.167 (0.97)	0.809 (1.90)	-1.256 (0.93)	-0.893 (0.30)	-7.21 (0.40)	-66.1 (1.85)
Municipality variables										
6–Hospitals/clinics per capita* 1,000	0.592 (1.53)	0.045 (0.08)	0.270 (0.86)	0.014 (0.02)	1.425* (2.78)	-1.167 (1.57)	-0.030 (0.06)	0.074 (0.63)		
7–Community % of people directly enrolled or beneficiaries of social security	0.497* (1.96)	0.79* (2.56)	-0.731 (1.24)	-2.05* (1.98)	0.482 (1.57)	-0.109 (0.26)	-2.115* (2.30)	-3.101 (1.87)		
8–Community % of households with electricity	0.151 (0.51)	0.011 (0.03)	0.130 (0.90)	-0.086 (0.36)	-0.034 (0.11)	0.243 (0.44)	0.239 (1.04)	-0.306 (0.71)		
9–Altitude (in mts above sea level)/100,000	-0.57 (0.25)	-2.08 (0.79)	-6.67 (1.65)	-10.56 (1.54)	-2.201 (0.79)	-3.95 (1.10)	-11.98* (1.91)	-27.04* (2.42)		
10–Distance to "capital" of "departamento" in km/1,000	0.206 (1.14)	0.272 (1.32)	0.441 (1.17)	-0.052 (0.07)	0.004 (0.02)	0.262 (0.87)	1.251* (2.16)	-1.098 (0.94)		
11–Community % of houses with basic services: electricity, water, sewage									7.002* (4.40)	0.495 (0.32)
12–Community % of houses with adequate number of rooms per person									10.84* (14.14)	11.70* (12.51)
13–(Non-labor income/1,000,000)* (Community % of houses with adequate number of rooms per person									9.60 (0.49)	76.50* (2.04)
Departamental variable										
14–Transfers per capita from central government to "departamento" for health	-2.474 (0.82)	-4.803 (1.25)	16.368 (0.70)	-28.591 (0.61)	-6.678 (1.88)	-2.524 (0.55)	14.257 (0.40)	23.118 (0.32)		
Individual regional variables[d]										
15–Dummy (lives in Atlantic Coast = 1)	0.052 (1.19)	0.079 (1.45)	-0.084 (1.02)	-0.001 (0.01)	-0.019 (0.36)	-0.083 (1.13)	-0.257* (2.07)	-0.432 (1.65)		
16–Dummy (lives in Pacific Coast = 1)	0.047 (1.02)	0.147* (2.89)	0.211* (2.79)	0.574* (4.34)	0.019 (0.33)	0.249* (3.42)	0.314* (2.59)	0.872* (4.03)		
Intercept	-1.780	-1.826	-1.816	-1.107	0.527	0.188	0.827	1.940	159.37	149.31
Test of joint significance Var. 3 to Var. 16	22.67*	34.07*	15.95	28.19*	1.68	3.41*	2.22*	2.99*	68.06*	43.05*
Prob > F or Prob > chi2	0.01	0.00	0.10	0.00	0.08	0.00	0.01	0.00	0.00	0.00
Log likelihood	-3965	-2613	-1224	-356						
Adjusted R squared	0.007	0.011	0.021	0.056	0.004	0.005	0.014	0.038	0.033	0.032
Number of observations	18,666	10,464	4,966	1,299	18,666	10,464	4,966	1,299	13,721	9,332

Sources: ENH-91 for columns (9) and (10); CASEN for all others.
[a] Econometric models used: probit for dummy disabled; OLS for number of days disabled and for height.
[b] z-statistics in brackets columns (1) to (4) and t-statistics in brackets for other columns.
[c] Monetary variables (5, 13, and 14) are in 1993 pesos for columns (1) to (8) and in 1991 pesos for columns (9) and (10). A 1991 peso is equivalent to 1.53 1993 pesos.
[d] Reference interior.

male sample; more distance to the capital of the *departamento* implies more days of disability. It is intuitive that distance is significant for a rural sample because urban areas usually have at least one health center, whereas rural individuals have to commute to find one. However, it is difficult to find an economic explanation for the gender difference in this result.

In addition to the other factors taken into account in Table 7, living on the Pacific Coast contributes positively to disability and to the number of days disabled for all females (rural and urban) and for rural males. People who live in that region experience an average of 0.25–0.87 additional day disabled. The dummy variable for the Atlantic Coast was significant in reducing the number of days disabled for the rural male sample, but it did not contribute in a special way to individual health in the other samples. When the models were estimated without the regional dummies, the other coefficients were very similar.[54]

The estimations for height by gender are shown in columns 9 and 10 of Table 7. Height increases with age until around 23 years, and then begins to decrease. The shape of a graph with height on the y axis and age on the x axis with the coefficients from Table 7 is an inverse U, which indicates that height is subject to diminishing returns to age—i.e., for older individuals an additional year implies a larger decrease in height than for younger individuals. This behavior was expected from the analysis of the descriptive statistics included in the third section. The height patterns are further explored in Table A3 in the Annex. Disaggregating by sex, a regression is first reported on age as a linear and then as a quadratic function to quantify the trend of improvement in height and nutrition, holding nothing else constant. The trend indicates that cohorts 1 year older have 0.06 cm less stature, and that is more or less the same for males and females. A woman with 1 additional year of schooling is expected to be 0.3 cm taller and a man is expected to be 0.4 cm taller, holding only age constant. When other individual variables such as nonlabor income, owner-occupied housing, and community characteristics are taken into account, the partial association between schooling and height decreases.

"Owner-occupied housing" is a significant determinant of height and has the expected positive sign. The wealthier an individual is, the better is his or her health status indicator. The "percentage of houses in the community with basic services" is significant to explain heights of individuals and it has a positive sign. To live in a community with a high level of basic services contributes to more height for the individual, although the coefficient is significant only for males. Similarly, the supply of adequate housing, measured by the "percentage of houses in the community with adequate number of rooms per person," is associated with better health outcomes for individuals, measured by height.

When wealth is interacted with public policies[55] to analyze the personal distribution of health benefits, the product of nonlabor income and the "percentage of houses with adequate number of rooms per person" is significant and positive, indicating that nonlabor income and the adequacy of houses in the community are "complements."[56] In parallel regressions run with the same explanatory variables but excluding the interaction term, nonlabor income was significant and positive, and the effect was greater for females than for males.[57]

Tests of joint significance of the identifying variables[58] imply that they are jointly significant. The hypothesis that the coefficients of the identifying variables in each model are jointly equal to 0 can be rejected at the 5% level. Only in columns 3 and 5 can the null hypothesis be rejected at the 10% level.

Hourly Earnings Equations with Instrumental Health Variables

In this section, the earnings function (Equation 1) is reestimated because the human capital health stocks (H) may be correlated with the earnings error or be measured with error, imparting bias to single equation estimates of the earnings equation. These problems are solved by estimating Equation 1 with IV methods. The estimated equation is

$$\log(w_i) = a + \sum b_j X_{ji} + \sum c_k C_{ki} + \sum d_h H_{hi}^* + f_i \quad (6)$$

where w_i is the hourly earnings, X_{ji} contains only exogenous endowments, C_{ki} are forms of human capital, and H_{hi}^* are the endogenous health status indicators. The health status variables are assumed to be endogenous because they result from a process that involves individual resource opportunities, local prices (O), and community prices and policies (P). H_i^* are computed using the estimated parameters from the preceding subsection

$$H_i^* = \hat{g} + \sum c_{\hat{l}} X_{li} + \sum h_{\hat{j}} O_{ji} + \sum r_{\hat{k}} P_k \quad (7)$$

---

[54] These regressions are not reported.

[55] The interaction is similar to the one between mother's education and program treatment mentioned by Rosenzweig and Schultz (1982a).

[56] See Schultz (1984): the fact that they are complements means that having adequate housing in the community does not reduce the lower health caused by a lack of nonlabor income.

[57] The regressions are not included in the paper. The estimated coefficient of "nonlabor income/10⁶" in the height female regression was 6.60 (t statistic = 2.68). For males, the coefficient was 1.72 (t statistic = 2.24).

[58] All except age and age squared.

TABLE 8. Hourly earnings equations, health instrumental variables; dependent variable, log (hourly earnings).

	Urban				Rural			
	Male		Female		Male		Female	
	(1)	(2)	(3)	(4)	(5)	(6)	(7)	(8)
Individual variables								
1–Age	0.070*	0.070*	0.075*	0.068*	0.026*	0.026*	0.036*	0.034*
	(21.3)	(21.3)	(15.5)	(13.2)	(4.49)	(4.50)	(2.29)	(2.09)
2–Age squared/1,000	–0.072*	–0.714*	–0.704*	–0.601*	–0.143*	–0.150*	–0.238	–0.201
	(14.8)	(15.1)	(11.4)	(9.0)	(1.85)	(1.93)	(1.22)	(1.00)
3–Years of education	0.087*	0.087*	0.106*	0.105*	0.075*	0.074*	0.100*	0.101*
	(62.1)	(61.6)	(47.9)	(47.2)	(18.1)	(17.97)	(11.8)	(11.73)
4–Dummy salaried worker	0.003	0.002	0.211*	0.209*	0.191*	0.190*	0.262*	0.259*
(person earns a wage = 1;	(0.2)	(0.11)	(9.6)	(9.53)	(7.32)	(7.19)	(3.77)	(3.67)
owns a business = 0)								
I.V. Health variables[a]								
6–Fitted number of days	8.756	–96.027*	–6.780	–90.633*	–32.930*	–3.555	–13.475*	0.545
disabled/1,000**	(0.98)	(3.98)	(1.14)	(4.36)	(5.04)	(0.09)	(2.04)	(0.03)
7–Fitted number of days disabled	51.104*		42.780*		–12.968		–7.965	
squared/1,000**	(4.45)		(4.22)		(0.79)		(0.74)	
Intercept	4.1	4.2	3.5	3.7	4.8	4.7	4.1	4.1
Critical values								
Max ln(w) attained at age:	49.81	48.81	53.05	56.18	89.90	85.59	75.70	83.67
Critical ln(w) attained at days:		9.40		10.59		–1.37		0.34
Adjusted R-squared	0.20	0.20	0.25	0.25	0.09	0.09	0.12	0.13
Joint test Var. 1 & Var. 2	450*	416*	232*	226*	59*	48*	16*	16*
Joint test Var. 6 & Var 7		13*		11*		15*		2*
No. of observations	18,666	18,666	10,464	10,464	4,966	4,966	1,299	1,299

Sources: ENH-91 for columns (13) to (16); CASEN for all others.

[a]Instrumental variables for health indicators based on models from Table 7.

*t-statistics for robust standard errors in brackets.

**Squared fitted variables are computed running first stage regressions on the quadratic term and using that auxiliary equation to predict squared fitted. Auxiliary regressions included in Table A-4.

The identifying instruments used to predict H^* are included in the environmental variables P and O.[59]

Table 8 reports the estimation results for the model with instrumental variables for health variables. This was done for rural and urban areas and by gender separately.[60] The pattern of effects of the health indicator changes significantly with the IV method, and health variables are now more significant and affect wages in the expected directions.

For the dummy variable disability, the effects become negative and significant for all the samples, although they are more significant for males than for females.[61] This is the expected sign for this variable and it was not observed in the estimations without IV methods shown in Table 5. The effect of number of days disabled on earnings is negative and significant for rural samples, and the size of the coefficients indicates that one additional day of disability reduces male earnings more significantly than female earnings. In the urban samples, the pattern for ln(w) depicted by the coefficients of the quadratic specification for number of days disabled is U-shaped. The returns to the number of days disabled decrease in the first 9 (for males)[62] or 11 (for females) days of disability. For more

[59] The squared endogenous variables are computed by running first-stage regressions on the quadratic term and using that auxiliary regression to predict the squared endogenous variable. The auxiliary regressions are included in Table A4 in the Appendix.

[60] Given that the percentage of domestic servants is only 4.6%, the model with disability and number of days disabled was estimated excluding domestic servants.

[61] The endogenous probability of disability for urban and rural females is significant at the 10% level.

[62] The critical values reported in the tables are calculated by differentiating totally the fitted equation of the model with respect to the variable of interest, equating the derivative to 0, and solving for the optimal value.

TABLE 8. *(continued)*

	Urban				Rural			
	Male		Female		Male		Female	
	(9)	(10)	(11)	(12)	(13)	(14)	(15)	(16)
Individual variables								
1–Age	0.067*	0.076*	0.038*	0.045*	0.049*	0.056*	0.038*	0.037*
	(22)	(16)	(6.9)	(3.1)	(13)	(13)	(7.2)	(6.7)
2–Age squared/1,000	–0.634*	–0.713*	–0.313*	–0.366*	–0.357*	–0.497*	–0.260*	–0.240*
	(16)	(11)	(4.7)	(2.1)	(7.1)	(8)	(3.5)	(3.0)
3–Years of education	0.087*	0.106*	0.076*	0.101*	0.091*	0.091*	0.090*	0.090*
	(62)	(48)	(19)	(11.9)	(62)	(62)	(47)	(46)
4–Dummy salaried worker	0.003	0.212*	0.201*	0.268*	–0.069*	–0.072*	0.141*	0.140*
(person earns a wage = 1;	(0.21)	(10)	(8)	(3.88)	(5.51)	(5.74)	(7)	(7)
owns a business = 0)								
5–Dummy domestic servant = 1					–0.381*	–0.372*	–0.370*	–0.370*
					(3.97)	(3.92)	(14)	(14)
I.V. Health variables[a]								
8–Fitted dummy	–0.281*	–0.144	–0.410*	–0.188				
(disabled = 1)	(3.17)	(1.73)	(3.35)	(1.75)				
9–Fitted height/100					7.973*	–477.4*	6.888*	56.10
					(14.2)	(3.63)	(9.28)	(0.65)
10–Fitted height squared/10^4**						142.92*		–15.36
						(3.69)		(0.57)
Intercept	3.7	3.2	3.8	3.6	–8.0	403.4	–5.6	–45.0
Critical values								
Max ln(w) attained at age:	53.03	53.11	60	61.37	68.76	56.71	73.03	76.8
Critical point of ln(w) attained at height:						167.02		182.64
Adjusted R squared	0.20	0.25	0.08	0.13	0.34	0.34	0.35	0.35
Joint test Var. 1 & Var. 2	526*	237*	44*	15*	736*	404*	288*	262*
Joint test Var. 9 & Var. 10						119*		48*
No. of observations	18,666	10,464	4,966	1,299	13,721	13,721	9,332	9,322

Sources: ENH-91 for columns (13) to (16); CASEN for all others.

[a]Instrumental variables for health indicators based on models from Table 7.

*t-statistics for robust standard errors in brackets.

**Squared fitted variables are computed running first stage regressions on the quadratic term and using that auxiliary equation to predict squared fitted. Auxiliary regressions included in Table A-4.

days of disability the returns reverse and increase. In fact, the bulk of the sample has fewer than 10 days of disability as shown in Figure 1. In the rural samples, the shape of ln(w) depicted by the quadratic specification for number of days disabled is decreasing and concave in all the relevant range,[63] which indicates that the effects on earnings of the number of days disabled are negative and are worse for a larger number of days. The education returns are approximately the same as those shown in Table 5.

When the endogeneity of health is taken into account, the estimated effects of being salaried for all the samples are equal to the ones shown in Table 5. Similarly, domestic servants continue to be paid less, but according to the IV methodology the coefficient's absolute value increases.

The IV models in the last four columns of Table 8 show that height is significant in the determination of wages in the linear and quadratic specifications for both males and females.[64] The size of the coefficients in the linear specifications of columns 13 and 15 is much larger than the corresponding OLS estimates from Table 5 (the male coefficient is 11 times larger, and the female coefficient is 15 times larger). This indicates that, when the endogenous determinants of height are taken into account, the effect of endogenous variation in height on productivity is increased substantially. The quadratic effects of height on hourly earnings estimated by instrumental variables are not defined precisely by our data for females or plausibly for males (Table 8). Therefore, the discussion here (and

---

[63] Although in rural samples both terms are not individually significant, they are jointly significant as indicated by the test reported in the table.

[64] Although for females both terms are not individually significant, they are jointly significant as indicated by the joint test reported in the table.

subsequent simulations) relies on the uniformly significant estimates of the linear specification by instrumental variables, which can be interpreted as the expected wage effects of height for the average person in our sample.[65]

Simulations with Health Production Functions and Hourly Earnings IV Equations

The last step of the research combined the estimates from the earnings function and the health outcome equations to simulate how changes in policy variables are likely to affect lifetime earnings. To apply this procedure, the simplifying assumption that the effects of health on wages are uniform over the life cycle is introduced. The effects of policy changes on the probability of having a disability,[66] on height, and on productivity are presented. This section is based on estimates from Tables 7 and 8.

Table 7 shows that most of the policy variables were not significant for the explanation of disability, which makes it difficult to draw many policy inferences from the model. Therefore, the only variable considered for simulations with disability was the coverage of affiliation to social security. Table 9 shows the results in the probability of being disabled for the different models when the percentage of individuals affiliated to social security in the *departamento* and area (urban or rural) is increased by 10%, 20%, and 30%. The second part of Table 9 shows the consequent changes in log earnings implied by such a policy.

As expected from the sign of the coefficients in Table 7, more affiliation to social security in rural areas decreases the probability of being disabled and increases productivity; the opposite holds in urban areas. According to the model described by Equation 5, and controlling for the other variables included in columns 1–4 of Table 7, an increase of 20% in the social security coverage in rural areas could reduce the probability of being disabled by 5.3% for rural females and by 2.1% for rural males. This particular change would reflect increases in the productivity for rural women of 0.7% and for rural men of 0.5%, controlling for the other variables included

in columns 9–12 of Table 8. Assuming that all other variables are held constant, all these conclusions hold. In addition, the link between social security and better health may not be causal. In urban areas, social security is associated with a greater tendency to report illness, and our indicator may be revealing only the formality of the labor markets in the subregions.

The effect on height and the consequent changes in earnings of performing diverse simulations are shown in Table 10. The first row shows the estimated model without variations. Subsequent rows show diverse simulations with "percentage of houses in the community with basic services" and "percentage of houses in the community with adequate number of rooms per person." Simulations confirm that both policies are positively associated with stature and earnings, as expected from Tables 7 and 8. Almost all the simulations produced a higher percentage effect on female height than on male height, but the related increases in earnings to each policy are higher for males than for females. This is consistent with the fact that the productivity effects of height for males are higher than those for females. The effect on earnings of increasing the provision of adequate housing is greater than the effect of increasing the provision of public services. Holding constant all the other variables included in the models, and assuming that it is possible to increase by one-third the "percentage of houses with adequate number of rooms per person," females' height would increase by 2.2% and males' height would increase by 1.9%, which in turn could imply increases in hourly earnings of 27% and 29%, respectively.

CONCLUSIONS

The purpose of this study was to understand how public and private investments in health in Colombia might be related to future earnings of individuals. There are no previous studies in Colombia that considered health as a determinant of an individual's income. Human capital had always been viewed from an educational perspective, although health is obviously an important component of individual human capital in increasing work productivity and enhancing the functioning of the economy as a whole. As with education, public policies can improve the health status of individuals. The study identified the magnitude of the returns to having good health status through the direct effect of health variables on earnings of individuals. One additional day of disability decreased male rural earnings by 32% and female earnings by 13%, having a disability in a given month decreased the earnings of urban males by 28% and of urban females by 14%, and having an additional 1 cm of stature in-

---

[65] The estimated values for height and height squared imply that earnings increase with height, as expected, for 99.9% of the female sample (those < 182 cm tall). However, the quadratic specification did not provide reasonable predictions for 33% of the male sample (those < 167 cm. tall). The estimated model exhibits negative income effects of height for that group, because the U-shaped curve of $\ln(w)$ against height reaches a minimum at 167 cm. This problem persisted when the sample was restricted to men older than 25, because younger men may not have reached their adult height and may receive low incomes.

[66] The results of the simulations with number of days disabled are very similar and are not included.

TABLE 9. Simulations of Policies by Area and Sex

| | Incidence of Disability | | | |
	Urban male	Urban female	Rural male	Rural female
Model	0.050	0.069	0.068	0.077
Coverage of social security (1 + 10%)	0.051	0.071	0.067	0.075
% change 1	2.40%	3.36%	−1.03%	−2.71%
Coverage of social security (1 + 20%)	0.052	0.073	0.067	0.073
% change 2	5.01%	7.01%	−2.06%	−5.30%
Coverage of social security (1 + 30%)	0.054	0.076	0.066	0.071
% change 3	7.41%	10.66%	−2.94%	−7.88%

| | Mean hourly labor earnings | | | |
	Urban male	Urban female	Rural male	Rural female
Model	535.500	448.855	293.536	262.146
Coverage of social security (1 + 10%)	533.415	447.332	294.241	263.934
% change 1	−0.39%	−0.34%	0.24%	0.34%
Coverage of social security (1 + 20%)	531.339	445.813	294.919	263.934
% change 2	−0.78%	−0.68%	0.47%	0.68%
Coverage of social security (1 + 30%)	529.271	444.300	295.62	264.860
% change 3	−1.16%	−1.01%	0.71%	1.04%

Sources: Model of Tables 7 and 8 and CASEN.

creased urban male earnings by 8% and urban female earnings by 7%.

At the descriptive level, illness is more frequent for women than for men, for less educated than for more educated persons, for rural than for urban residents, and for older individuals. Corresponding patterns were found with height, although this sample was only for urban individuals. The well educated are almost 9 cm taller than those with no years of education, and mean height is lower for older age groups. Investments in health affect an individual's productivity, and the impact is greater than was found in one African study. A Mincerian log-earnings equation that included health indicators as a parallel form of human capital was estimated. The initial OLS regressions with number of days disabled and disability exhibited a weak correlation between health status variables and earnings. When health status variables are treated as endogenous and estimated by instrumental variables, both variables become significant and have the expected signs. The regressions with height showed the correct sign and high significance even without the IV correction for health, but the coefficients increased significantly with IV methods. The linear returns to height are increasing. Correcting for the selection bias introduced when only individuals who are earning positive wages are analyzed made little difference in the hourly earnings equation estimates.

Significant and positive effects of height have been estimated. They were greater than those found in other countries. A taller man receives hourly earnings 8% higher per additional centimeter in height and a woman receives hourly earnings that are 7% higher per additional centimeter. Contrary to results observed in other studies, the returns to education are almost invariant to the introduction of health in the earnings equations. They change from 9.8% without height to 9.1% with height for urban men and from 9.6% without height to 9.0% with height for urban women. They are identical when the dummy for disability or the number of days disabled is included in the IV estimates of the earnings function.

Social security coverage and altitude were among the most important determinants of incidence of disability and number of days disabled in rural areas. In those areas where the coverage of social security is low, more social security implies fewer disabilities and also fewer days disabled. On the contrary, in urban areas, higher levels of social security are associated with reporting disabilities more frequently. This led to the conclusion that increasing social security in rural areas could be associated with a lower incidence or duration of illness in these regions. However, social security may not necessarily improve the health of individuals and it may be associated with the tendency of respondents to report illnesses more often, as is the case in urban areas.

A general result that does not depend on the measure of health status used is that wealthier individuals (those who have higher nonlabor incomes, own the house where they live, or live in a house or apartment), controlling for age, community characteristics, and geographic location tend to have better health. Also, a complementarity be-

TABLE 10. Simulation of policies, by sex.

Simulations	Height							ln (hourly earnings)			
	Female			Male			Female		Male	
	Mean	Change in comm.	Change (%)	Mean	Change in comm.	Change (%)	Mean	Change in real earnings (%)	Mean	Change in real earnings (%)
1–Mean values at original model[a]	160.90 (1.21)			169.40 (1.22)			7.2784 (0.476)		7.4982 (0.440)	
2–(Community % of houses with lack of one basic service: electricity, water, sewage) * (1–33%) and (community % of houses with adequate number of rooms per person) *(1+50%)	164.42 (1.70)	3.53	2.19	172.63 (1.45)	3.22	1.90	7.5216 (0.491)	27.54 0.476	7.7553 (0.451)	29.32
3–(Community % of houses with lack of one basic service: electricity, water, sewage) * (1–50%) and (community % of houses with adequate number of rooms per person) * (1+ 50%)	166.24 (2.02)	5.34	3.32	174.28 (1.59)	4.88	2.88	7.6469 (0.500)	44.56	7.8876 (0.458)	47.60
4–(community % of houses with lack of one basic service: electricity, water, sewage) * (1–33%)	160.90 (1.21)	0.00	0.00	169.45 (1.17)	0.05	0.03	7.2786 (0.476)	0.03	7.5025 (0.438)	0.43
5–(community % of houses with adequate number of rooms per person) * (1+33%)	164.42 (1.70)	3.52	2.19	172.57 (1.49)	3.17	1.87	7.5214 (0.491)	27.51	7.7511 (0.454)	28.77
6–(community % of houses with lack of one basic service: electricity, water, sewage) * (1–50%)	160.90 (1.20)	0.01	0.00	169.48 (1.16)	0.08	0.05	7.2287 (0.476)	0.04	7.5045 (0.437)	0.63
7–(community % of houses with adequate number of rooms per person) * (1+50%)	166.23 (2.03)	5.34	3.32	174.21 (1.65)	4.80	2.84	7.6465 (0.501)	44.51	7.8813 (0.462)	46.68

Sources: Models from Tables 7 and 8 and ENH-91.
[a] Standard deviations in parentheses.

tween the nonlabor income (wealth) of the individual and the number of rooms per person in the houses of the community where the person lives was found in the production of health. The interaction of these two variables positively affects the health status of individuals.

Individual wealth and favorable environmental conditions, such as the provision of public services and adequate housing in the community, were the most important determinants of health in urban areas. Under the assumptions specified in the models, policies oriented to increase the coverage of basic services in the households (electricity, potable water, or sewerage) were found to have a negligible effect on height and, through height, on productivity. An increase in the supply of adequate housing would translate into better health conditions and productivity for individuals. These changes, in general, would benefit male earnings more than female earnings.

Finally, it should be noted that the quality of information available about public health interventions is a limitation of the study. The answers to the questions "Were you disabled in the last month?" and "How many days were you disabled in the last month?" are subjective and may exhibit recall errors. Although height may also be subject to measurement errors, the study showed that it offers a better measure of health status, revealing the value of using anthropometric measures as adult health indicators. Despite a large effort of collecting data at the *departamento* and municipality levels to describe the individuals' environment and merging it with the household surveys data for the analysis, most of these indicators could not account for the variation in individual health indicators. Although several patterns are suggestive, variables that were expected to be correlated with health outcomes, such as coverage of vaccination programs for different diseases, supply of hospitals in the region, number of hospital beds in each region, and number of primary and secondary schools, were not significant in explaining the available health indicators. This fact may reveal the poor quality of the information collected from sources other than the surveys and the need for better indicators of the quality and prices of health services. It may reveal also that the health services offered may be of poor quality or that they are not relevant in improving the adult health indicators used in the study.

Future research should extend this analysis of height in combination with household survey measures of acute and chronic illnesses and weight-to-height ratios (BMI), which could be jointly explained by local policy and environmental factors. With these data, a firmer case may be made for investing in particular health programs and policies that would be expected to raise labor productivity by improving the Colombian population's current health status.

REFERENCES

Behrman J. The economic rationale for investing in nutrition in developing countries. *World Development*. 1993; 21(11): 749–771.

Behrman J, Deolalikar AB. Health and nutrition. In: Chenery HB, Srinivasan TN, eds. *Handbook of Economic Development*, Vol. 1. Amsterdam: North Holland; 1988.

Deolalikar AB. Nutrition and labor productivity in agriculture: estimates for rural South India. *Review of Economics and Statistics*. 1988; 70(3): 406–413.

Económica Consultores. *Estudio para la implementación del sistema de cargos a los usuarios de carreteras*. Bogotá: Economic Consultors; February 1996.

Encuesta CASEN. *Material de soporte*. Bogotá: DNP; December 1993.

Fogel RW. Economic growth, population theory and physiology: the bearing of long term processes on the making of economic policy. *American Economic Review*. 1994; 84(3):369–395.

Greene W. *Econometric Analysis*. Englewood Cliffs: Prentice Hall; 1997.

Heckman J. Sample selection bias as a specification error. *Econometrica*. 1979; 47(1):153–161.

Instituto Geográfico Agustín Codazzi. *Diccionario geográfico de Colombia*. Bogotá: Instituto Geográfico Agustín Codazzi; 1996.

Johansson SR. The health transition: the cultural inflation of morbidity during the decline of mortality. *Health Transition Review*. 1991;1:39–68.

Leibovich J, Rodriguez LA, Nupia O. *El empleo en el sector rural colombiano: qué ha pasado en los últimos años? qué se puede prever?* Documento CEDE 97-08. Bogotá: CEDE; 1997.

Martorell R, Habicht JP. Growth in early childhood in developing countries. In: Falkner F, Tanner JM, eds. *Human Growth*, Vol. 3. New York: Plenum Press; 1986.

Mincer J. *Schooling, Experience and Earnings*. New York: Columbia University Press; 1974.

Ribero R, Meza C. Earnings of men and women in Colombia: 1976–1995. *Archivos de macroeconomía*. Bogotá: Departamento Nacional de Planeación; 1997. Mimeograph.

Rosenzweig MR, Schultz TP. Market opportunities, genetic endowments and intrafamily resource distribution: child survival in rural India. *American Economic Review*. 1982a; 72(4): 803–815.

Rosenzweig MR, Schultz TP. *Determinants of fertility and child mortality in Colombia: interactions between mother's education and health and family planning programs*. Final Report. New Haven: Economic Growth Center; 1982b.

Rosenzweig MR, Schultz TP. Estimating a household production function: heterogeneity, the demand for health inputs and their effects on birthweight. *Journal of Political Economy*. 1983; 91(5): 723–746.

Rosenzewig MR, Wolpin K. Heterogeneity, intrafamily distribution and child health. *Journal of Human Resources*. 1988; 23(4):437–461.

Schultz TP. 1984. Studying the impact of household economic and community variables on child mortality. *Population and Development Review*. 1984; 10(Suppl.):215–235.

Schultz TP. *Wage Rentals for Reproducible Human Capital: Evidence from Two West African Countries*. Working Draft. New Haven, CT: Yale University; 1996.

Schultz TP. Assessing the productive benefits of nutrition and health: an integrated human capital approach. *Journal of Econometrics*. 1997; 77(1):141–158.

Schultz TP, Tansel A. Wage and labor supply effects of illness in Cote d'Ivoire and Ghana: instrumental variable estimates for days disabled. *Journal of Development Economics*. 1997; 53(2):251–286.

Sahn DE, Alderman H. The effect of human capital on wages, on the determinants of labor supply in a developing country. *Journal of Development Economics*. 1988; 29(2):157–183.

Strauss J, Thomas D. Human resources: empirical modeling of household and family decisions. In: Behrman J, Srinivasan TN, eds. *Handbook in Development Economics*, Vol. 3A. Amsterdam: Elsevier Science; 1995.

Strauss J, Thomas D. Health and wages: evidence on men and women in urban Brazil. *Journal of Econometrics*. 1997; 77(1):159–186.

Strauss J, Thomas D. Health, nutrition and economic development. *Journal of Economic Literature*. 1998; 36(2):766–817.

United Nations Development Program. *Human Development Report*. New York: Oxford University Press; 1998.

TABLE A-1. Descriptive statistics, ENH-91 survey.

	All	Women	Men
Individual variables			
1 - Age	33.9	32.8	34.7
	(10.38)	(9.93)	(10.61)
2 - Age squared	1260	1175	1319
	(777)	(726)	(805)
3 - Height (in cm)	165.91	160.87	169.41
	(7.91)	(6.77)	(6.65)
4 - Height squared	27590	25924	28743
	(2618)	(2173)	(2253)
5 - ln (hourly wages)	7.380	7.236	7.480
	(0.79)	(0.80)	(0.76)
6 - Non-labor income (in 1991 pesos)	3997	3503	4497
	(58062)	(27682)	(73014)
7 - Education	8.57	8.75	8.51
	(4.23)	(4.30)	(4.18)
8 - Dummy wage earner =1	0.711	0.759	0.677
9 - Dummy domestic servant =1	0.053	0.127	0.002
10 - Owner occupied housing[a]	0.687	0.697	0.680
Municipality variables			
11 - % of houses in community with basic services (electricity, water, and sewage)	0.977	0.978	0.977
12 - % of houses in community with favorable number of persons per room	0.885	0.890	0.882
8 - Var. 6 * Var. 12	3655	3230	3950
	(54171)	(26363)	(66978)

Source: ENH-91 (labor force participants, with height >135 cm, ages 18-60).

Standard deviations in parentheses.

[a] Dummy: owns house or apartment where lives = 1; rented or other = 0.

TABLE A-2. Descriptive Statistics, CASEN Survey.[a]

	Urban		Rural	
	Male	Female	Male	Female
Individual variables				
1–ln (hourly labor earnings)	6.28	6.11	5.68	5.57
	(0.89)	(1.00)	(0.88)	(1.15)
2–Age	36.63	35.75	38.07	38.96
	(12.55)	(11.33)	(13.92)	(13.26)
3–Age squared	1499	1406	1643	1694
	(1033)	(910)	(1169)	(1126)
4–Years of education	7.04	7.94	3.45	4.27
	(4.26)	(4.40)	(3.00)	(3.71)
5–Dummy wage earner =1	0.63	0.59	0.55	0.38
6–Non-labor income (in 1993 pesos)	9823	10329	3874	4941
	(109298)	(61026)	(31092)	(28131)
7–Type of housing[b]	0.94	0.95	0.97	0.96
Health variables				
8–Dummy disabled = 1	0.0503	0.0696	0.0693	0.0847
9–Number of days disabled	0.42	0.49	0.58	0.67
	(2.58)	(2.65)	(2.96)	(3.06)
10–Number of days disabled squared	6.80	7.25	9.12	9.79
	(62.9)	(62.8)	(71.4)	(69.4)
Municipality variables				
11–Hospitals per capita * 10^5	1.36	1.26	3.69	3.06
	(3.93)	(3.75)	(9.60)	(8.63)
12–% enrolled in social security	0.248	0.254	0.066	0.066
13–% of houses with electricity	0.983	0.985	0.718	0.745
14–Altitude (mts)	776.74	823.79	104.09	1154.18
	(835)	(865)	(928)	(999)
15–Kms to capital	57.71	54.79	104.73	96.15
	(90.6)	(93.1)	(87.1)	(85.0)
Departamental variables				
16–Transfers for health per capita * 10^3	8.56	8.78	7.42	7.37
	(5.65)	(6.06)	(1.25)	(1.29)
Regional variables[c]				
17–Dummy Atlantic Coast	0.34	0.30	0.32	0.28
18–Dummy Pacific Coast	0.15	0.18	0.20	0.28

Sources: CASEN, Instituto Geográfico Agustín Codazzi, Ministerio de Salud, author's calculations.
Standard deviations in parentheses.
[a] Samples exclude domestic service.
[b] Type of housing: lives in house or apartment = 1; lives in room or other = 0.
[c] Reference interior.

TABLE A-3. Height regressions, labor force ages 25–55.

Dependent variable:	Height							
	Female				Male			
	(1)	(2)	(3)	(4)	(5)	(6)	(7)	(8)
Individual variables								
1–Age	–0.061*	0.208*	0.187*	0.169	–0.064*	0.012	–0.053	–0.055
	(6.05)	(2.23)	(2.05)	(1.87)	(8.44)	(0.17)	(0.76)	(0.78)
2–Age squared/1,000		–3.544*	–2.702*	–2.63*		–0.986	0.340	0.277
		(2.91)	(2.26)	(2.21)		(1.05)	(0.38)	(0.31)
3–Education			0.304*	0.251*			0.391*	0.350*
			(16.95)	(13.20)			(27.24)	(22.51)
4–Non-labor income/10^6				–47.62				–11.28
(in 1991 pesos)				(1.22)				(0.62)
5–Dummy owner occupied housing				0.287				0.043
(owns house or apartment where				(1.69)				(0.33)
lives = 1; rents or other = 0)								
Municipality variables								
6–% of houses in community with				–2.989				0.754
basic services (electricity, water, sewage)				(1.77)				(0.42)
7–% of houses in community with favorable				9.66*				5.76*
number of persons per room				(8.96)				(6.60)
8–Var. 4* Var. 7				52.51				12.87
				(1.26)				(0.66)
Intercept	163.1	158.2	155.2	150.2	171.8	170.4	167.6	162.2
Adjusted R squared	0.005	0.006	0.044	0.055	0.006	0.006	0.069	0.074
No. of observations	7,260	7,260	7,260	7,260	10,940	10,940	10,940	10,940

Source: ENH-91.
t-statistics in parentheses.

TABLE A-4. Quadratic health production functions.

Dependent health variable:	Quadratic of number of days disabled				Quadratic of Height	
Region:	Urban		Rural		Urban	
Gender:	(1)	(2)	(3)	(4)	(5)	(6)
Individual variables						
1–Age	–0.270	0.418	–0.645	–1.584	29.43*	37.59
	(1.22)	(1.30)	(1.47)	(1.73)	(2.28)	(2.42)
2–Age squared/1,000	6.604*	–2.571	13.16*	26.42*	–666*	–793*
	(2.47)	(0.64)	(2.51)	(2.46)	(4.00)	(3.83)
3–Dummy type of housing (rents or owns house or apartment =1; rents room or rooms or other, e.g., squatter =0)	–1.167	–4.130	–6.319	–0.686		
	(0.59)	(1.41)	(1.01)	(0.07)		
4–Dummy owner occupied housing (owns house or apartment where lives = 1; rents or other = 0)					99.65*	99.59*
					(2.44)	(2.05)
5–Non-labor income/10⁴ (a)	50760	187534	–330618	–350236	7.980	34.669*
	(1.20)	(1.86)	(1.01)	(0.52)	(1.50)	(3.50)
Municipality variables						
6–Hospitals/clinics per capita* 1,000	33.30*	–30.93	–3.76	26.72		
	(2.66)	(1.75)	(0.31)	(1.05)		
7–Community % of people directly enrolled or beneficiaries of social security	8.57	–6.69	–50.38*	–65.09		
	(1.14)	(0.67)	(2.27)	(1.72)		
8–Community % of households with electricity	–2.17	12.01	4.16	0.001		
	(0.28)	(0.92)	(0.75)	(0.00)		
9–Altitude (in mts above sea level)/100,000	–36.78	–91.40	–272	–581*		
	(0.54)	(1.07)	(1.79)	(2.27)		
10–Distance to capital of *departamento* in kms/1,000	–3.23	4.766	30.65*	–35.16		
	(0.59)	(0.67)	(2.20)	(1.31)		
11–Community % of houses with basic services: electricity,water, sewage					2422*	120
					(4.49)	(0.24)
12–Community % of houses with adequate number of rooms per person					3668*	3745*
					(14.13)	(12.48)
13–(Non-labor income/10⁴)* (community % of houses with adequate number of rooms per person)					29.63	258*
					(0.45)	(2.14)
Departmental variable						
14–Transfers per capita from central government to *departamento* for health	–161.4	–9.75	82.21	1914		
	(1.86)	(0.09)	(0.10)	(1.15)		
Individual regional variables(b)						
15–Dummy (lives in Atlantic Coast = 1)	–0.89	–2.74	–6.82*	–8.35		
	(0.70)	(1.57)	(2.27)	(1.40)		
16–Dummy (lives in Pacific Coast = 1)	0.024	5.109*	5.533*	14.68*		
	(0.02)	(2.95)	(1.89)	(2.97)		
Intercept	9.55	–9.59	18.87	25.27	29020	25980
Adjusted R-squared	0.0033	0.003	0.0106	0.0264	0.0329	0.0305
No. of observations	18,666	10,464	4,966	1,299	13,721	9,332

Sources: ENH-91 for columns (5) and (6); CASEN for all others. Different sources for variables 6, 9, 10, and 14.

t-statistics in parentheses.

(a) Monetary variables (5, 13, and 14) are in 1993 pesos for columns (1) to (4) and in 1991 pesos for columns (5) and (6). A 1991 peso is equivalent to 1.53 1993 pesos.

(b) Reference interior.

LINKING HEALTH, NUTRITION, AND WAGES: THE EVOLUTION OF AGE AT MENARCHE AND LABOR EARNINGS AMONG ADULT MEXICAN WOMEN

Felicia Marie Knaul[1]

INTRODUCTION

A nation's potential to achieve economic growth and development is reflected in the health and nutritional status of its population. For the individual, particularly at low levels of income, health may be an essential determinant of productive capacity in the labor market and, hence, of earnings and the capacity to escape poverty.

The relationships among health, nutrition, and income have been important elements in theories of economic development, particularly as expressed in nutrition-based efficiency wages (Leibenstein, 1957; Rosenzweig, 1988; Strauss and Thomas, 1998). Economic history also has been advanced considerably by recent efforts to further the analysis of the relationship between long-term changes in the health of populations and the process of economic development and structural transformation (Fogel, 1994; Steckel, 1995). Recently, knowledge of the link between health and income has been enriched by empirical evidence of the causal impact of health on wages and productivity among poorer populations (Strauss and Thomas, 1998). The relationship between labor productivity and health is now being explored in an integrated human capital framework (Schultz, 1997; Schultz and Tansel, 1997; Schultz, 1996; Strauss and Thomas, 1997). Models of economic growth have been extended to include the importance of health as a human capital input (Barro, 1995). These breakthroughs are a product of advances in economic theory and in the quality of data. The surge in research on this topic also reflects an increased recognition of the opportunities and challenges for formulating relevant and effective health policies.

This study uses a human capital framework to evaluate the impact that investments in health and nutrition in Mexico have on labor market productivity. The research extends existing literature by proposing age at menarche as an effective indicator for analyzing the impact of health and nutritional investments during childhood and adolescence on productivity in the labor market. As in the case of adult height and body mass index (BMI), indicators that have been widely used in the analysis of the health–productivity relationship, menarche is a variable that reflects the secular increase in the level of economic development of many countries in the region (Brundtland and Walløe, 1973; Marshall, 1978; Malcolm, 1978; Wyshak and Frisch, 1982; Wyshak, 1983; Manniche, 1983; Wellens et al., 1990; Hulanicka and Waliszko, 1991; Liestøl and Rosenberg, 1995). Over the past 150 years, age at menarche has shown a steady decrease of approximately three-to-four months per decade in many countries. This decrease is a reflection of a variety of socioeconomic factors, particularly nutritional status in childhood. Despite the parallels between menarche and adult height as indicators of cumulative health status, age at menarche apparently has not been previously incorporated into the analysis of the impact of health on economic development.

This chapter considers the correlates of age at menarche in the framework of a reduced form health production function. Particular emphasis is placed on the importance of policy-sensitive health variables as determinants of age at menarche and, hence, of female health in the long term. Hourly wages are used to measure the impact on labor market productivity of investment in health and nutri-

[1]Director of Development and of the Program on Health Economics, Centro de Investigación y Docencia Económicas (CIDE), Carr. México-Toluca 3655, Lomas de Santa Fe, Deleg. Alvaro Obregon, 01210, México, DF, México. Tel: 525-727-9840/9813/9800; Fax: 727-9878; email: knaul@dis1.cide.mx.

tion early in the life cycle. Age at menarche is presented as a proxy for certain aspects of the health and nutritional components of human capital. The integrated human capital framework that underlies the theoretical model was developed by Schultz (1997) and was applied in works such as that of Schultz (1996), Schultz and Tansel (1997), and Strauss and Thomas (1997).

The chapter's first section provides a brief introduction to the recent evolution of health in Mexico. The next section discusses menarche as an indicator of health and nutritional status. The third section provides an overview of the data used in the analysis. The fourth section summarizes the model and the estimation strategy following Schultz (1996) and Schultz and Tansel (1997). The fifth section provides descriptive statistics, with particular emphasis on the distribution of menarche by cohort, level of education, and hourly wages. The results of the first-stage, reduced form estimates of the health production function are given in the sixth section. The seventh section presents the instrumental variable estimates of the wage regressions, emphasizing the relationship between age at menarche and wages. Conclusions and policy recommendations are given in the final section.

The model uses an instrumental variable approach given the significant degree of measurement error that is inherent in retrospective information about menarche. The instruments used to identify menarche are based on the availability of personal health services, public services, housing quality, average levels of education, and access to educational facilities in the community. A number of variables are included in the wage function to control for variation that is related to genetic and other determinants of menarche. These variables are expected to be uncorrelated with the reproducible component of health, human capital.

It is important to note that the measure of the impact of age at menarche on labor market productivity is a lower-bound estimate of the welfare impact of ill health (Schultz and Tansel, 1997). First, age at menarche measures only a few of many dimensions of health. In particular, it is a cumulative measure reflecting investments in early nutritional status and other investments in childhood health. In addition, labor market productivity and wages reflect only one aspect of the myriad implications of adult ill health in terms of personal and family welfare.

It is useful to clarify that, given the nature of the data, in this chapter menarche is considered as the onset of the first menstrual cycle. Puberty is a collective term that summarizes a set of morphological and physiological processes that are the result of complex developmental processes in the central nervous and endocrine systems. In women, these processes include the adolescent growth spurt, the development of secondary reproductive organs

and sex characteristics, changes in body composition, and development of the circulatory and respiratory systems leading to increases in strength and endurance. Menarche is a relatively late event in physical development that typically occurs after the adolescent growth spurt and after the peak in growth (Marshall, 1978; Tanner, 1962).

TRANSFORMATION OF HEALTH AND NUTRITION IN MEXICO

Mexico is a particularly interesting case for studying the evolution of age at menarche. Although the country is well into its epidemiologic transition, the process has been characterized as "protracted and polarized" (Frenk et al., 1989). This is a reflection of inequalities that include both income and access to resources such as health services. Mexico faces a combined challenge. "Pretransitional" diseases—many of which are infectious or based on nutritional deficiencies—that are related to infant and maternal mortality and preventable with relatively inexpensive public health interventions are juxtaposed with an increasing health burden from chronic, noninfectious illness. Pretransitional diseases disproportionately affect the poor (Frenk et al., 1989; Frenk et al., 1994c).

As has been the case in many Latin American countries, Mexico's decline in mortality has occurred quickly. Life expectancy almost doubled between the early 1900s and 1950, and it is currently over 70 years. Infant mortality has dropped considerably, from 323 per 1,000 live births in 1910 to nearly 40 in the past decade (Frenk et al., 1989; Bobadilla et al., 1993). Similarly, the proportions of deaths related to maternal mortality and malnutrition have declined substantially (Frenk et al., 1994b).

Although historical data on nutrition are scarce, there is evidence that the prevalence of malnutrition has been rising in some rural areas and declining in others. Overall, the proportion of rural children 1–5 years old with normal height for age increased from 49% in 1974 to 52% in 1996. Further, both mortality and morbidity attributable to nutritional deficiencies declined based on data from 1990 to 1996 (Salud Pública de México, 1998; Avila et al., 1998). Figures for the Region are both more accessible and more dramatic. The prevalence of nutritional deficiency dropped from affecting 19% of the population of Latin America and the Caribbean in 1969–1971 to 15% in 1990–1992, and it is projected to reach 7% in 2010 (Food and Agriculture Organization, 1996).

Health indicators for Mexico, although clearly demonstrating a tendency to improve, are less advanced than they should be when considered as a function of the country's economic development level. The reduction in the proportion of deaths attributable to infectious diseases has been slower than in many other Latin American countries. The number went from 30% in 1960 to 13% in 1985. By comparison, in Argentina, Cuba, Costa Rica, and Chile the number is now well below 10% (Frenk et al., 1994c). Similarly, the ratio of deaths from infectious and parasitic diseases to deaths from noncommunicable diseases approximates unity, whereas the values are below 0.5 for several other countries with similar levels of per capita income.

The differences within and among regions and municipalities reflect the high degree of inequality in both health status and distribution of health services. Infant mortality in the southern, poorer states was about 147 per 1,000 live births in the early 1960s and 92 in the 1980s. In the wealthier, northern region the numbers are 92 and 28, respectively. The ratio of infant mortality between the southern and northern regions increased from 1.6 to 3.3 over the same period (Bobadilla et al., 1993). The differences within states also suggest important inequalities based on rural versus urban residence.

The health situation that has resulted from this prolonged and polarized epidemiologic transition places a heavy burden on a relatively extensive but inefficient health system. The Mexican system is dualistic. The poor and uninsured have access to the public health system run by the Secretariat of Health. In contrast, the insured, working population have the right to use the Mexican Social Security Institute, which covers close to half the labor force and its families. Despite this coverage, many people use and pay out of pocket for private services. This is an indicator of overlap in, inefficiencies of, and dissatisfaction with the system (Zurita et al., 1997; Knaul et al., 1997; Frenk et al., 1994b).

Further, the distribution of health services parallels and hence often intensifies the existing inequalities in the health status of the population. For example, Frenk et al. (1995, 1997) showed that there are approximately 200 inhabitants per physician in Mexico City, a number that exceeds the average in many developed countries. However, the numbers are much higher in the poorer states and in rural areas. In Oaxaca there are an estimated 1,120 inhabitants per doctor, and in Chiapas there are 1,370. As a partial response to the deficiencies in the health system, reforms have been initiated at the Instituto Mexicano del Seguro Social (IMSS) and a system-wide process of decentralization is well under way (Frenk, 1997).

MENARCHE AS A MEASURE OF HEALTH AND NUTRITIONAL STATUS

Fogel (1994) and Steckel (1995) highlight the secular improvements in mortality and morbidity and their relationship to a complex set of factors associated with economic development. These factors include improvements in nutritional status, medical technology, access to health care, education, public health facilities, and hygiene.

Traditionally, height and weight have been used as predictors of morbidity and mortality risk among children. More recently, adult height and BMI have been put forward as indicators of the probability of dying or of developing chronic diseases at middle and older ages (Fogel, 1994; Strauss and Thomas, 1997; Schultz, 1996) and as measures of living standards (Steckel, 1995).

Adult height and BMI measure different aspects of nutrition and health. Adult height is considered an indicator of nutritional status during infancy, childhood, and adolescence. BMI is a measure of current nutritional status. This evidence was analyzed and extended by Fogel (1994), who documented the secular increase in average height and BMI in several European countries between the seventeenth and nineteenth centuries. This evidence is used to develop an argument for the importance of physiological factors in economic growth.

The research summarized here adds another dimension to the existing literature on the importance of health as a reproducible form of human capital. In this chapter, age at menarche is used as an indicator of the result of investments in nutrition and health during childhood and adolescence. This parallels the work that other researchers have undertaken using adult height as an indicator. The logic of the association between menarche or adult height and investments in health and nutrition is based on the idea that, in a fixed population that does not experience variation in its mix of biological groups, changes over time in average height or age at menarche may be attributed to changes in reproducible human capital investments and changes in disease environments (Schultz, 1996; Fogel, 1994; Steckel, 1995). Further, several studies have shown the significant impact on labor productivity of investment in health and nutrition as measured by height and BMI in an integrated human capital framework. These include the studies of Schultz (1996) for Côte d'Ivoire and Ghana and of Thomas and Strauss (1997) for urban Brazil.

Several authors have pointed to the importance of average age at menarche as an overall, comparative indicator of population health, timing of maturation, and nutritional status (Hediger and Stine, 1987; Malcolm, 1978). Further, there is a close link between adult height, the timing of the adolescent growth spurt, height for age, and age of menarche that has been documented in a variety of countries and settings (Malcolm, 1978). Trussel and Steckel (1978) used data on height velocity for female slaves transported within the United States in the 1800s to predict probable age at menarche. Díaz de Mathman,

Ramos Galván, and Landa Rico (1968a and 1968b) found that malnourished Mexican adolescents were significantly older at menarche than the well nourished. In a study of Japanese girls, Nagata and Sakamoto (1988) found that age at menarche was an important predictor of adult height.

Some evidence suggests that age at menarche may be an important complementary indicator to adult height and possibly a more accurate tracer of early nutritional status in certain cases. Specifically, catch-up growth may allow certain individuals to attain a normal height, given the expectations of their genetic group, despite having suffered from malnutrition or poor health during childhood (Floud, 1994). Catch-up growth reduces the effectiveness of adult height as a measure of cumulative health status to the extent that malnutrition and ill health are expected to have effects on productivity that are independent of completed height. A delay in menarche, on the other hand, may be a more dependable tracer of malnutrition and ill health during childhood and adolescence because it is a one-time event that occurs during puberty. For example, Eveleth (1978) citing the study by Dreizen et al. (1967) suggests that girls with chronic malnutrition in a poor, rural area of the United States were delayed in age at menarche and skeletal maturation compared with a control group. The completed height of these two groups was not significantly different, although the malnourished group was shorter than the control group during the period of adolescent growth. Laska-Meirzejewska (1970) found that age at first menstruation was more sensitive to external conditions related to socioeconomic status and family well-being than height or weight among a sample of Polish girls. Further, Liestøl and Rosenberg (1995) suggested that menarcheal age, possibly related to changes in weight, may be more sensitive than height to regional differences in poverty among schoolchildren in Oslo.

Both age at menarche and adult height have demonstrated secular improvements. These improvements are likely to be closely related to increased nutritional standards (Trussell and Steckel, 1978). Marshall (1978) evaluated a group of studies of age at menarche and concluded that, despite differences in data quality, they were remarkably consistent in illustrating an average decline of three-to-four months per decade over the past 100 years. The secular decline is also evident over the past 100–150 years in a variety of developed countries based on aggregate trends (Wyshak and Frisch, 1982). The estimated rate of decline is between two and three months per decade. Brundtland and Walløe (1973) cited evidence from North America, Japan, and Europe to show that girls have been maturing faster over the past 50 years—at a rate of about four-to-five months per decade. More recent stud-

ies have confirmed this tendency for well-nourished women in the United States born since 1920 (Wyshak, 1983), in Denmark born since the 1940s (Manniche, 1983), in Flemish women in the nineteenth century (Wellens et al., 1990), in Poland since about 1950 (Hulanicka and Walizko, 1991), and in Norway among schoolchildren since the 1920s (Brundtland and Walløe, 1973; Liestøl and Rosenberg, 1995). Further, these studies suggest that the trend is coming to a halt among some well-nourished groups of high economic status in developed countries, coincident with a threshold age at menarche (Brundtland and Walløe, 1973).

The determinants of age at menarche can be divided into genetic and environmental factors, and the latter are widely thought to reflect nutritional differences. The literature on adolescent growth widely concurs in establishing the link between malnourishment in infancy and childhood, later age at menarche, and a slowdown in growth (Díaz de Mathman, Landa Rico, and Ramos Galván, 1968a and 1986b; Marshall, 1978; Eveleth, 1978; Frisch and Revelle, 1970; Maclure, 1991; Liestøl, 1982; Trussell and Steckel, 1978). Environmental factors such as socioeconomic status, urban residence, number of siblings, birth order, racial differences, climate, altitude, physical activity, psychological stress, season of year, and presence of a related male in the family have all been put forward, with the first two being the most consistently associated with menarche (Eveleth, 1978; Marshall, 1978; Malcolm, 1978; Moisan et al., 1990; Weir et al., 1971; Komlos, 1989; Ulijaszek et al., 1991; Bojlén and Weis, 1971; Valenzuela et al., 1991; Delgado and Hurtado, 1990; Cumming, 1990; Treloar and Martin, 1990; Graber et al., 1995; Bielicki et al., 1986). Racial differences also figure prominently in many of these studies. These partially reflect variation in socioeconomic and climatic factors but also may have an important genetic component.

Heredity-related or genetic factors may dominate among well-nourished populations (Stark et al., 1989) and appear to be more important among later cohorts (Treloar and Martin, 1990). This is supported both by important population differences and by studies comparing twins with other siblings. These studies show much larger differences in age at menarche between nontwins (Eveleth, 1978; Marshall, 1978).

In summary, literature from a variety of countries demonstrates a secular decline in the age at menarche throughout the world. This research suggests that, although a variety of environmental and genetic factors may make the analysis less precise, menarche occurs earlier among healthier and better-nourished girls and adolescents. For the purposes of the research presented below, the crucial hypothesis developed in this section of the chapter is that age at menarche is a plausible proxy for measuring part of the differences in adult labor market productivity among women that result from investments in nutrition and health during childhood and adolescence.

DATA

The main data source for this study is the Encuesta Nacional de Planificación Familiar [National Family Planning Survey] (NFPS), undertaken by Consejo Nacional de Población (CONAPO) in 1995. The NFPS includes an individual, a household, and a community questionnaire. The individual survey is directed toward the target population of women ages 15–54 who are living permanently or temporarily in the household included in the survey. This part of the NFPS was answered directly by each woman and includes detailed fertility and marital histories as well as socioeconomic characteristics and work activity. The household questionnaire considers socioeconomic characteristics, family structure, work activities, and condition of the dwelling. The community survey was carried out in sites (primarily those with fewer than 5,000 inhabitants)[2] and was directed at a community leader. This part of the NFPS contains information on basic characteristics of the community including information on access to and use of health and educational facilities.

The sampling frame of the NFPS is designed to overrepresent the poorest, most rural states. In particular, nine states account for 90% of the sample. The information for the other 23 and most populous states is given by the remaining observations, which amount to about 1,000 cases in the overall sample of women and 300 female wage earners. The survey includes expansion factors that are designed to restore the balance between states and to provide appropriate estimates for the country as a whole. Still, given the small number of observations for the 23 undersampled states, the analysis of age at menarche using the expansion factors proved to be somewhat unstable. As a result, the information provided here is based on the unexpanded numbers, which implies that the estimates do not necessarily reflect the distributions within the population as a whole.[3] To account for the important geographic differences in socioeconomic status and the availability of health services, the regressions include ei-

ther a dummy variable for rural versus urban residence (rural = 1) and another for the overrepresented states (Chiapas, Guanajato, Guerrero, Hidalgo, Mexico, Michoacán, Oaxaca, Puebla, and Veracruz = 1) or a full set of state dummies.

It is important to highlight that, in the NFPS, women who are interviewed in the individual survey self-report all variables.[4] This clearly improves the quality of the data in the sense that self-reported responses are likely to be more correct. In particular, the labor market variables are reported both as part of the household survey, and in many cases by a proxy respondent, and then repeated by the individual as own-respondent. Comparison of the two responses suggests that they differ substantially. For this reason, the data in this research are based on the self-reported information.[5]

There are two severe restrictions in terms of the data available from the NFPS. First, the only measure of adult health is menarche so that it is impossible to be more encompassing of the impact of different aspects of health status on wages. Further, the data include no information on place of birth or migration.

In addition to the information available from the community segment of the NFPS, this research uses two sources of municipality-level information. The first is the Indicadores Socioeconómicos e Indice de Marginación Muncipal generated by CONAPO in conjunction with the Comisión Nacional del Agua in 1993 and based on the results of the XI Censo General de Población undertaken by the Instituto Nacional de Estadística, Geografia e Informática (INEGI) in 1990. These indicators are disseminated as the Sistema del Indice de Marginación Municipal (SIMM). These data were compiled with the purpose of developing an indicator of marginality applicable to all the municipalities in Mexico and include, as proportions of the inhabitants of each municipality, the illiterate adult population, the adult population without complete primary education, those without electricity, those

---

[2] While the questionnaire and manuals report that the community segment was exclusively directed at sites with a maximum of 2,500 inhabitants, the data analysis shows that a large proportion contain between 2,500 and 5,000 inhabitants according to responses of community leaders.

[3] The descriptive figures using expansion factors are available from the author upon request.

[4] The fact that only self-reported information is accepted in the survey also generates a sampling problem. Approximately 10% of women ages 18–54 identified in the household survey are excluded from the individual data that include age at menarche. Most are excluded because they could not be located for the interview. This introduces a particular form of selection bias into the research, because the women who were identified in the household survey and not found for the individual interview are more likely to be younger, working, more educated, and earning a higher income (see Annex Table 1). This bias cannot be explicitly dealt with using the econometric techniques applied in this paper given that age at menarche, as the key variable, is missing for these women. Given that women with these characteristics tend to be younger at menarche according to the available sample, the results of the impact of menarche on productivity may be biased downward.

[5] It would be interesting to conduct a more careful analysis of these differences in the future as a means of bounding the possible error in household surveys where proxy respondents are common.

whose homes have earthen floors, those who lack toilet and drainage facilities, those without running water, those who live in overcrowded homes, individuals in sites with fewer than 5,000 inhabitants, and the working population earning less than two minimum salaries per month.[6]

The second source of information at the municipality level is a database jointly developed by researchers at the Colegio de México, CONAPO, and Johns Hopkins University based on the records of the Secretariat of Health (Secretaría de Salud) and IMSS (Wong et al., 1997). This database also includes information on private sector health services and personnel taken from the Economic Census undertaken by INEGI. The information on altitude comes from the Sistema de Información Municipal en Bases de Datos (SIMBAD) compiled by INEGI and is based on cartographic data (INEGI, 1995). All three data sets were merged with the NFPS at the level of the municipality, with information available for both urban and rural areas.

THEORETICAL AND EMPIRICAL FRAMEWORK FOR MODELING HEALTH PRODUCTION AND LABOR PRODUCTIVITY

Schultz (1996, 1997) modeled household demand for human capital as a derived demand for the services of these human capital stocks. Summarizing this work, household demand for input j for individual i is given as:

$$I_{ij} = \alpha_j Y_i + \beta_j X_i + \mu_{ij} \qquad j = H \text{ or } M, E, R, \text{ and } B \quad (1)$$

where the distinction between the Y and X variables is critical. The Y variables affect the demand for human capital through the impact on wage structures and hence via the incentive for investing in human capital as well as through other channels. By contrast, the X variables affect the demand for human capital without affecting wage opportunities. The error term is given by μ.

The inputs in an integrated framework include indicators of early investments in nutrition and health (H for adult height and M for age at menarche) (Fogel, 1994; see also discussion above), education (E) (Becker, 1993; Mincer, 1974; Griliches, 1977), migration from region of birth (R) (Schultz, 1982), and BMI (B) as an indicator of adult nutritional status and current health (Fogel, 1994; Strauss and Thomas, 1997). In this chapter, and given data limitations, only age at menarche and education are considered.

The girl and her family maximize a single period utility function that includes health (h^*), proxied by menarche (m^*), the non-health-related consumption bundle (C), and annual time allocated to nonwage activities (H_2)

$$U = U(h^*, C, H_2) \quad (2)$$

Equation 2 is maximized subject to the budget, time, and health production constraints

$$RI = HI^*P_1 + C^*P_2 = W^*H_1 + V \quad (3)$$

$$T = H_1 + H_2 \quad (4)$$

where RI is market income, P values are market prices, W is the wage rate, and V is annual household income from nonhuman wealth. Total available time (T) is divided into wage work (H_1) and nonwage activities (H_2).

Cumulative health status is produced over an individual's lifetime and begins with parents' and own investment in nutrition, disease-preventing interventions and practices, and health-conserving behaviors. These health inputs (HI) and heterogeneous endowments of the individual (G) unaffected by family or individual behavior combine to determine an individual's cumulative health status (h^*), proxied by age at menarche (m^*)

$$h^* = f(m^*) \quad (5)$$

where

$$m^* = m^*(HI, G, \varepsilon) \quad (6)$$

In Equation 6, ε is the error term in the health function. The estimates of the determinants of age at menarche are used as the first stage of the estimation of the wage function.

Expanding on the Mincerian semilogarithmic framework (Mincer, 1974), the hourly wage of an individual is a function of her cumulative health status as proxied by age at menarche, acquired skills related to education, experience as a quadratic function of aging, the vector of exogenous variables (Y) that are included additively, and other unobserved forms of human capital transfers and genetic endowments

$$W_i = \sum_{j=1}(d_j I_{ij}) + tY_i + \phi_i \quad (7)$$

This chapter includes only reduced form estimates of the health production function in Equation 2.

The econometric strategy is based on an errors-in-variables model identified with instrumental variables. This parallels Schultz (1996), Schultz and Tansel (1997), and Strauss and Thomas (1997). The two-stage, instrumental variables approach is designed to correct for the downward bias of the estimated effect of health on wages due to the errors in measuring age at menarche. Reported age

---

[6] The minimum salary is a government-imposed floor on wages that applies in the formal sector of the economy.

at menarche may diverge from true age at menarche by measurement error e

$$m_i = m_i^* + e_i \qquad (8)$$

where e is assumed to be a random variable that is uncorrelated with the other determinants of health or modeled aspects of behavior. Note that it is the correlation between ϕ and e that gives rise to bias due to heterogeneity or simultaneity in estimating the wage function. The correlation between the error in the wage function and unobserved health heterogeneity leads to simultaneous equation bias if the observed health inputs are related to the unobserved health heterogeneity. To correct for this problem, it is necessary to include in the health demand function variables that affect health input demand, such as prices or access to health services, but are not correlated with health heterogeneity. These variables generate a series of exclusion restrictions that permit identification of the unbiased wage function.

There is ample evidence to support the hypothesis that age at menarche is measured with considerable error, particularly using the type of retrospective data available for this research. The literature on measuring age at menarche highlights the issue of recall error in these types of data. Of the existing means of determining age at menarche, the cross-sectional retrospective method is considered inferior to longitudinal (repeated questioning of adolescents) or status quo (proportion of adolescents who have menstruated by a given age) methods (Marshall, 1978; Brundtland and Walløe, 1973). Several studies have measured the recall error by comparing the results from these different methods. Most notably for this study, Cravioto et al. (1987) found that, among adolescents from rural Mexico, the correlation coefficient between age at menarche from longitudinal data and from recall data collected four years after menarche was only 0.61. Similarly, only 70% of the adolescents could recall the age at menarche within one year of the actual date. In a study of Swedish teens, Bergsten (1976) found that, four years after menarche, only 63% could recall age at menarche within three months of the correct date. Hediger and Stine (1987) discussed studies showing that recall capacity falls off rapidly four-to-five years after the event and then stabilizes. They highlight the finding by Bean et al. (1979) that, in a group of U.S. women, an average of 34 years after the event, about 90% were able to recall age at menarche within one year. In their own work, Hediger and Stine (1987) found that, using information on a group of U.S. adolescents, about half the sample have low recall ability and the other half remember relatively accurately for several years after the event. They suggested that the probability of recall is not as closely related to the length of time since the event as in other studies.

Recall bias is likely to be associated with three other types of error in the data used in this study. First, age at menarche is reported in completed years so that there will be a consistent downward bias in the mean age. Women are likely to state age based on the preceding birthday, even if they began to menstruate in the second half of the year (Marshall, 1978). As the data from the NFPS does not record month at menarche it is impossible to correct for this bias directly.

Second, there are many conflicting feelings associated with adolescence and therefore with menstruation that may induce young women to provide inaccurate information, particularly if menarche was very early, very late, or especially traumatic. It is difficult to judge the nature or direction of the bias as some women may experience negative feelings and embarrassment, causing them to downplay late or early events, and others may do the same because of the positive feelings associated with particular cultural or religious practices (Hediger and Stine, 1987; Amann, 1986; Ruble and Brooks-Gunn, 1982). To the extent that older women are less likely than teens to suffer from embarrassment, recall data such as those used here may be more accurate.

Another source of error may be due to women not clearly identifying the onset of menstruation. The particular question used in the NFPS is related to how old the person was when she first menstruated. The exact wording is "Cuántos años tenía usted cuando le bajó la regla por primera vez?" Given the uneven pattern that is common at the onset of menstruation, it is possible that the women might not associate the first incidence of bleeding with menstruation if it was either very mild or not closely followed in time by another occurrence. There may also be some misinformation and confusion associated with the differences between menstruation, other aspects of puberty, and events such as fertility, pregnancy, and marriage.

Finally, another source of error may be related to "telescoping." Women may tend to report a later, or an earlier, age at menarche as they grow older or as the event becomes more distant in time. This is related to the perception that an event occurred "a certain number of years in the past." Although the direction of the error may be randomly distributed, it is possible that the accuracy of recall is related to some other factor such as intelligence, education, or literacy. Further, these factors also may be related to a woman's ability to interact with the health system. Therefore, this source of error may be more problematic than those outlined above, as it may be systematically correlated with the instrument set. Unfortunately, additional data on the accuracy of recall are necessary to evaluate the severity of this problem.

As mentioned above, in order to control for the bias due to simultaneity and measurement error, the econometric analysis in this paper is based on an instrumental variables approach. The instrument set consists of community health infrastructure and water and sanitation conditions as well as the level of education in the community. These variables are assumed to affect the demand for health human capital inputs and to be uncorrelated with unobserved health heterogeneity or measurement error, thus identifying the wage equation. The instruments are selected by using the results of the literature review, the descriptive analysis, and the regressions of the production function of health measured by age at menarche. The specification of the instrumental variables approach to the errors in variables is evaluated with Hausman tests (Hausman, 1978; Greene, 1997). In addition, the robustness of the instrumental variable estimate is explored by varying the instrument set.

The other human capital inputs that can be measured with the NFPS are education and postschooling—potential years of experience. Education is analyzed by using both a linear specification in years and dummy variables for levels. In the latter, 0 years of education is the excluded category and the dummies represent some or complete primary education (1–6 years), some or complete secondary education including preparatory and technical schools (7–12 years), and higher education including nonuniversity training (13 or more years). Experience in the wage equations is formulated in the traditional Mincerian fashion as age minus years of education minus 6 and is included as a quadratic (Mincer, 1974).

Another potential source of bias in the analysis of the impact of health on wages, as measured by age at menarche, results from what Schultz (1996) referred to as aggregation. This bias arises when inputs that have different productive effects on wages are combined in a single indicator. In a cross section, the fraction of the variance in menarche that can be explained by environmental factors may have either a smaller or a larger impact on productivity than the fraction that is largely unaccounted for and based in part on genetic variability. Aggregating the two sources of variation in the single measure of age at menarche may provide misleading results about the impact on productivity of changes in variables that affect only the environmental aspects of menarche.

This form of bias is partially offset by including, in both the wage and human capital demand functions, a series of variables that are related to the genetic component of age at menarche and to environmental factors. These controls are included in order to avoid relying on intergroup genetic variation to identify the wage effects of the reproducible component of health human capital (Schultz, 1996). The independent, exogenous control variables are selected based on the results of the literature review and the findings for the determinants of age at menarche discussed below. Individual characteristics include age and place of residence. Using the information from the rural site survey included in the NFPS, the proportion of the population who do not speak Spanish (this information is not available for individuals) and distance in km to the nearest and most frequented market are also used. As mentioned above, this information is available only for small, rural communities. For the larger municipalities and cities, these two variables are coded as zero. The controls also include altitude in m above sea level for each municipality, a dummy for rural residence, and another for the poorer states that are overrepresented in the sample.

Because the proportion of women who declared that age at menarche was below age 10 or above age 18 is very small, this sample is restricted to women who declared that age at menarche was between 10 and 17 years. In addition, this restriction makes it possible to exclude from the production function and wage equations women ages 17 and younger. The restriction of age at menarche to 10–17 is useful for the later extension to the wage function as it guarantees a completed profile of menarche for the women ages 18 and over at the time of the survey. The exclusion of these youths from the wage equation is also supported by the fact that many are still in school and not earning a wage. This restriction reduces the sample by only 1%. (See Table 1.)

Just under 30% of the adult women in the sample work and earn a positive wage, which suggests the need to identify, and correct for, sample selection bias using full information maximum-likelihood estimates of the two-stage technique originally developed by Heckman (1979). Unfortunately, the available data do not include sufficient information on exogenous determinants of labor force participation to identify the selection equation. The only exogenous measures of wealth included in the survey are the physical characteristics of the home, and the sample correction term is repeatedly insignificant when identified based on these variables. For this reason, the analysis does not include a correction for sample selection. Based on the selection-corrected regressions that were undertaken, this omission is unlikely to bias the findings about the impact of age at menarche on productivity and wages.[7] The results of the sample selection corrected model are presented in the Annex.

---

[7] The instrumental variable wage equations were also calculated with a selection equation for labor force participation. The selection term was identified by including a series of arguably endogenous variables in the participation equations. In particular, a dummy variable for marriage as well as a series of indirect indicators of wealth (measured by physical characteristics of the home and access to services) were included in the probit regression. The results

TABLE 1. Mean and standard deviation (SD), women ages 18–54, menarche between ages 10 and 17 years.

Variable	All		Wage earners	
	Mean	SD	Mean	SD
Hourly wages (ln)			1.477032	1.04837
Menarche (years)	13.146	1.343	13.127	1.373
Menarche (ln)	2.571	0.102	2.569	0.105
Menarche squared	174.629	35.714	174.193	36.435
(Menarche) × (years of education)	75.819	53.797	91.732	60.431
Community level policy variables				
Public health services				
% of population with dirt floor	33.958	24.135	30.742	22.902
% of population without toilet or drainage facilities	34.654	24.050	31.877	24.372
% of population living in overcrowded conditions	65.289	10.590	63.673	10.665
% of population without running water	30.755	23.415	27.988	22.292
Personal health services				
Distance (km) to nearest nonprivate health center (urban = 0 km)[a]	2.429	6.579	1.308	4.445
Dummy distance to health center missing (1 = missing values)[c]	0.137	0.343	0.083	0.275
Number of physicians per capita in *localidad* or municipality (×100)	0.001	0.001	0.001	0.001
Dummy for the presence of a community health center in *localidad*	0.679	0.467	0.743	0.437
Educational capital				
% of population over age 15 with incomplete primary education	48.881	17.657	45.751	17.915
% of population over age 15 who are illiterate	20.763	13.808	19.196	13.448
Distance (km) to nearest secondary school (urban = 0 km)	12.622	17.864	8.717	15.813
Dummy distance to school missing (1 = missing)[c]	0.361	0.480	0.254	0.435
Dummy for no secondary school in the *localidad*	0.454	0.498	0.318	0.466
Other human capital variables				
Education in years	5.811	4.115	7.049	4.631
Experience (age – education – 6)	18.983	11.971	18.740	11.872
Experience^2	503.653	529.992	492.070	516.056
Controls for ethnicity and residence				
% of population in *localidad* who do not speak Spanish (×100)	0.042	0.150	0.023	0.104
Dummy for missing values (1 = missing value)[c]	0.025	0.156	0.022	0.145
Altitude (km above sea level)	1.408	1.452	1.401	1.451
Dummy for missing values (1 = missing value)[c]	0.016	0.127	0.013	0.113
Dummy rural-urban (rural = 1)	1.588	0.492	0.452	0.498
Dummy oversampled states (oversampled = 1)[b]	0.918	0.274	0.921	0.270
Distance (km) to most common market (urban = 0)	10.016	15.102	7.652	13.969
Dummy distance to market missing (1 = missing values)[c]	0.020	0.139	0.008	0.087
Age of woman	31.779	9.846	32.779	9.584
n	10,839		3,158	

[a]See text for explanation.

[b]Oversampled states: Chiapas, Estado de México, Guanajuato, Guerrero, Hidalgo, Michoacán, Oaxaca, Puebla, and Veracruz.

[c]Applies only to rural areas as the variable is assumed to be 0 for urban areas.

It is important to mention two general points about the regression analysis. First, all the standard errors are calculated using the robust, White heteroskedasticity con-

of including the sample selection term derived from this analysis have very little impact on the magnitude, sign, or level of significance of the menarche variable in the wage equations. The analysis was again repeated using only the measures of the physical characteristics of the home. When this estimation strategy is used, the sample selection term is repeatedly insignificant, which suggests that the identifying variables are too weak to permit a precise estimation of the characteristics of exclusion from the labor force. Schultz and Tansel (1997), using data from Cote d'Ivoire and Ghana, found that the selectivity correction term is insignificant in predicting the impact of disabled days on productivity.

sistent, estimator (White, 1980; Greene, 1997). Further, all the instrumental and exogenous control variables that suffer from a small number of missing values are recoded with the median value. A dummy value for each variable is added to signal that the observations originally had a missing value. This guarantees comparability across regressions as the number of observations remains constant.

The wage regression uses hourly wages as the dependent variable. The adjustment to hourly wages is done by converting hours worked, when reported by day or month, to hours worked per week using days worked last week. Similarly, when labor earnings are reported

FIGURE 1. Distribution at menarche, ages 18–54.

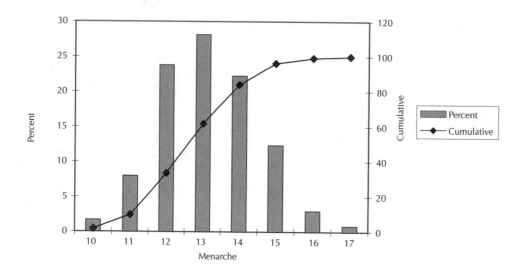

by a period other than the week, they are first adjusted to weeks and then divided by hours worked per week.[8]

The means and standard deviations (SDs) of all variables are reported in Table 1 for the full sample of 18- to 54-year-old women as well as for those with positive wages and for the sample of women living with their mothers. Given the sampling features of the survey discussed above, the numbers are presented without expansion factors.

PATTERNS IN THE AGE AT MENARCHE IN MEXICO

The mean age in the sample of women in the NFPS who experienced menarche between ages 10 and 17 is 13.1 years with an SD of 1.3 (Figure 1, Table 2). The distribution of age at menarche is concentrated at ages 12, 13, and 14 years. Further, only 1.2% of the sample of 521 youths aged 15 said they had not yet menstruated. The average age of 13.1 years coincides relatively closely with figures collected for the 1960s and 1970s for certain European countries, although in several other developed countries, including the United States, average ages ap-

proach 12.5 years (Marshall, 1978). By comparison, Díaz de Mathman, Landa Rico, and Ramos Galván (1968a and 1968b) reported an average age of 12 years (confidence interval, ±13 months) among well-nourished young women and an average age of 13.4 years (confidence interval, ±10 months) among poorly nourished young women from Mexico City. The overall average age was 12.8 years (confidence interval, ±16 months). Using the status quo method, Jacobo and Malacara (1985) found an average age at menarche of 12.8 years (confidence interval, ±1.3 years) in a population of urban, Mexican adolescents with no significant difference based on socioeconomic status.

There is a small but consistent negative correlation between menarche and age cohort (Table 3). The time

TABLE 2. Distribution of age at menarche.

Menarche	Frequency	%	Cumulative (%)
10	184	1.69	1.69
11	871	7.99	9.68
12	2,596	23.82	33.50
13	3,066	28.13	61.63
14	2,423	22.23	83.86
15	1,345	12.34	96.20
16	323	2.96	99.17
17	91	0.83	100.00
Total	10,899	100.00	

Mean = 13.14
SD = 1.34
Kurtosis = 2.81
Observed = 10,899

---

[8]It is important to note that the information on hours refers to the principal job, whereas labor earnings refers to all jobs. There is no way to adjust for this difference, as the survey does not mention the total number of jobs. Still, the proportion of women in the National Urban Employment Surveys (undertaken by INEGI on a quarterly basis) who report a second job is very low.

TABLE 3. Age at menarche by age cohort, level of education, and rural-urban residence.

| | | Age at menarche | | | | | |
		Mean	Mode	SD	Skewness	Kurtosis	Observed
Age cohort							
	18–24	13.03	13	1.32	0.30	2.88	3,258
	25–34	13.10	13	1.35	0.19	2.92	3,537
	35–44	13.23	13	1.34	0.15	2.79	2,556
	45–54	13.35	14	1.36	–0.07	2.66	1,546
Education (years)							
	0	13.27	13	1.31	0.03	2.79	1,574
	1–6	13.23	13	1.31	0.16	2.82	5,574
	7–12	12.99	13	1.38	0.30	2.89	3,127
	13+	12.83	12	1.41	0.35	2.80	616
Residence							
	Rural	13.00	13	1.37	0.21	2.81	4,483
	Urban	13.24	13	1.73	0.18	2.80	6,416

trend in age at menarche across birth cohorts is measured with more precision following Schultz (1996), by regressing menarche on age and controlling for the proportion of the population in a community that does not speak Spanish—the only information available on ethnic background. The ordinary least squares (OLS) linear trend suggests a rate of decline of slightly less than one month per decade in Mexico ($b = 0.011$, $t = 8.54$). The finding of a long-run decline is consistent with other studies summarized above that show a secular decline over the past 100–150 years in a variety of countries (Wyshak and Frisch, 1982; Marshall, 1978). Still, the rate of decline is one-quarter to one-half the reported fall in developed countries.[9]

Increases in education are also associated with a slightly more pronounced decline in age at menarche (Table 3). Women with no formal education report an average age of menarche of 13.3 years compared with 13.2, 13.0, and 12.8 years for women with at least some primary, secondary, and higher education, respectively. This partly explains the cohort effect, as education levels have increased substantially in Mexico during the past decades. Still, the inverse relationship between menarche and education is also evident within cohorts (Table 4).

Rural residence is associated with older onset menarche. The average age is 13.2 compared with 13.0 years in urban areas.[10] This is a lower-bound estimate, as it is based on current residence. It is likely that half the sample of women living in urban areas at the time of the survey were rural residents during infancy and childhood or at the time of menarche. The higher number is related to a variety of factors including the greater prevalence of malnutrition and the scarcity of health services in rural areas as well as selective migration, poverty, and educational achievement.

Menarche shows a weak but steadily declining pattern with respect to the distribution of hourly labor income (Figure 2, Table 5). Women in the lowest wage quartile have a reported mean age at menarche of 13.3 years compared with 13.0 in the highest decile. It is interesting to note that the average age at menarche is virtually identical among labor force participants and those who do not work.

In summary, the tabulations show that, in cross-sectional data, menarche tends to be inversely related to age, education, and wages, and it tends to be lower in urban areas. Although the trends tend to be small, the patterns are consistent both overall and within cohorts. The findings coincide with the expected link to malnutrition and to the socioeconomic determinants of age at menarche cited above.

DETERMINANTS OF AGE AT MENARCHE AND THE INSTRUMENT SET

A reduced-form, health production function is estimated in this section to evaluate individual, community, and regional determinants of age at menarche. The variables include both exogenous controls and variables that are excluded in the second stage and used as instruments in the wage equation.

The instrument set is composed of 11 variables related to the accessibility of public and health services, the quality of housing, and the level and availability of educa-

---

[9] A large part of this divergence is likely to be attributable to differences in data collection strategies.

[10] Although there are only six cases of 15-year-olds who have not menstruated, it is interesting to note that the proportion is higher in rural areas.

TABLE 4. Age at menarche by age cohort and level of education.

Age cohort	Mean age at menarche	SD	Skewness	Kurtosis	Observed
18–24					
Education (years)					
0	13.11	1.21	–0.08	2.65	171
1–6	13.14	1.28	0.32	2.95	1,403
7–12	12.95	1.36	0.32	2.84	1,481
13+	12.81	1.35	0.57	3.12	186
25–34					
Education (years)					
0	13.20	1.30	0.08	3.02	379
1–6	13.21	1.30	0.19	2.94	1,755
7–12	12.97	1.40	0.31	2.98	1,125
13+	12.84	1.41	0.20	2.58	268
35–44					
Education (years)					
0	13.30	1.32	0.10	2.91	509
1–6	13.25	1.33	0.13	2.70	1,544
7–12	13.17	1.35	0.25	2.99	351
13+	12.80	1.51	0.50	2.89	125
45–54					
Education (years)					
0	13.33	1.34	–0.06	2.53	514
1–6	13.39	1.33	–0.09	2.79	851
7–12	13.23	1.55	0.15	2.40	132
13+	12.97	1.42	–0.13	2.58	37

FIGURE 2. Age at menarche by hourly wage, ages 18–54.

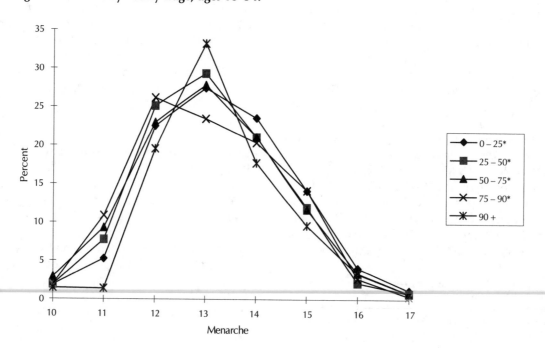

TABLE 5. Wage percentiles.

	0–25	26–50	51–75	76–90	91+
Mean	13.25	13.08	13.18	13.02	12.99
SD	1.30	1.36	1.42	1.39	1.43
Skewness	0.17	0.11	0.14	0.30	0.23
Kurtosis	2.68	2.79	2.74	2.85	2.68
Observed	770	835	762	476	313

tional resources. This assumes that the present distribution of services and resources is correlated with the distribution that prevailed at the time when, and in the place where, a woman grew up and experienced menarche. The first four instruments are indicators of the lack of availability of basic services in the community and poor quality of housing. These factors should be associated with an older age at menarche as they indicate higher health risks and poverty. The variables included in the instrument set are the proportion of individuals in each municipality whose homes have an earthen floor, who do not have indoor drainage or sanitary facilities, who live in overcrowded conditions, and who do not have access to running water. This information is from SIMM.

Increasing availability and access to health services should be negatively correlated with age at menarche. Three instruments are used as indicators of the availability or accessibility of personal health services. The first variable is distance in km from the site to the nearest health center using data from the NFPS. The sign is expected to be positive. This variable is somewhat difficult to interpret given the multiplicity of providers of personal health services discussed in the first section of this paper. Services may be provided through the Secretariat of Health, the social security system, state and other public welfare systems, pharmacies, and, to a lesser degree in rural areas, private clinics and individual physicians and practitioners. The survey includes information on all the public and social security clinics, although no information is given about distance to private clinics. The variable is designed to measure the distance to the nearest public or social security clinic. Although the uninsured theoretically are unable to use social security clinics, many of the units in rural areas form part of the IMSS system, which is open to the general public and targeted toward the poor and uninsured.[11]

The other two instrumental variables for the accessibility of personal health services are related to the presence of trained practitioners. The number of physicians per capita is constructed by combining the information

from the community survey of the NFPS with the information on municipalities. Thus, physicians per capita is calculated for all individuals living in sites using the NFPS and for residents of larger conglomerates using the information at the level of the municipality.[12] This variable enters into the second set of instruments in addition to the variables for earthen floors, drainage, and distance to clinics.[13] A dummy variable indicating the presence of a community health worker at the level of the site is derived from the NFPS data. This variable is expected to be particularly important in the smaller and poorer communities. Both variables are expected to be negatively related to age at menarche.

Education is considered an important input in enhancing the ability of the individual and the family to make more efficient use of health technology (World Bank, 1993). Given the externalities that apply to public health services, the impact of education is likely to operate at the level of both the individual and the community. For this reason, measures of the level of education and access to educational services of the community constitute another group of instruments. The average level of education is measured as the proportion of the population with incomplete primary schooling and the proportion over age 15 who report that they are illiterate according to SIMM data. Access to education, under the assumption that the present allocation of educational services is related to earlier patterns, is measured by the distance in kilometers to the nearest secondary school and a dummy if the site has no secondary school. These data come from the community model of the NFPS. Each of these measures is expected to be associated with being older at menarche.

The empirical results suggest that, as hypothesized, the public service and housing variables are significant in the regression of wages on age at menarche (Table 6). The largest and most significant effect is through the presence of sanitary facilities and the proportion of the population living in housing with earthen floors. The marginal impact of overcrowding and running water is insignificant. Of particular interest are the findings that the personal health service variables have almost no significant

---

[11] For a more detailed discussion of the organization and usage patterns of the different parts of the system see Frenk *et al.* (1994b) and Secretaría de Salud (1994).

[12] Physicians include only those individuals who have completed their medical training and obtained a license. Students undertaking their social service are not counted.

[13] Another instrumental variable for health services that was explored in the composite indicator of accessibility of health services was developed by Wong *et al.* (1997). This indicator uses factor analysis to optimally combine information on health personnel, clinics, and hospitals within a 10-km radius of the political center (*cabecera*) of each municipality. The coefficients are somewhat difficult to interpret given that the women under consideration in this study may not live in the *cabeceras* and the results of the instrumental variable regressions do not differ substantially from those reported below.

TABLE 6. Determinants of age at menarche by residence.[a]

Independent variables	All	Urban	Rural
Community level policy variables (instrumental variables)			
Public services and quality of housing			
% of population with earth floor (×100)	0.473	1.233	0.297
	(3.61)	(4.04)	(2.02)
% of population without toilet or drainage facilities (×100)	0.404	0.630	0.397
	(3.50)	(2.42)	(2.98)
% of population living in overcrowded conditions (×100)	0.150	0.343	−0.023
	(0.57)	(0.79)	(0.07)
% of population without running water (×100)	0.028	−0.326	0.074
	(0.31)	(1.58)	(0.68)
Personal health services			
Distance (km) to nearest nonprivate health center (urban = 0 km) (×100)	0.091		0.125
	(0.35)		(0.48)
Dummy distance to health center missing (1 = missing values)[a]	−0.097		−0.087
	(2.15)		(1.90)
Number of physicians per capita in *localidad* or municipality (1/100)	−0.288	−0.264	−0.369
	(1.61)	(0.63)	(1.76)
Dummy for the presence of a community health worker in *localidad*	0.037		0.029
	(1.03)		(0.77)
Educational capital			
% of population over age 15 with incomplete primary education (×100)	−0.167	−0.399	−0.343
	(0.71)	(0.90)	(1.11)
% of population over age 15 that is illiterate (×100)	−0.284	−1.428	0.316
	(1.08)	(3.04)	(0.97)
Distance (km) to nearest secondary school (urban = 0) (×100)	0.148		0.195
	(1.44)		(1.85)
Dummy distance to school missing (1 = missing values)[b]	−0.049		−0.046
	(1.07)		(1.00)
Dummy for no secondary school in the *localidad*	−0.096		−0.083
	(1.56)		(1.35)
Other human capital variables			
Education in years (×10)	−0.122	−0.247	0.012
	(3.18)	(4.56)	(0.21)
Age of woman (×100)	−0.147	0.172	−0.159
	(0.16)	(0.12)	(0.13)
(Age of woman)² (×100)	0.014	0.005	0.018
	(1.04)	(0.24)	(1.06)
Controls for ethnicity and residence			
% of population in *localidad* who do not speak Spanish	−0.038		−0.071
	(0.37)		(0.65)
Dummy for missing values (1 = missing values)[b]	−0.447		−0.464
	(4.24)		(4.30)
Altitude (km above sea level)	0.009	−0.015	0.008
	(0.92)	(0.55)	(0.72)
Dummy values for altitude missing (1 = missing values)[b]	−0.096		−0.142
	(0.91)		(1.30)
Dummy rural-urban (rural = 1)	0.250		
	(4.35)		
Dummy oversampled states (oversampled = 1)[c]	0.126	0.137	0.129
	(2.48)	(1.95)	(1.68)
Distance (km) to most common market (urban = 0) (×100)	−0.372		−0.318
	(2.97)		(2.39)
Dummy distance to market missing (1 = missing values)[a]	0.292		0.323
	(2.50)		(2.76)
Constant	12.659	12.796	12.903
	(60.93)	(37.41)	(47.33)
F statistic	15.16	11.87	7.53
R^2	0.03	0.03	0.03
n	10,831	4,459	6,372

(Continued)

TABLE 6. (continued)

Independent variables	All	Urban	Rural
Wald test of joint significance			
All community-level policy variables	9.26	7.8	5.77
	(0.00, 13)	(0.00, 7)	(0.00, 13)
Public service and quality of housing variables	9.77	6.46	4.89
	(0.00, 4)	(0.00, 4)	(0.00, 4)
Personal health service variables	1.91	0.4	1.68
	(0.12, 4)	(0.53, 1)	(0.15, 4)
Educational capital variables	2.39	6.81	1.71
	(0.04, 5)	(0.00, 2)	(0.13, 5)
Age and age^2	16.63	2.71	17.96
	(0.00, 2)	(0.07, 2)	(0.00, 2)

[a]Dependent variable: age at menarche (restricted to 10–17), OLS regressions (absolute value of t in parentheses). Sample: women ages 18–54; menarche between ages 10 and 17.

[b]Applies only to rural areas because the variable is assumed to be 0 for urban areas.

[c]Oversampled states: Chiapas, Estado de México, Guanajuato, Guerrero, Hidalgo, Michoacán, Oaxaca, Puebla, and Veracruz.

[d]Wald test of joint significance, F statistic with probability at 10% significance and degrees of freedom in parentheses.

[e]Standard errors calculated using robust (Huber, White, Sandwich) estimator of variance provided with STATA.

impact. Only the variable for physicians is significant at the 10% level in rural areas. The sign, as hypothesized, is negative. The variables measuring the average level of education in the community are also generally insignificant. One surprising result is the negative, significant coefficient on illiteracy in the urban areas. This could be related to multicolinearity. The measure of distance to the nearest secondary school is positive and significant in the rural equation. The rest of the measures are generally insignificant.

Based on the results of the F tests reported at the bottom of the table, the instrument set is jointly significant for the regression on the full sample as well as for each of the rural and urban areas. Further, the public service and housing variables are also jointly significant in each of the regressions. The group of personal health service variables is much weaker and is significant at the 11% level only for the full sample. The educational capital variables are also weak, although they are jointly significant at the 4% level for the full sample.

The coefficients on the control variables support the descriptive results presented in the first section. Education, and especially age, are also important determinants of menarche. Coincident with the descriptive results, menarche decreases with level of education and occurs earlier among younger cohorts. It is somewhat challenging to interpret the role of the education variable given that menarche and secondary school are likely to be coincident. It is probable that this variable is measuring issues related to the educational capital of the family in which the women grew up. Further, the fact that all the education variables, at the level of both the woman and the community, are significant only in the urban areas may be related to differential migration. It is probable

that more educated women are more likely to move from rural to urban areas.

The age variable is presented using a quadratic specification in order to more closely approximate the specification used later in the wage equation. Although each of the terms in the quadratic specification is insignificant, the Wald tests of joint significance show that age is an important determinant of menarche. The linear specification (not presented in the table) suggests that an increase of 1 year in age is associated with an increase of 1 month in the age at menarche for the complete sample. The effect is larger and more significant in rural areas, reaching approximately 1.5 months per year. In urban areas, the effect is only 0.5 month.

The results for the control variables for ethnicity and residence also reinforce the descriptive results. Age at menarche is older in rural areas and older in the oversampled, poorer states.[14] The variable for distance to the nearest market is negative and significant, again suggesting that more urbanized areas have younger ages of menarche. Further, ease of contact with other populations and with a flow of goods and services may reflect both higher incomes and better access to health care services. Finally, the term for the missing values on the variable for the proportion of the population that does not speak Spanish is negative and significant. This is likely to re-

---

[14] The regressions on the determinants of menarche were repeated excluding the dummy for missing values of the variable for the population who do not speak Spanish. The variable for not speaking Spanish remains insignificant and negative, and the other variables in the regression show no significant change either in sign or in magnitude. The only notable impact is that the variable indicating missing values for distance to the nearest market becomes insignificant, which suggests some degree of multicollinearity between the indicators of missing values.

flect the fact that the information is missing for a few larger *municipios* that are registered in the NFPS as sites yet are registered with much larger populations in other sources.

The findings of this section underscore the importance of a variety of individual factors in explaining the evolution in age at menarche. There is a strong, positive association with the age of the women, rural residence, and living in a poorer state. This is likely to reflect the important improvements over time and with economic development of nutritional and health status. Further, the community-level variables have a significant overall effect on age at menarche. Still, personal health services show a negligible impact, and public services and housing are the dominant determinants.

WAGE REGRESSIONS

This section develops the empirical estimates of the impact of investment in the health and nutrition of women on wages by using variation in the age at menarche as a proxy for health and nutrition. Although previous sections of this paper developed arguments to support the existence of an important link between childhood and adolescent nutritional status, labor market productivity, and age at menarche, the functional form of the associations is not clear. There may be a linear relationship between wages and menarche, but it is also possible that this linkage involves returns to scale or is mediated by complementarity between health and education. Given this potentially nonlinear relationship, a variety of specifications of the menarche variable in the wage equation are explored in this section. In particular, the regressions are run using a linear, a logarithmic, a quadratic, and an interaction with education as different specifications for the menarche variable.

The results of the instrumental variable estimates of the impact of age at menarche on the wage equations for the full sample are given in Table 7. As a point of reference, the OLS result is given for the double-logarithmic specification and the menarche variable is insignificant.[15] This, contrasted with the significant results for the instrumental variable regressions, suggests the presence of downward attenuation bias due to errors of measurement.

The first column of the instrumental variable regressions refers to the double-logarithmic, the second column refers to the linear, and the third column refers to the quadratic specification of the functional relationship between menarche and wages. The fourth column presents the results including a linear term for menarche and an interaction term with years of education. The final column includes both a quadratic specification of the menarche variable and the education interaction term.

The effect of age at menarche, in both the double-logarithmic (column 1) and the semilogarithmic specifications (column 2), is negative and significant. The quadratic function (column 3) also shows an inverse relationship between menarche and wages. Further, the three functions give very similar results in terms of the marginal impact of menarche on wages. The coefficients in the semilogarithmic equation indicate that a decrease of one year in the age at menarche is associated with an increase of 26% in hourly wages. The results of the double-logarithmic specification suggest that a fall of 1% in menarche results in an increase of 3.54% in wages. This number is very similar to the coefficient for the linear specification in that a decline of 1 year in menarche is equivalent to a change of 7.63% at the mean age of menarche of 13.15 years, resulting in a wage increase of 24%. Further, the quadratic specification suggests that a change of 1 year in menarche is associated with a 23% difference in wages at the mean age at menarche.

The quadratic specification of the menarche variable gives especially interesting results. The coefficient on the linear term is negative and significant and that of the squared terms is positive and significant. This suggests some nonlinearity in the variable and that the gains to investments in childhood nutrition and health have a greater payoff at higher levels of nutritional status. In other words, the impact on wages is more pronounced at younger ages of menarche that correspond to healthier, better nourished women. The function reaches a minimum between ages 13 and 14 and demonstrates a range with a positive slope between ages 14 and 17.

The finding of higher returns among healthier and better nourished women contrasts with previous work and must be interpreted with caution. Strauss (1986), for example, evaluated the impact of health on productivity in Sierra Leone and found decreasing returns to scale using calories as a measure of health. Further, the low explanatory power of the instruments, the lack of previous research using age at menarche, and the nature of the survey and its sample used in this research suggest the need to be careful in interpreting the result of increasing returns. Still, the finding does suggest many interesting hypotheses for further study. First, it is possible that menarche is a variable that is very nonlinear in terms of

---

[15] Other OLS regressions were also run, but they are not reported. The relationship between menarche and wages is negative and significant in a simple OLS regression with no other control variables. Adding education and experience to the human capital equation reduces the impact of menarche and renders the coefficient statistically insignificant.

TABLE 7. Wage functions[a] with various specifications of the menarche variable estimated by instrumental variables;[b] sample, women ages 18 to 54, menarche between ages 10 to 17 (absolute value of *t* in parentheses).

Independent variables	OLS	Instrumental variable				
		(1)	(2)	(3)	(4)	(5)
Menarche (estimated by instrumental variables)						
ln(menarche)	0.089	−3.524				
	(0.56)	(2.44)				
Menarche			−0.261	−7.258	−0.569	−6.688
			(2.35)	(2.26)	(2.31)	(2.01)
Menarche squared				0.266		0.240
				(2.18)		(1.84)
(Menarche) × (years of education)					0.047	0.019
					(1.44)	(0.49)
Other human capital variables						
Education in years	0.135	0.130	0.131	0.117	−0.484	−0.127
	(29.51)	(24.50)	(25.06)	(13.04)	(1.13)	(0.26)
Experience (age − education in years − 6) (×10)	0.34	0.375	0.375	0.363	0.336	0.349
	(6.60)	(6.41)	(6.41)	(5.18)	(5.06)	(4.78)
Experience^2 (×1,000)	−0.414	−0.438	−0.435	−0.503	−0.324	−0.452
	(3.44)	(3.34)	(3.33)	(3.25)	(1.97)	(2.46)
Control for ethnicity and residence						
% of population in *localidad* who do not speak Spanish	−0.527	−0.503	−0.498	−0.655	−0.546	−0.659
	(2.24)	(2.11)	(2.09)	(2.45)	(2.23)	(2.51)
Dummy for missing values (1 = missing values)[c]	−0.033	−0.164	−0.165	−0.007	−0.060	0.020
	(0.24)	(1.09)	(1.09)	(0.04)	(0.35)	(0.10)
Altitude (km above sea level)	0.012	−0.013	−0.013	−0.012	−0.003	−0.008
	(0.72)	(0.79)	(0.79)	(0.68)	(0.14)	(0.42)
Dummy for missing values (1 = missing values)[c]	0.077	−0.098	−0.091	−0.107	−0.151	−0.130
	(0.46)	(0.53)	(0.49)	(0.47)	(0.79)	(0.57)
Dummy rural–urban (rural = 1)	−0.025	0.062	0.061	0.007	0.064	0.014
	(0.56)	(1.06)	(1.03)	(0.10)	(1.05)	(0.19)
Dummy oversampled states (oversampled = 1)[d]	−0.132	−0.038	−0.041	−0.046	−0.046	−0.047
	(2.56)	(0.57)	(0.62)	(0.54)	(0.69)	(0.59)
Distance (km) to most common market (urban = 0) (×100)	0.026	−0.020	−0.030	0.259	−0.105	0.200
	(0.17)	(0.12)	(0.17)	(1.13)	(0.57)	(0.77)
Dummy distance to market missing (1 = missing values)[c]	−0.163	−0.145	−0.140	−0.300	−0.267	−0.335
	(0.75)	(0.65)	(0.62)	(1.21)	(1.07)	(1.33)
Constant	0.021	9.170	3.546	49.147	7.599	46.251
	(0.05)	(2.51)	(2.53)	(2.35)	(2.36)	(2.18)
n = 3,155						
R^2	0.26					
F statistic	99.61	83.12	84.22	51.29	73.41	53.81
Hausman test		6.714	6.177	5.648	7.242	9.503
[$P > \chi^2$, degrees of freedom (df)]		(0.01, 1)	(0.01, 1)	(0.01, 2)	(0.03, 2)	(0.001, 3)
Overidentification test		33.37	33.92	34.51	32.65	23.58
($P > \chi^2$, df = 13)		(0.00)	(0.00)	(0.00)	(0.00)	(0.04)

F test for joint significance of instruments using sample of positive wage earnings: 3.77 ($P > F = 0.00$, df = 13)

[a]Standard errors are calculated using robust (Huber, White, Sandwich) estimator of variance provided with STATA. There is no correction for sample selection as the inverse Mills ratio is insignificant using available identifying variables. Hourly positive wages of salaried and unsalaried workers using weekly wages as the base.

[b]The instrumental variables are % of population in municipality with earth floor in their homes and distance to the nearest nonprivate health center. % of population without running water, % of population over age 15 with incomplete primary education, % of population over age 15 who are illiterate, distance (km) to nearest nonprivate health center (urban = 0 km), dummy distance to health center missing (1 = missing values), number of physicians in *localidad* or municipality, dummy for the presence of a community health center in *localidad*, distance (km) to nearest secondary school (urban = 0), dummy distance to school missing (1 = missing values), dummy for no secondary school in the *localidad*, controls for ethnicity and residence, % of population in *localidad* who do not speak Spanish, dummy for missing values (1 = missing value), altitude (km above sea level), dummy for missing values (1 = missing value), dummy rural–urban (rural = 1), distance (km) to most common market (urban = 0), dummy distance to market missing (1 = missing values), dummy oversampled states (oversampled = 1). Dummies for missing values are included for distance to nearest health clinic and for distance to nearest secondary school.

[c]Applies only to rural areas because distance is assumed to be 0 for urban areas.

[d]Oversampled states are Chiapas, Estado de México, Guanajuato, Guerrero, Hidalgo, Michoacán, Oaxaca, Puebla, and Veracruz.

the investment in health and nutrition required to gain a reduction at younger ages. Specifically, it may be the case that a small investment in health or nutrition results in a reduction from age 17 to age 16 but that further reductions around the age of 13 are related to much greater investment in nutritional and health status. Further, it may be that the earlier gains are related to genetic or other factors not well measured in the model. It is also possible that labor market productivity gains related to investment and nutrition are associated with a higher payoff at the upper end of the productivity distribution. Finally, the cross-sectional nature of the data may drive part of the results in the quadratic specification, suggesting that longitudinal data will be needed to develop a stronger explanation of nonlinearities in the health, nutrition, labor market productivity nexus.

The last two specifications of the wage function include the interaction of age at menarche with years of schooling. The instrument set remains the same, and the linear term on years of education is treated as exogenous, whereas the menarche variable and the interaction term are treated as endogenous. The interaction term is added under the hypothesis that improvements in nutrition and health may operate through the individual's capacity to obtain educational capital (Mook and Leslie, 1986). The results of introducing this term are much weaker (Table 7, columns 4 and 5). The menarche variable retains its negative sign and significance in both the semilogarithmic (column 4) and the quadratic specifications (column 5). The magnitude of the coefficient increases with the addition of the interaction term in the semilogarithmic case, yet the coefficients for the quadratic are similar to column 3 without the interaction term. The coefficients on the interaction term are insignificant. Further, the coefficient on the exogenous, years of education variable becomes insignificant. These results may reflect the need to endogenize both education and menarche as well as to use additional variables to measure health inputs. Neither of these techniques is feasible with the existing data set.

The results for the other variables in the regressions are consistent with human capital theory. The experience terms display increasing returns to scale in all the regressions. The returns to education vary between 12% and 13%. The insignificance of the rural and of the oversampled state dummies is surprising given the results of the first stage of the regression. Still, this may be due to differential rural-to-urban migration or to the special characteristics of the sample of the NFPS. When the regressions are repeated on the urban and rural samples separately, the impact of menarche is stronger for the urban areas. Given that the urban areas and the more urbanized states are underrepresented in the sample, it is possible that these types of differences are understated. It is also possible that the other independent variables explain a large part of the rural-urban differences in wages.

The Hausman tests are generally significant and reject the hypothesis of exogeneity. This is a particularly strong finding given that Hausman tests may be indecisive if the OLS estimates are imprecise or if the instrumental variables do not explain a significant portion of the variance in the endogenous variable of interest (Staiger and Stock, 1997). Still, the overidentification tests reject the equality of coefficients, which suggests some misspecification of the instrumental variables.

Although the set of instruments is jointly significant even for the restricted sample of positive wage earners, it is important to highlight the limitations of these variables. First, the explanatory power of the overall regression is very low. Although this is not unusual in estimates of health production functions (see, for example, Schultz and Tansel, 1997), it is worrisome. Recent studies on the validity of instrumental variable estimation with weak instruments suggest that results may be biased (Bound et al., 1995). Further, the available instruments for this study are all indicators of community-level factors and refer to current conditions. In the absence of information on migratory histories, it is impossible to analyze how closely these are correlated with the conditions in the place and at the time when the women were growing up. Given these considerations, the robustness of the findings is tested by repeating the analysis with a variety of instrument sets including state-level fixed effects by including information on the mother for a subset of the women under study and by restricting the sample to younger cohorts. The results of these robustness tests are summarized below.

The sign of the menarche variable is quite robust to varying the instrument set, although the magnitude of the impact of menarche on wages increases when the number of instruments is reduced. These results are presented for the double-logarithmic specification in Table 8. Further, the differences in the strength and magnitude of the coefficient underscore the unimportance of the personal health service variables (line 3) and the contrasting strength of the public service and housing variables (line 2) as determinants of age at menarche. These results coincide with the findings from the estimates of the health production function presented in the previous section. If the instruments are limited to the four public service and housing variables (line 2), the effect of a 1% increase in age at menarche increases to 6.36%. The effect is 6.53% if only type of flooring and drainage facilities are used as instruments (line 5). If personal health services and educational capital are included, the effect is 4.76% (line 10).

TABLE 8. Impact of a 1% increase in age at menarche on hourly wages with varying instrument set.[a]

Instrument set	Coefficient of menarche (logarithmic specification)[a]	t statistic for the coefficient
1. Complete set	−3.52	−2.44
2. Public services and housing quality (including all four instruments)	−6.36	−3.25
3. Personal health services (including all three instruments)	−1.68	−0.36
4. Education level and educational services (including all four instruments)	−5.63	−2.53
5. Public services and housing quality (including only flooring and drainage)	−6.53	−3.17
6. Public services and housing quality (including only flooring)	−8.42	−3.33
7. Public services and housing quality (including only drainage)	−4.65	−2.18
8. Public services and housing quality (including all four instruments) and education level and educational services (including all four instruments)	−3.75	−2.50
9. Public services and housing quality (including all four instruments) and personal health services (including all three instruments)	−5.61	−3.16
10. Personal health (including all three instruments), education level and educational services (including all four instruments)	−4.67	−2.35

[a]The model is identical to column 2 of the instrumental variable estimates presented in Table 7 with the exception of the variation in the instrument set. The dependent variable is the natural logarithm of hourly wages. Menarche is also presented as the natural logarithm.

The results of the quadratic specification are also robust to varying the instrument set, although they are much more sensitive than in the case of the linear or logarithmic specification. Specifically, the coefficients lose individual significance with the exclusion of a large number of the instruments. They are robust in terms of significance and magnitude to the exclusion of any part of the instrument set other than the educational access and capital variables as well as to dividing the sample between the rural and urban areas.

The robustness of the instrumental variable wage equation was also tested by adding a full set of state dummies to the equations (Table 9). This latter specification provides a test for the validity of the instrumental variable instruments. Although the full set of dummies absorbs a substantial degree of the geographic variation that is not attributable to the accessibility of health services and local levels of education, the coefficient on the menarche variable is stable in sign, magnitude, and significance.

To further test the strength of the model, both the analysis of the determinants of age at menarche and the wage equations were repeated for the sample of women who live with their mothers. For this small sample, it is possible to identify education of the mother and, for the further reduced sample of those whose mother is between 15 and 54 years old, her age at menarche. Although these are very select groups, the analysis provides additional insight into the importance of family-level genetic and socioeconomic determinants of age at menarche. The sign and significance of the menarche variable is robust to this respecification.[16]

The analysis was also repeated for the restricted sample of younger cohorts. This provides a strategy for testing the sensitivity of the results to issues related to differential migration. In particular, these regressions provide insight into the importance of using instruments based on current conditions at the community level, which are likely to differ from the situation experienced by the women under study when they experienced childhood and adolescence. Further, given that the probability of migration increases over time, it is also more likely that younger cohorts reside in the place where they experienced puberty. The results of the wage regressions are very stable both to restricting the sample to women ages 44 and younger as well as to a further reduction to include only women between the ages of 18 and 30. The signs, magnitudes, and levels of significance of the impact of age at menarche on wages are similar to the results for the complete sample. This is true for all five specifications of the instrumental variable wage regression and for both age groups. Considering the quadratic specification, for example, the coefficients are −9.9 (t statistic = 2.4) and 0.36 (t statistic = 2.3) and −8.9 (t statistic = 2.5) and 0.33 (t statistic = 2.5) for women ages 18–44 and 18–30, respectively.

The findings of this section support the hypothesized relationship between investments in health and nutrition, measured through age at menarche, and labor market productivity. The finding of higher wages among women who are younger at menarche is robust to including a number of control variables as well as to changes in functional form and in the instrument set.

CONCLUSIONS

This paper proposes age at menarche as a factor that can be used to estimate labor market returns to childhood

---

[16] These results are available from the author.

TABLE 9. Wage function[a] with varying specifications of the menarche variable and including full set of state dummies,[b] estimated by instrumental variables;[c] sample, women ages 18–54, menarche between ages 10 and 17 (absolute value of *t* in parentheses).

Independent variables	OLS	Instrumental variable				
		(1)	(2)	(3)	(4)	(5)
Menarche (estimated by instrumental variables)						
ln(menarche) (restricted to 10–17)	0.116	−3.264				
	(0.73)	(1.57)				
Menarche			−0.238	−5.303	−0.632	−3.474
			(1.51)	(1.43)	(2.17)	(0.86)
Menarche squared				0.190		0.110
				(1.37)		(0.71)
Menarche and years of education					0.055	0.041
					(1.67)	(1.10)
Other human capital variables						
Education in years	0.132	0.128	0.129	0.119	−0.593	−0.414
	(28.09)	(22.12)	(22.91)	(12.39)	(1.38)	(0.86)
Out-of-school experience	0.035	0.038	0.038	0.038	0.034	0.035
	(6.86)	(6.54)	(6.56)	(5.78)	(5.00)	(5.13)
Experience² (×100)	−0.043	0.000	0.000	0.000	0.000	0.000
	(3.62)	(3.42)	(3.42)	(3.33)	(1.87)	(2.09)
Controls for ethnicity and residence						
% of population in *localidad* who do not speak Spanish	−0.423	−0.417	−0.414	−0.485	−0.478	−0.503
	(1.76)	(1.71)	(1.70)	(1.89)	(1.88)	(1.98)
Dummy for missing values (1 = missing value)[e]	−0.043	−0.167	−0.166	−0.070	−0.052	−0.025
	(0.32)	(1.02)	(1.01)	(0.35)	(0.28)	(0.13)
Altitude (km above sea level)	−0.027	−0.028	−0.028	−0.027	−0.012	−0.016
	(1.39)	(1.47)	(1.47)	(1.39)	(0.57)	(0.72)
Dummy for missing values (1 = missing value)[e]	−0.059	−0.188	−0.179	−0.269	−0.231	−0.270
	(0.34)	(0.97)	(0.93)	(1.16)	(1.15)	(1.23)
Dummy rural-urban (rural = 1)	−0.030	0.046	0.044	0.030	0.059	0.047
	(0.68)	(0.67)	(0.64)	(0.40)	(0.80)	(0.62)
Distance to most common market (km) (×100)	0.046	0.001	−0.007	0.193	−0.126	0.021
	(0.29)	(0.01)	(0.04)	(0.82)	(0.64)	(0.07)
Dummy distance to market missing (1 = missing value)[e]	−0.188	−0.172	−0.167	−0.296	−0.293	−0.335
	(0.86)	(0.77)	(0.75)	(1.24)	(1.16)	(1.36)
Constant	−0.164	8.450	3.189	36.623	8.372	26.466
	(0.39)	(1.59)	(1.58)	(1.50)	(2.20)	(1.02)
n = 3,155						
R²	0.2711					
F statistic	45.43	40.69	41.50	28.15	35.22	38.04
Hausman test		6.176	6.050	4.024	4.546	6.536
[$P > \chi^2$, degrees of freedom (df)]		(0.13, 1)	(0.01, 1)	(0.13, 2)	(0.10, 2)	(0.09, 3)
Overidentification tests		29.22	29.64	22.73	24.93	24.28
($P > \chi^2$, df = 13)		(0.01)	(0.01)	(0.05)	(0.02)	(0.03)

F test for joint significance of instruments using positive wage earners: 1.87 ($P > F = 0.0291$, df = 13)

[a]Standard errors are calculated using robust (Huber, White, Sandwich) estimator of variance provided with STATA. There is no correction for sample selection as the inverse Mills ratio is insignificant using available identifying variables.

[b]Individual state dummies are included but not reported.

[c]The instrumental variables are % of population in municipality with earth floor in their homes and distance to the nearest nonprivate health center. % of population without running water, % of population over age 15 with incomplete primary education, % of population over age 15 that is illiterate, distance (km) to nearest nonprivate health center (urban = 0 km), dummy distance to health center missing (1 = missing values), number of physicians in *localidad* or municipality, dummy for the presence of a community health center in *localidad*, distance (km) to nearest secondary school (urban = 0), dummy distance to school missing (1 = missing values), dummy for no secondary school in the *localidad*, controls for ethnicity and residence, % of population in *localidad* who do not speak Spanish, dummy for missing values (1 = missing value), altitude (km above sea level), dummy for missing values (1 = missing value), dummy rural-urban (rural = 1), distance (km) to most common market (urban = 0), dummy distance to market missing (1 = missing values), dummy oversampled states (oversampled = 1). Dummies for missing values are included for distance to nearest health clinic and for distance to nearest secondary school.

[d]Oversampled states are Chiapas, Estado de México, Guanajuato, Guerrero, Hidalgo, Michoacán, Oaxaca, Puebla, and Veracruz.

[e]Applies only to rural areas because the variable is assumed to be 0 for urban areas.

investments in health and nutrition. Measurement error, combined with simultaneity, however, suggests the need to use instrumental variable techniques when estimating such wage functions.

The retrospective recall data available for this study show that average age at menarche has been decreasing in Mexico over the past 40–50 years. The decline has been somewhat slower than in the developed world. Factors associated with this decline include urbanization, increased levels of education, and improved living conditions. In particular, variables that measure access to public services and the quality of housing appear to have an important impact. The proportion of the community with earth flooring in their homes and the proportion who lack toilet or drainage facilities are particularly strong correlates of menarche. Access to personal health services appears to have little marginal impact on the age at menarche.

The findings reported here suggest that nutrition and cumulative health status, measured by age at menarche, have a significant effect on the labor market productivity of Mexican women. Younger ages at menarche are associated with higher wages. The overall effect is masked in an OLS wage equation because of errors of recall, rounding by year, and misreporting of the variable. The instrumental, errors-in-variables model suggests that a decline of one year in age at menarche is associated with a wage increase of 23%–26%. This value is consistent using a double-logarithmic, semilogarithmic, or quadratic specification of the menarche variable. The results suggest the possibility of higher returns to some health investments among the healthier segments of the population. This finding deserves further research as it contrasts with the existing evidence that suggests that health has a larger return at lower levels of health and that the importance of health investments as inputs into labor productivity will decline with economic development (Strauss and Thomas, 1998).

Future research should use other data sets to include other human capital inputs. It will also be interesting to broaden the conceptualization of female health by considering additional measures of health and nutrition. These should be compared and combined with age at menarche. Further, it will be important to include additional information on the origin and migration patterns of the women in order to better identify the impact of health, education, and other public services as well as poverty and living conditions during infancy and childhood on health outcomes.

The results of this paper lend support to the importance of investing in health and early nutrition, particularly through sanitation and housing conditions, in order to improve individual and family well-being and to reduce poverty. Health has an important, independent effect as an investment in human capital in addition to education. Further, the findings suggest that, for the purposes of economic analysis, age at menarche should be considered a complement to adult height as a measure of secular changes in the health and nutritional condition of women.

REFERENCES

Amann GM. Sexual socialization during early adolescence: the menarche. *Adolescence*. 1986; 21(83):703–710.

Avila A. La desnutrición infantil en el medio rural. *Salud Pública de México*. 1998; 40:150–160.

Barro R. *Economic Growth*. New York: McGraw Hill; 1995.

Bean JA, Leeper JD, Wallace PB. Variations in the reporting of menstrual histories. *American Journal of Epidemiology*. 1979; 109(2):181–185.

Becker GS. *Human Capital*. Chicago: University of Chicago Press; 1993.

Bergsten BA. A note on the accuracy of recalled age at menarche. *Annals of Human Biology*. 1976; 3(1):71–73.

Bielicki T, Waliszho A, Hulanicka B. Social-class gradients in menarcheal age in Poland. *Annals of Human Biology*. 1986; 13(1): 1–11.

Bobadilla JL, Frenk J, Lozano R. The epidemiologic transition and health priorities. In: Jamison D. (ed.) *Disease Control Priorities in Developing Countries*. Oxford: Oxford University Press for the World Bank; 1993.

Bojlén K, Weis BM. Seasonal variation in the occurrence of menarche in Copenhagen girls. *Human Biology*. 1971; 43(4):493–501.

Bound J, Jaeger D, Baker R. Problems with instrumental variables estimation when the correlation between the instruments and the endogenous explanatory variable is weak. *Journal of the American Statistical Association*. 1995; 90(430):443–450.

Brundtland G, Walloe L. Menarchal age in Norway: halt in the trend towards earlier maturation. *Nature*. 1973; 241:478–479.

Cravioto P, Cravioto J, Bravo G. Age of menarche in a rural population: accuracy of records four years later. *Boletín Médico del Hospital Infantil de México*. 1987; 44(10):589–593.

Cumming DC. Menarche, menses and menopause: a brief review. *Cleveland Clinical Journal of Medicine*. 1990; 57(2):169–175.

Delgado HL, Hurtado E. Physical growth and menarche in Guatemalan adolescents. *Archives Latinoamerican of Nutrition*. 1990; 40(4):503–517.

Díaz de Mathman C, Ramos GR, Landa RV. Crecimiento y desarrollo en adolescentes femeninos: edad de la menarquía. *Boletín Médico del Hospital Infantil de México*. 1968a; 25:787–793.

Díaz de Mathman C, Ramos GR, Landa RV. Crecimiento y desarrollo en adolescentes femeninos: menarquía y crecimiento. *Boletín Médico del Hospital Infantil de México*. 1968b; 25:795–802.

Dreizen S, Spirakis CN, Stone RE. A comparison of skeletal growth and maturation in undernourished and well-nourished girls before and after menarche. *Journal of Pediatrics*. 1967; 70:256.

Eveleth P. Population differences in growth: environmental and genetic factors. In: Falkner F, Tanner JM, eds. *Human Growth: A Comprehensive Treatise*, Vol. 2. New York: Plenum Press; 1978.

Floud R. The heights of Europeans since 1750: a new source for European economic history. In: Komlos J, ed. *Stature, Living Standards, and Economic Development: Essays in Anthropometric History*. Chicago: The University of Chicago Press; 1994.

Fogel RW. Economic growth, population theory and physiology. *American Economic Review*. 1994; 84(3):369–395.

Food and Agriculture Organization of the United Nations. *The State of Food and Agriculture*. Rome: Food and Agriculture Organization of the United Nations; 1996.

Frenk J. Reformar sin deformar: la necesidad de una visión integral en la transformación del sistema de salud mexicano. In: Frenk J, ed. *Observatorio de la salud: necesidades, servicios y políticas*. México, DF: Fundación Mexicana para la Salud; 1997.

Frenk J, Bobadilla JL, Sepúlveda J. Health transition in middle-income countries: new challenges for health care. *Health Policy and Planning*. 1989; 4(1).

Frenk J, González-Block MA, Lozano R. *Economía y salud: propuestas para el avance del sistema de salud en México. Informe final*. México, DF: Fundación Mexicana para la Salud; 1994b.

Frenk J, Lozano R, Bobadilla JL. La transición epidemiológica en América Latina. *Notas de Población*, Santiago de Chile. 1994c; XXII(60).

Frenk J, Duran-Arenas I, Vázquez-Segovia A. Los médicos en México, 1970–1990. *Salud Pública de México*. 1995; 37:19–30.

Frenk J, Knaul F, Vázquez-Segovia A. *Trends in Medical Employment: Persistent Imbalances in Urban México*. México, DF: Centro de Investigación y Docencia Económicas; 1997.

Frisch R, Revelle R. Height and weight at menarche and a hypothesis of critical body weights and adolescent events. *Science*. 1970; 169:397–398.

Graber J, Brooks-Gunn J, Warren J. The antecedents of menarcheal age: heredity, family environment and stressful life events. *Child Development*. 1995; 66:346–359.

Greene WH. *Econometric Analysis*. Englewood Cliffs, NJ: Prentice Hall, 1997.

Griliches Z. Estimating the return to schooling: a progress report. *Econometrica*. 1977; 45(1):1–22.

Hausman JA. Specification tests in econometrics. *Econometrica*. 1978; 46(6):1251–1272.

Heckman JJ. Sample selection bias as a specification error. *Econometrica*. 1979; 47(1):153–162.

Hediger ML, Stine RA. Age at menarche based on recall information. *Annals of Human Biology*. 1987; 14(2):133–142.

Hulanicka B, Waliszko A. Deceleration of age at menarche in Poland. *Annals of Human Biology*. 1991; 18(6):507–513.

Instituto Nacional de Estadística, Geografía e Informática (INEGI). *Anuarios Estadísticos Estatales, 1995*. México, DF: INEGI; 1995.

Jacobo M, Malacara JM. Correlation of menarche with age and various somatometric indexes. *Boletín Médico del Hospital Infantil de México*. 1985; 42(1): 37–41.

Knaul F, Parker S, Ramírez R. El prepago por servicios médicos privados en México: determinantes socio-económicos y cambios a través del tiempo. In: Frenk J, ed. *Observatorio de la salud: necesidades, servicios y políticas*. México, DF: Fundación Mexicana para la Salud; 1997.

Komlos J. The age at menarche and age at first birth in an undernourished population. *Annals of Human Biology*. 1989; 16(5):559–562.

Laska-Mierzejewska T. Effect of ecological and socio-economic factors on the age at menarche, body height and weight of rural girls in Poland. *Human Biology*. 1970; 42(2):284–292.

Leibenstein H. *Economic Backwardness and Economic Growth: Studies in the Theory of Economic Development*. New York: Wiley and Sons; 1957.

Liestøl K. Social conditions and menarcheal age: the importance of early years of life. *Annals of Human Biology*. 1982; 9(6):521–537.

Liestøl K, Rosenberg M. Height, weight and menarcheal age of schoolgirls in Oslo. An update. *Annals of Human Biology*. 1995; 22(3):199–205.

Maclure M. A prospective cohort study of nutrient intake and age at menarche. *American Journal of Clinical Nutrition*. 1991; 54(4): 649–656.

Malcolm L. Protein-energy malnutrition and growth. In: Falkner F, Tanner JM, eds. *Human Growth: A Comprehensive Treatise*, Vol. 2. New York: Plenum Press; 1978.

Manniche E. Age at menarche: Nicolai Edvard Ravn's data on 3385 women in mid-19th century Denmark. *Annals of Human Biology*. 1983; 10(1):79–82.

Marshall WA. Puberty. In: Falkner F, Tanner JM, eds. *Human Growth: A Comprehensive Treatise*, Vol. 2. New York: Plenum Press; 1978.

Mascie, Taylor CGN, Boldsen JL. Recalled age of menarche in Britain. *Annals of Human Biology*. 1986; 13(3):253–257.

Mincer J. *Schooling, Experience and Earnings*. New York: Columbia University Press; 1974.

Moisan J, Meyer F, Gingras S. A nested case control study of the correlates of early menarche. *American Journal of Epidemiology*. 1990; 132(5):953–961.

Moock P, Leslie J. Childhood malnutrition and schooling in the Terai region of Nepal. *Journal of Development Economics*. 1986; 20:33–52.

Nagata H, Sakamoto Y. A comparison of height growth curves among girls with different ages of menarche. *Human Biology*. 1988; 60(1):33–41.

Rosenzweig M. Labor markets in low income countries. In: Chenery H, Srinivasan TN, eds. *Handbook of Development Economics*, Vol.1. Amsterdam: North-Holland Press; 1988.

Ruble D, Brooks-Gunn J. The experience of menarche. *Child Development*. 1982; 53:1557–1566.

Salud Pública de México. Aspectos relevantes sobre la estadística de deficiencias de la nutrición. *Salud Pública de México*. 1998; 40(2):206–215.

Schultz TP. Lifetime migration within educational strata. *Economic Development and Cultural Change*. 1982; 30(3):559–593.

Schultz TP. *Wage Rentals for Reproducible Human Capital: Evidence from Two West African Countries*. Working Draft; New Haven: Yale University, mimeo; 1996.

Schultz TP. Assessing the productive benefits of nutrition and health: an integrated human capital approach. *Journal of Econometrics*. 1997; 77(1):141–158.

Schultz TP, Tansel A. Wage and labor supply effects of illness in Côte d' Ivoire and Ghana: instrumental variable estimates for days disabled. *Journal of Development Economics*. 1997; 53(2):251–286.

Secretaría de Salud. *Encuesta nacional de salud II*. México, DF: Secretaría de Salud; 1994.

Staiger D, Stock J. Instrumental variables regression with weak instruments. *Econometrica*. 1997; 65(3):557–586.

Stark O, Peckham CS, Moynihan C. Weight and age at menarche. *Archives of Disease in Childhood*. 1989; 64(3): 383–387.

Steckel RH. Stature and the standard of living. *Journal of Economic Literature*. 1995; 33(4):1903–1940.

Strauss J. Does better nutrition raise farm productivity? *Journal of Political Economy*. 1986; 94(2):297–320.

Strauss J, Thomas D. Health and wages: evidence on men and women in urban Brazil. *Journal of Econometrics*. 1997; 77(1):159–186.

Strauss J, Thomas D. Health, nutrition and economic development. *Journal of Economic Literature*. 1998; 36(2):766–817.

Tanner JM. *Growth at Adolescence*. Oxford: Blackwell Scientific Publications; 1962.

Treloar SA, Martin NG. Age at menarche as a fitness trait: nonadditive genetic variance detected in a large twin sample. *American Journal of Human Genetics*. 1990; 47(1):137–148.

Trussel J, Steckel R. The age of slaves at menarche and their first birth. *Journal of Interdisciplinary History*. 1978; 8(3):477–505.

Ulijaszek SJ, Evans E, Miller DS. Age at menarche of European, Afro-Caribbean and Indo-Pakistani schoolgirls living in London. *Annals of Human Biology*. 1991; 18(2):167–175.

Valenzuela CY, Nuñez E, Tapia C. Month at menarche: a re-evaluation of the seasonal hypothesis. *Annals of Human Biology*. 1991; 18(5):383–393.

Weir J, Dunn JE, Jones EG. Race and age at menarche. *Communications in Brief*. 1971; 111(4):594–596.

Wellens R, Malina RM, Beunen G. Age at menarche in Flemish girls: current status and secular change in the 20th century. *Annals of Human Biology*. 1990; 17(2):145–152.

White H. A heteroskedasticity-consistent covariance matrix estimator and a direct test for heteroskedasticity. *Econometrica*. 1980; 48: 817–838.

Wong R, Parker S, de la Vega S. *Household Health Expenditures in Mexico: The Influence of the Local Health Sector*. Presented at the Annual Meeting of the Population Association of America; Washington, DC, March 1997.

World Bank. *Investment in Health, World Development Report*. Washington, DC: World Bank; 1993.

Wyshak G, Frisch R. Evidence for a secular trend in age of menarche. *New England Journal of Medicine*. 1982; 306(17):1033–1035.

Wyshak G. Secular changes in age at menarche in a sample of US women. *Annals of Human Biology*. 1983; 10(1):75–77.

Zurita B, Nigenda G, Ramírez T. Encuesta de satisfacción con los servicios de salud 1994. In: Frenk J, ed. *Observatorio de la salud: necesidades, servicios y políticas*. México, DF: Fundación Mexicana para la Salud; 1997.

ANNEX

TABLE 1A. Differences between women included in the individual questionnaire and those not interviewed.

Variable	Included	Excluded
Age		
Mean	31.91	30.18
Median	30	27
Observed	11,058	1,392
Groups		
18–24	3,246	564
25–35	3,615	389
35–44	2,604	244
45–54	1,588	195
Education		
Mean	5.80	6.57
Median	6	6
Observed	11,049	1,374
Labor force participation		
Mean	0.29	0.37
Observed	11,058	1,392
Weekly wages		
Mean	263.47	265.31
Median	140	175
Observed	3,273	535

TABLE 2A. Wage functions[1] with sample selection correction for labor force participation. Log menarche estimated with instrumental variables;[2] sample, women ages 18–54, menarche between ages 10 and 17 (absolute value of z in parentheses).

Independent variables	Probit for labor force participation	OLS wage function[5]	Instrumental variable wage function
Menarche			
ln(menarche)	0.162	0.080	–3.639
	(1.25)	(0.50)	(2.53)
Other human capital variables			
Experience (age – years of education – 6)	0.039	0.030	0.037
	(8.79)	(3.19)	(3.51)
Experience squared (×100)	–0.046	–0.035	–0.042
	(4.91)	(2.43)	(2.56)
Education in years	0.084	0.127	0.132
	(16.92)	(6.73)	(6.46)
Controls for ethnicity and residence			
% of population in *localidad* who do not speak Spanish	–0.359	–0.446	–0.480
	(3.23)	(2.27)	(1.86)
Dummy for missing values (1 = missing value)[3]	0.375	–0.087	–0.173
	(3.41)	(0.56)	(1.00)
Altitude (km above sea level)	0.012	–0.015	–0.015
	(1.20)	(1.26)	(0.92)
Dummy for missing values (1 = missing value)[3]	0.123	0.099	–0.077
	(1.09)	(0.64)	(0.41)
Dummy rural-urban (rural = 1)	–0.277	–0.003	0.050
	(7.55)	(0.04)	(0.58)
Dummy oversampled states (oversampled = 1)[4]	0.134	–0.145	–0.033
	(2.77)	(2.17)	(0.43)
Distance (km) to most common market (urban = 0) (×100)	–0.142	0.075	0.024
	(1.27)	(0.49)	(0.14)
Dummy distance to market missing (1 = missing values)[2]	–0.668	–0.095	–0.157
	(4.80)	(0.38)	(0.56)
Identification of labor force participation			
If house has interior sewage connection (sewage = 1)	0.039		
	(1.14)		
Number of bedrooms per family member	0.304		
	(4.52)		
If house has own kitchen (kitchen = 1)	–0.119		
	(2.79)		
If house has interior running water (water = 1)	–0.058		
	(1.76)		
Inverse Mills ratio[5]		–0.129	0.032
		(0.43)	(0.10)
Constant	–1.950	0.294	9.409
	(5.71)	(0.39)	(2.62)
F statistic	848.81	83.70	33.82
[$P > F$, degrees of freedom (df)] (values for χ^2 given for probit model)	(0.00, 16)	(0.00, 13)	(0.00, 13)
R^2	0.26		
n	10,774	3,133	3,133
Hausman statistic: $H = 7.22$, df = 1, $P > \chi^2 = 0.01$			

[1]Standard errors are calculated using robust (Huber, White, Sandwich) estimator of variance provided with STATA. Hourly positive wages of all salaried and unsalaried workers, using weekly hours and wages as the base and dividing by weekly hours.

[2]The instrumental variables are % of population with earth floor, % of population without toilet or drainage facilities, % of population living in overcrowded conditions, % of population without running water, % of population over age 15 with incomplete primary education, % of population over age 15 who are illiterate, distance (km) to nearest nonprivate health center (urban = 0 km), dummy distance to health center missing (1 = missing values, rural), number of physicians in *localidad* or municipality, dummy for the presence of a community health center in *localidad*, distance (km) to nearest secondary school (urban = 0), dummy distance to school missing (1 = missing, rural), dummy for no secondary school in the *localidad*, controls for ethnicity and residence, % of population in *localidad* who do not speak Spanish, dummy for missing values (1 = missing value, rural), altitude (meters above sea level), dummy for missing values (1 = missing value, rural), dummy rural–urban (rural = 1), distance (km) to most common market (urban = 0), dummy distance to market missing (1 = missing values, rural), dummy oversampled states (oversampled = 1). Dummies for missing values are included for distance to nearest health clinic and for distance to nearest secondary school.

[3]Applies only to rural communities, because the variable is assumed to be 0 for urban areas.

[4]Oversampled states: Chiapas, Estado de México, Guanajuato, Guerrero, Hidalgo, Michoacán, Oaxaca, Puebla, and Veracruz.

[5]The inverse Mills ratio is entered into the instrumental variable wage equation by a two-step procedure.

HEALTH AND PRODUCTIVITY IN PERU: AN EMPIRICAL ANALYSIS BY GENDER AND REGION[1]

Rafael Cortez[2]

INTRODUCTION

This study aims to measure the association between health and wages in Peru, in order to then explore the impact that health has on productivity. It also seeks to assess the consequences of omitting the variable health from the estimates of other variables included in the wage equation. Finally, it examines the impact that availability of public health care services has on productivity, all of the above based on the existence of a relationship of simultaneity between earnings and self-reported health status.

In the study of economic growth and distribution of wealth, increasing importance is being attached to human capital factors as determinants of economic growth and wage rates. However, only recently have the returns on investment in health begun to be studied in developing countries. Recent studies (Schultz, 1997; Schultz and Tansel, 1997; Thomas and Strauss, 1997) confirm the idea that health is a form of human capital that influences wage levels and, therefore, the capacity of individuals to generate sustained and rising income over time, with immediate positive consequences on the level of expenditure and living standard of their household members.

The earliest studies that associated health with productivity were carried out in the framework of the efficiency wage hypothesis (Pitt, Rosenzwei, and Hassan, 1990; Behrman and Deolaliker, 1988; Sahn and Alderman, 1988). These were the first studies that looked at developing countries and linked nutrition with productivity.

Recently, literature on economics has placed greater emphasis on the measurement of health status through the use of indicators included in household surveys. These health indicators include adult height data, reported morbidity rates, days disabled, and days ill. These variables are subject to measurement errors, given the biases that result from self-reporting. Such biases are obviously correlated with the educational level of the respondent, household income, and other unobserved variables.

The inclusion of the health indicator in the wage equation represents an attempt to measure the returns to health in the labor market and, at the same time, facilitate the evaluation of the effects that public investment policies have on health status and, consequently, on income. Within this analytical framework, Thomas and Strauss (1997) used the results of the Brazilian household survey, which contains information on adult height. The authors conclude that greater height has a positive effect on individual productivity. Another interesting finding from their study is that, when the health variable was included, the estimated returns to education were 45% lower for men with no education and 30% lower for men with secondary or higher education.

Schultz and Tansel (1997) used instrumental variable estimates for days of disability to estimate wage equations in Ghana and Côte d'Ivoire. Their principal finding was that health status is an explanatory factor in wage level and that better health status also is associated with longer productive life.

This study estimated the effects of health on productivity in Peru. For that purpose, a health indicator based on days of illness reported by adults in the 15 days prior

[1] This study was conducted as part of the Latin American Research Network project "Productivity of Household Investment in Health," sponsored by the Inter-American Development Bank (IDB). The author is grateful for the contribution of César Calvo, who assisted in the research, and for the valuable comments of Dr. Paul Schultz of Yale University, Dr. Bill Savedoff of IDB, and all the participants in the seminar "Impact of Public and Private Investment in Health on Productivity." The author alone is responsible for any errors or omissions.

[2] Professor and investigator at Centro de Investigación de la Universidad del Pacífico and Post-doctoral Fellow of the Economic Growth Center of the Economics Department of Yale University.

to the interview was used. The data for the study were derived from Peru's 1995 National Household Survey.

First, the wage functions for adults by sex and geographic area (rural and urban) were estimated, with the health variable instrumented as one of the human capital variables. Second, the study analyzed the impact that public investment in health has on wages. The estimation process corrected for the selection bias and controlled for endogeneity and measurement error in the health status indicator. The health variable equation used a set of identifiers such as health infrastructure (number of health care facilities per capita), housing infrastructure (hours of water supply, availability of adequate sewerage, and type of flooring in the housing unit), and price of health inputs, which directly affect health but do not directly influence the determination of wages.

Given the nature of the indicator, the health equation was estimated using a tobit model censored at zero. The instruments used were robust, and an inverse relationship was found between age and health status, which is consistent with the fact that morbidity rates and number of days ill generally rise with age. Access to adequate housing infrastructure had a positive effect on health; conversely, low living standards at the community level have a negative effect on individual health status for community residents. In rural areas, non-labor income levels were not significant.

The wage equation was estimated using a two-stage procedure (Heckman, 1979; Lee, 1983) and corrected for the selection bias resulting from the inclusion of non-participants in the labor market. The wage equations showed that the rate of return to education was overestimated if the health variable was omitted and that the difference was greater for the female population than for the male population in urban areas. The difference in rates of return (wage equation without health versus wage equation with health [IV]) was 9.5% and 1.3% for urban and rural men, respectively, and 15.7% and 1.3% for urban and rural women, respectively. The results clearly show the positive effect of health on productivity; the coefficients were significant and indicated that the impact of more healthy days on wages was greater in rural populations than in urban ones.

Section 2 describes the database for the study—the 1995 Peruvian National Household Survey—which includes demographic, social, economic, and health information on 98,984 individuals in 19,975 households. It also presents a brief overview of the health and well-being of the Peruvian population. Section 3 deals with how to measure health and correct for measurement error, and Section 4 is about the simultaneity between health and productivity. Section 5 describes the model of analysis, which is based on the conceptual framework suggested by

Becker (1965). Section 6 explains the econometric estimation model, which takes account of the relationship of simultaneity that exists between health and wages, the problem of omission of variables, and measurement error. Section 7 summarizes the empirical findings of the study, and Section 8 presents the conclusions and some policy recommendations.

BASIC DESCRIPTION OF THE DATABASE

The data for this study were drawn from Peru's 1995 National Household Survey (NHS), which included socioeconomic and demographic information on 19,975 households. The information was compiled between October and December of that year by the National Statistics and Informatics Institute (INEI). A total of 98,984 individuals were surveyed.[3]

Using information from the NHS, Table 1 provides a basic profile of health and poverty conditions in Peru. Because of the study's focus on the productive impact of health, the data in column 1 of the table relate only to persons aged from over 17 and under 70 years old—i.e., potential wage-earners. According to Table 1, 36.0% of this population lives in poverty, and 13.2% live in extreme poverty.[4]

Health status is measured on the basis of morbidity rates and average number of days ill (in the 15 days preceding the survey). The latter data are also illustrated in Figure 1. In both cases, Table 1 shows a negative correlation between poverty and health. Morbidity rates among the population living in extreme poverty (31.6%) are clearly higher than the rates in the non-poor population (25.9%). The average morbidity rate for the working-age population is 27.0%.

The association between higher poverty and poor health captures several effects of the interaction of the two variables and constitutes the subject of this study. Even as a first approximation to the problem, Table 1 reveals that poverty is also associated with lower rates of health service usage among ill individuals. The rate is markedly lower among the extremely poor (26.2%) compared to the non-poor (42.9%). Health service usage might partly explain the negative association between poverty and health.

Table 2 shows the important role that the public sector plays in providing health services. On average, 60.0% of the population that seeks medical attention in case of illness does so in a public health care facility. The percent-

---

[3] The population group analyzed in the study included 51,545 persons over 17 and under 70 years of age.
[4] The NHS yielded lower percentages of poverty for the population as a whole: 32.6% and 12.6%, respectively.

FIGURE 1. Distribution of days ill.

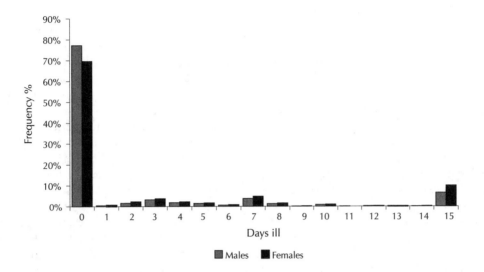

TABLE 1. Health conditions, health care, and poverty levels in Peru: population over 17 and under 70 years of age.

Poverty levels	Percentage of the population	Reported morbidity rate	Average number of days of reported illness	Health care rates
Non-poor	64.0%	25.9%	2.58	42.9%
Poor	22.8%	27.5%	2.74	32.8%
Extremely poor	13.2%	31.6%	2.88	26.2%
Total	–	27.0%	2.65	38.0%

Source: National Household Survey, Peru, 1995.
Table prepared by the author.

age is higher for the poor population (63.2%) and even higher for the population living in extreme poverty (66.0%). Hence, reliance on public health care services is greater among lower-income households. On the few occasions that these households do seek medical care, they receive a greater proportion of such care from ministry of health establishments.

In this context, public investment in health is essential to improve health conditions in the country. Presumably, poverty would also be alleviated by investing in health, if health leads to higher earnings and if it can be shown that health yields positive and substantial returns. Table 3

TABLE 2. Percentages of the total number of ill persons who receive medical attention at different health service providers, by poverty level in the population.

Health service provider	Total	Poverty levels		
		Non-poor	Poor	Extremely poor
Public providers	60.0	57.9	63.2	66.0
Ministry of Health post or center	26.3	22.5	31.1	38.7
Social security hospital	16.6	18.0	15.3	11.2
Ministry of Health hospital	12.6	12.4	12.9	13.3
Other	4.5	5.0	3.8	2.8
Private providers	40.0	42.1	36.8	34.0
Pharmacy	17.8	17.6	19.7	15.1
Private physician	9.9	11.5	7.7	4.8
Private clinic	4.1	4.9	2.7	2.6
Traditional healer	0.9	0.8	1.1	1.2
Other	7.3	6.3	5.6	10.3
Total	100.0	100.0	100.0	100.0

Source: National Household Survey, Peru, 1995.
Table prepared by the author.

TABLE 3. Relationship between self-reported health status and hourly wage.

Hourly wage quintiles	Morbidity rates (%)	
	Males	Females
1	29.0	35.1
2	21.4	29.5
3	20.4	28.0
4	21.4	25.7
5	19.3	28.3

Source: National Household Survey, 1995.
Table prepared by the author.

describes the relationship to be tested through the design and estimation of an explicit model: the association between health status and poverty (see Figure 2). The results of the NHS show a positive relationship between individual health status and productivity (measured by hourly wage).

The population in the highest hourly wage quintiles experiences the lowest rates of illness. Among males, the rate falls from 29.0% to 19.3% between the highest and lowest quintiles, while among women the difference between quintiles is less marked: 35.1% in the highest quintile versus 28.3% in the lowest (see Figure 2). The following sections use parametric methods to estimate the relationship between health and productivity. This approach affords the possibility of assessing the consequences of greater or lesser public investment in health (for a specific population group) and estimating the returns to health.

MEASURING HEALTH: SELF-REPORTED HEALTH STATUS AND MEASUREMENT ERROR

Measuring health is difficult for several reasons. Some indicators are not objective, some are associated with only one dimension of health, and some do not measure a complete range of conditions. By analyzing the measurement process, it is possible to pinpoint the main problems and devise methods for dealing with them. In particular, the model selected can correct for the problem of bias introduced by measurement errors and the loss of information due to downward censoring of the indicator.

Recent economic literature has used health indicators such as standardized anthropometric measures of height and/or weight (i.e., Rosenzweig and Schultz, 1983; Rosezweig and Wolpin, 1986; Barrera, 1990; Pitt, Rosenzweig, and Hassan, 1990; Schultz, 1996) and self-reported illness or disability (Wolfe and Behrman, 1984; Pitt and Rosenzweig, 1985; Schultz and Tansel, 1997). At a more aggregate level, average values of the foregoing variables have been used, as have mortality or survival rates (Rosenzweig and Schultz, 1982; Pitt, Rosenzweig, and Gibbons, 1995).

In comparison with other forms of human capital, health status is especially difficult to measure. Health status (H*) can be considered a latent variable that is not observable and that is approximated by imperfect indicators (H), such as days of illness, days during which the individual was unable to work due to illness, and others. When these indicators are obtained from household sur-

FIGURE 2. Reported morbidity rate by income level.

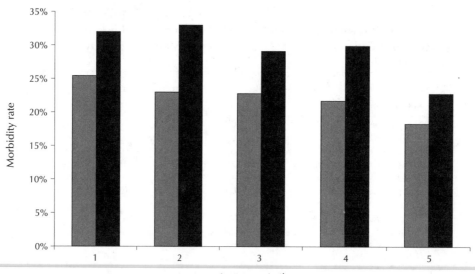

veys, they are self-reported values and they are therefore contaminated by measurement errors. The problem is that if measurement errors κ ($\kappa = H - H^*$) are not reduced, the estimated effect of health on another variable, such as wage, can be expected to be biased toward zero.

Measurement errors are especially significant when the available information on health status is self-reported. Self-perception of health (or illness) may be correlated with certain personal characteristics. For example, people with more education or greater access to health services may be more likely to detect and report symptoms of illness. In an equation in which health is a variable to be explained, these effects might confound the direct impact of education or medical care.[5] Another possible consequence of the subjectivity of self-reporting of health is the presence of heteroskedasticity in the health equation, since the variability of the measurement error would also depend on some of its explanatory variables.

In addition, there is an inevitable underestimation of the severity of recent illness, which may not be fully resolved at the time of the survey interview.[6] Using a dichotomous variable (i.e., occurrence or non-occurrence of illness) or a variable of non-recent illness avoids this possible distortion, but all sensitivity to the severity or nature of the illness is lost. In any case, the longer the recall period used in the survey (e.g., last week or during the last three months), the more reliably true health status will be approximated. To a certain extent, a lengthier recall period increases the number of observations and therefore reduces the sensitivity of the indicators to temporal or random factors.

Going back further in time is also desirable because of the impact that earlier health conditions generally have on current health status. In accordance with the intrapersonal variations proposed by Behrman (1990), the human body can maintain similar levels of productivity in the short term, despite adverse health conditions. With data from the south of India, Deolalikar (1988) observed that current nutrition indicators lose significance when indicators that reflect longer-term nutritional status are included.

---

[5] Butler et al. compared self-reporting of arthritis with objective diagnosis. The authors found that correct reporting was more likely among male wage-earners with a secondary education. The probability of reporting an illness appeared to rise with severity of the illness, income, and age. On the other hand, Wolfe and Behrman (1984), with data from Nicaragua, found that women with the most schooling were less likely to report the occurrence of parasitic diseases.

[6] Assuming that the duration of the illness (D) perfectly reflected its severity, a survey would find $D^* = Min\{D; L\}$, where L is the time elapsed between the onset of the illness and the moment when the survey is conducted. If, in addition, the time of onset were related to some individual characteristic (e.g., occupation, place of residence), the estimate of the impact of this characteristic would be even more biased in a health equation.

In practice, the problem of selecting the best indicator of health status is usually "solved" by the lack of a better alternative in the majority of household (or individual) surveys available.[7] Peru's 1995 National Household Survey offers two possible indicators: a dichotomous variable of recent occurrence of illness and number of days that a person was affected by the illness or condition. In the first case, it must be assumed that the illness is a situation caused by poor health status. In other words, if H^* is the true and unobservable indicator of health status, then:

$$G = 1, \quad \text{if } H^* < H^C,$$
$$\text{and} \quad G = 0, \quad \text{if } H^* \geq H^C,$$

where G is the dichotomous variable and H^C is a certain critical level of health. Below that level, the individual gets sick.

Using number of days ill as an indicator of health status requires this additional assumption—the weaker the individual's health (i.e., the less capacity he/she has for recovery), the longer the period of illness will be. In this case, the duration of the illness (D) would be negatively dependent on H^*:

$$D = D(H^*), \quad \text{if } H^* < H^C, \quad \text{where } D' < 0,$$
$$\text{and} \quad D = 0, \quad \text{if } H^* \geq H^C.$$

It is important to bear in mind that the description of health by means of days of illness would be censored for values higher than H^C. Despite differences in the health status of individuals who have not been ill, the indicator D attributes the same value (zero) to all of them (see Figure 2). However, the indicator "days ill" takes account of interpersonal differences in health better than the dichotomous variable and it is therefore employed in this study to calculate the health indicator used in the wage equation.

An additional distortion associated with the use of days of illness as the basis for the health indicator is rooted in the fact that individuals tend to round their responses. As a result, differences between individuals whose illness had a duration close to the same round number of days (3, 5, 10, 15) are lost. The tendency toward rounding is especially marked when the illness is lengthy. A precise response is more likely when the illness lasts only a few days.

---

[7] In the empirical sphere, investigators in the field of economics have a limited number of health indicators at their disposal and generally choose the one that has the least measurement error. The evidence does not show any conclusive divergence among the most frequent indicators. Haddad, Kennedy, and Sullivan (1994) compared databases from the Philippines, Brazil, Ghana, and Mexico and found that both absolute occurrence of illness and the number of days ill are "useful" approximations to indicators based on weight and height.

The relationship between health status and days ill ($D=D(H^*)$) may not be linear. It is therefore advisable to test several transformations of D in order to generate a health indicator H. Of course, all these transformations imply an inverse relationship between the two variables and recognize upward censoring in the indicator H. The upper limit would be $H^s = D^{-1}(0)$.

SIMULTANEITY BETWEEN HEALTH AND PRODUCTIVITY

Estimating the impact of health on productivity is a complex undertaking because the interactions between wage and health are not limited to this impact. Just as health is a form of human capital that enhances the level of productivity, wage level (W) also affects health.

The income effect is the most obvious means by which productivity contributes to better health status (considering health a normal good): the capability to earn more permits an individual to consume more health "inputs" (e.g., foods or drugs). However, greater productivity may generate certain incentives that affect individuals' behavior. For example, productivity may encourage an individual to work harder, which, in turn, may affect his/her health negatively, or a family might opt to utilize a greater portion of its disposable income to strengthen the health of the most productive member of the household.

The concept of endowment figures prominently in the literature on the subject. The term refers to a set of unobservable characteristics inherent in individuals that affect their health and, therefore, their productivity. These are unalterable features (a certain physical constitution, for example) that are exogenous and random. It is generally assumed that endowments (μ) are a component of the error term of the equations of the variables they affect. In this case, simultaneity between two variables does not occur only in the presence of explicit effects of one variable on the other. The correlation of their error terms also distorts the estimates. If ε_W and ε_{H^*} are the error terms of equations that explain wage and health, a problem of simultaneity would occur if Cov $(\varepsilon_W, \varepsilon_{H^*})$ were not equal to zero.

Thus, φ_W and φ_{H^*} being the true error terms, $\varepsilon_W = \mu_W + \varphi_W$, y $\varepsilon_{H^*} = \mu_{H^*} + \varphi_{H^*}$. Hence, even if the terms φ_W and φ_{H^*} are distributed independently, Cov $(\varepsilon_W, \varepsilon_{H^*})$ = Cov (μ_W, μ_{H^*}). The relationship between μ_W and μ_{H^*} may be the result of the fact that the same endowment (a particular skill or physical ability, or a psychological trait) both engenders greater productivity and enables the individual to maintain better health status. In addition, such a relationship may be linked to individual behavior. For example, if an individual is endowed with qualities that greatly enhance productivity (μ_W), he/she has an incentive to invest in reinforcing those qualities (or in compensating for them within the family unit) through unobservable variables captured by μ_{H^*} (e.g., special efforts to promote health).

THE MODEL

According to Becker (1965), household decisions can be seen as the result of maximization of a utility function, whose variables are consumer goods (C^i), consumer goods that improve health (Y), health status (H^i), and amount of leisure (l^i). It is assumed that household decisions are unitary (i.e, the head of the household imposes his/her preferences on the rest of the individuals) and that the household faces time and full-income constraints. Summarizing, the model is expressed as follows.

A household has n members and is run by the household head, who seeks to maximize the utility function:

$$U = U (C^i, Y^i, H^i, l^i) \ i = 1,2,\ldots,n \tag{1}$$

The utility function is assumed to have the desired conditions, i.e., the function is continuous, strictly increasing, and quasi-concave, and twice-continuously differentiable in all its arguments.

The first constraint is the health production function:

$$H^i = H^i(C^i, Y^i, l^i, X^{-i}, Z^i, Z^{-i}, F, u^i, u^{-i}) \ I = 1,2,\ldots,n \tag{2}$$

where C^i, Y^i, and l^i represent, respectively, level of consumption of goods, health inputs, and leisure for an individual i. X^{-i} denotes the level of consumption, health, and leisure of other members of the household, and Z^{-i}, u^{-i} are the vectors of observed and unobserved characteristics of these individuals, respectively; F denotes availability of health or welfare programs and community infrastructure.

The second constraint is the full-income (S) constraint, which indicates that all available resources of the household are being devoted to the purchase of goods and services and to leisure activities.

$$\sum_{j=1}^{J}\sum_{i} p_j c_j^i + \sum_{k=j+1}^{K}\sum_{i} p_k Y_k^i + \\ \sum_{i} wl^i = \sum_{i} wT^i + V = S \tag{3}$$

V represents non-labor income, p_j and p_k represent the prices of consumer goods and health inputs, T^i is the total amount of time available, and w is the wage rate.

The reduced-form health demand function would be as follows:

$$H^i = h (P_c, P_y, S, F, Z^i, u^i) \quad (4)$$

where P_c and P_y are the prices of the consumer goods important for health and health inputs, respectively.

The wage equation (6) is estimated on the basis of the framework used by Mincer (1974) and therefore takes into account the presence of an equation that explains the decision to participate in the labor market (7), which should make it possible to correct for the wage function's problem of selection bias. The wage function depends on individual characteristics (age, sex), human capital variables (years of schooling and work experience), and regional variables that describe the characteristics of the labor market.

Owing to (a) errors in the measurement of health and (b) its simultaneity with respect to wage or endogeneity of the variable health, the estimate must be corrected through the use of instrumental variables. The latter requires that the variables that explain wage be included in the equation used to instrument the health indicator H:

$$H = \beta_0 + \beta_1 X_H + \beta_2 X_W + \varepsilon_H, \quad (5)$$

where the error term e_H captures the measurement error κ ($\varepsilon_H = \varepsilon_{H*} + \kappa$).

In this context, the acceptance of health as a form of human capital leads to its inclusion among the explanatory variables of productivity. The wage equation would thus take the form:

$$\ln(W) = \alpha_0 + \alpha_1 X_W + \alpha_H H^* + \varepsilon_W, \quad (6)$$

where X_W is a group of relevant variables; H* denotes corrected individual health status; and ε_W is a random error term. A semilogarithmic specification is used because it is the type most commonly employed in empirical studies on the returns to human capital.

The wage equation (6) has a selection bias which must be corrected by using the Heckman procedure, or two-stage estimation (Heckman, 1979; Lee, 1983). The dichotomous equation that expresses the decision to participate in the labor market (L) includes as explanatory variables wage, health, and a set of variables X_L, which identify the system. In the estimate, wage is not directly included because it is not observable when the individual does not participate in the labor market; it is therefore replaced by the explanatory variables X_W. Similarly, health is replaced by a set of instrumental variables X_H.

$$L = L (W, H^*, X_L)$$
$$L = L (X_W, X_H, X_L) \quad (7)$$

The set of equations (5), (6), and (7) make up the system of equations to be estimated. Health is predicted in equation (5)—which is estimated using a tobit model due to censorship of the health indicator H—and is included in the wage equation (6).

THE ECONOMETRIC ESTIMATION STRATEGY

Following the practice generally used in previous empirical studies, the sample is divided by sex, so that specific equations are estimated for males and females. To take account of differences between urban and rural en-

FIGURE 3. Labor participation by years of schooling.

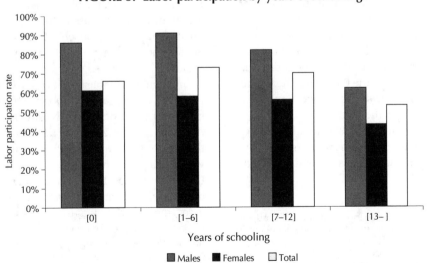

FIGURE 4. Labor participation by age.

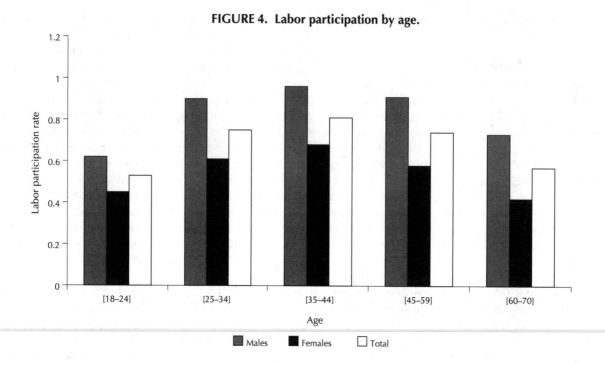

vironments, the wage functions for males and females are estimated separately in each geographic area. Determination of the explanatory variables X_W, X_H, and X_L also follow the practice customarily found in the literature. Annex I shows the definitions and sample moments for all the variables used in the estimates in the study.

In addition to the health variable, the wage equation includes age, years of schooling, and the quadratic terms of both. These terms take account of possible non-linearities in the impacts of these variables. The variable X_W incorporates two additional variables: residence in the country's capital city and local unemployment rate. The aim in including the latter variable is to capture inter-district differences in labor markets.

For exploratory purposes, the wage equation was estimated without including health. The results show that the signs of the human capital coefficients and individual characteristics are predicted by the theory that health has an effect on productivity. These results were robust to changes in the equation specification.[8]

With regard to the determinant variables of health X_H, it should be noted that the literature suggests that there are unobserved characteristics μ_H, associated with indi-vidual heterogeneity, which would be incorporated in the error term $\varepsilon_H = \varphi_{H^*} + \mu_H + \kappa$.

Moreover, equation (5) is a function of demand and not a function of health production and, therefore, the vector X_H should incorporate income and prices of health-related products as explanatory variables. These variables influence the quantity of health "inputs" (e.g., nutrients, medical services) consumed by the family unit.

When families demand health inputs for their members, they are aware of their endowments and other un-observed characteristics μ_H. The level of consumption of these inputs is therefore probably correlated with the error term ε_H. In fact, health demand only can include factors that, while they affect the production of health, are not determined by households, at least in the short term. Such is the case with age, education, food prices, supply of public services, etc.

Among the variables that explain health, access to State-provided health care is important to a subsequent analysis of the impact of public investments in personal health. Access to health services is not measured on the basis of the services received by each individual because to do so would introduce the endogenous nature of those services. Use is a decision based on, among other variables, the individual's income, opportunity cost of time (in both cases, measured by wage), and health status.

To simplify the analysis, the number of per capita public health care facilities in each district was introduced into the health equation (5). This variable makes it possible to more directly assess the impact of public invest-

---

[8] Replacing age by potential experience maintained the adjustment in the regression. The coefficients of the variables were modified in accordance with the linear relationship between experience, age, and years of schooling (EXPERIENCE = AGE − SCHOOLING − 6). The specification that incorporates age was chosen, as it also captures part of the impact of the work experience.

FIGURE 5. Hourly wage by years of schooling.

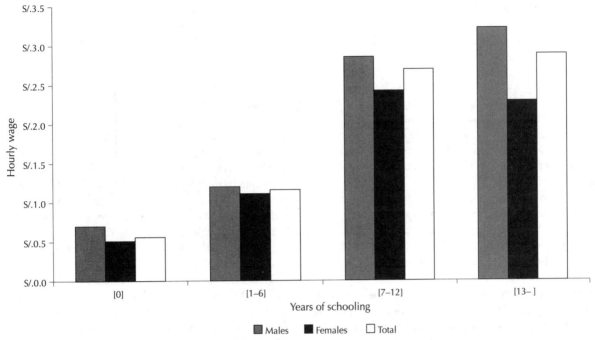

FIGURE 6. Wage by age group.

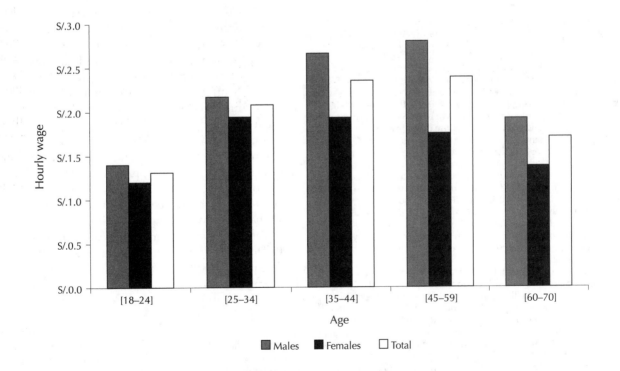

ment on health in terms of the supply side. The quadratic term of this variable was also included in order to observe possible non-linear effects.[9]

Analysis of the Results

The sample used in the regressions includes only individuals over 17 and under 70 years of age—i.e., adults who are potential participants in the labor market. The probit equation of participation in the market is shown in Annex II. Wald tests indicate that the set of instruments, X_L, is significant in the four samples comprising men and women in urban and rural areas.

Table 4 shows the regressions that include health as a dependent variable. The transformation $H = 1/(1 + D)$ was used as a health indicator. This transformation proposes an inverse relationship between the duration of illness and the health indicator. It is upwardly censored at $1 = [1/(1+0)]$.

An advantage of the proposed health indicator is that it shows a marginally declining impact for a larger number of days ill. This is desirable owing to respondents' tendency to round their answers when they do not remember exactly how many days their illness lasted, which is more likely when the illness has been prolonged. The indicator H reduces the importance of variations in reported days ill as the number of days rises.[10]

The results of the health equation (see Table 4) are predicted by the theory. In the case of age, both the linear and the quadratic terms obtain negative coefficients in most cases. In general, aging is associated with deteriorating health status, and it also accelerates that deterioration. The final effect of age on health is always negative, except in the sample of rural men.

The variables indicative of wealth are significant only in some cases. Per capita non-labor family income is significant only for women, and for women in rural areas an unexpected negative coefficient was obtained. This result is difficult to explain, but it is, nevertheless, consistent with the concept of health as a normal good. Hours of access to the public drinking water supply system and availability of adequate floors have a positive and significant impact on health among the population in urban areas. In this case, in addition to the effect associated with wealth, there appears to be a direct impact on the production of health.

Education yields a positive impact that is probably associated with better use of knowledge and available inputs, which enable better care of health. In general, the education coefficients in Table 4 would be downwardly biased if it were true that individuals with more schooling tend to report symptoms of illness more frequently.

As for the impact of prices of health inputs, with the exception of milk, increases in food prices significantly reduce health demand in all the samples. The positive coefficient for milk price might be explained by its correlation with the prices of other foods not included in the estimate.[11]

Conditions in the community affect the health status of individuals. Quality of housing construction (non-dirt floors), provincial poverty index, and local unemployment rate show a positive impact on health. Health is presumably affected by the living conditions in which the individual develops. In addition, residence in the city of Lima and the coastal region has a positive impact on health, controlling for local level of poverty and access to public health services, which might be associated with the use of other inputs (e.g., private services) and other conditions (e.g., climatic factors).

In rural areas, the number of public health facilities per capita has a positive and significant impact on health status. Table 4 evaluates the implicit effect on the coefficients of the linear and quadratic terms at the sample mean. The negative coefficient of the quadratic term indicates declining returns on public investment in health. In urban areas, the impacts are negative, and among women

---

[9] The introduction of the number of public health care facilities into equation (5) raises a problem of endogeneity. Presumably, the State does not distribute its services randomly, with no criteria whatsoever. Sen (1995) presents a brief description of the political economy of the distribution of the benefits of social programs. Beyond the desire to target those who most need these benefits—as suggested by Rosenzweig and Wolpin (1986) and Pitt, Rosenzweig, and Gibbons (1995)—there are problems to be overcome, including political feasibility and the influence of the most powerful groups. The theory of pressure groups models this phenomenon. On the other hand, the theory of altruism gives formal expression to the desire to compensate the neediest members of society. In particular, if the public infrastructure is placed preferentially in localities with the fewest health resources, the correlation between the error term ε_H and the number of public facilities would be a number other than zero, and their impact on health would be downwardly biased. This endogeneity of public health infrastructure necessitates the use of instrumental methods. For the sake of simplicity, this analysis has not been undertaken here, though the possibility of downward biasing of the results is recognized.

[10] Other transformations were tried, and it was found that those that showed marginally declining impacts for D (reported days ill) had higher levels of likelihood. The following showed the highest levels: $H_a = -\div D$, $H_b = -\ln(1 + D)$, and $H = 1/(1 + D)$. The latter transformation yielded the highest values for the logarithm of the likelihood function in all samples (Annex III). It was therefore preferred to the alternatives. The results presented in the following sections were robust to changes in the selection of the health indicator as long as the indicator preserved the characteristic of marginally reducing the impact of D.

[11] Only some consumer prices were available for all the country's departments. The data in this case were obtained from the 24 departmental statistical compendiums for 1995 published by the National Statistics and Informatics Institute (INEI).

TABLE 4. Health equation by sex and region: censored tobit.[a]

Independent variables	Males Urban	Males Rural	Females Urban	Females Rural
Constant	3.020*	1.408***	2.367***	1.572***
	[10.54]	[3.74]	[10.84]	[4.98]
Individual traits	*180.3****	*70.7****	*280.5****	*128.5****
Age [10⁻²]	−0.578	0.105	−1.163***	−1.537**
	[−1.11]	[0.13]	[−2.93]	[−2.25]
Age squared [10⁻⁴]	−0.871	−1.584*	−0.192	0.093
	[−1.36]	[−1.68]	[−0.39]	[0.12]
Human capital variables	*49.7****	*22.5****	*56.1****	*13.2****
Years of schooling [× 10⁻²]	3.827*	5.899***	2.296***	−0.480
	[2.62]	[3.26]	[2.63]	[−0.36]
Years of schooling squared (× 10⁻¹)	−0.071	−0.275**	−0.024	0.178
	[−0.76]	[−2.05]	[−0.39]	[1.64]
Household assets				
Non-labor income	0.018	−0.017	0.041***	−0.097*
	[1.35]	[−0.53]	[3.55]	[−1.85]
Housing infrastructure	*16.4****	*6.1*	*26.4****	*8.6****
Hours of water supply [× 10⁻⁴]	1.538	3.762*	−0.155	2.907*
	[1.25]	[1.86]	[−0.16]	[1.75]
Adequate sewerage system	0.006	0.049	0.013	−0.113
	[0.22]	[0.57]	[0.61]	[−1.63]
Non-dirt floor	0.276*	0.093	0.283***	0.124*
	[3.66]	[1.22]	[4.96]	[1.93]
Regional variables	*13.9****	–	*21.2****	–
Residence in the coastal region	−0.130*	0.131**	−0.101***	0.228***
	[−2.98]	[2.31]	[−3.05]	[4.86]
Residence in Lima	0.182*	–	0.176***	–
	[3.64]		[4.60]	
Community variables	*9.7****	*6.2***	*17.4****	*6.7***
Poverty indicator	−0.978**	−7.095**	−0.711*	−1.214
	[−1.99]	[−2.20]	[−1.76]	[−0.45]
Unemployment rate	−1.095**	−1.036*	−1.361***	−1.236**
	[−2.22]	[−1.74]	[−3.65]	[−2.57]
Health infrastructure	*2.3*	–	*6.7***	–
Number of health care facilities per capita	−0.321	0.139**	−0.797**	0.089*
	[−0.66]	[2.15]	[−2.18]	[1.70]
Number of health care facilities per capita squared	0.224	−0.014**	0.699**	−0.012***
	[0.48]	[−2.50]	[1.99]	[−2.73]
Food prices	*101.2****	*17.0****	*97.4****	*14.4****
Price of rice	−0.977*	−0.410***	−0.718***	−0.322***
	[−9.32]	[−2.92]	[−9.08]	[−2.77]
Price of tomatoes	−0.285*	−0.092	−0.198***	−0.088
	[−6.64]	[−1.37]	[−6.03]	[−1.53]
Price of milk	0.276**	0.607***	0.286***	0.475***
	[2.08]	[3.26]	[2.77]	[2.92]
∂H/∂ [facilities]	−0.304	0.135**	−0.740**	0.085*
	[−0.68]	[2.14]	[−2.20]	[1.67]
Ln (likelihood function)	−12,209	−4,174	−16,107	−4,721
Chi-square	483.3***	–	755.4***	–
Prob [H*<1]	22.7%	29.1%	32.7%	38.0%
Number of observations	18,787	5,633	20,435	5,671

[a] Dependent variable: H = 1/(1+ number of days ill).

[*t*-statistic in brackets] and joint significance test italicized.

(*) Statistically significant at 10% confidence level; (**) Statistically significant at 5% confidence level; (***) Statistically significant at 1% confidence level.

this effect is statistically significant. These results might be explained by the possible presence of heteroskedasticity in the health equation, as discussed in section 3.[12] Only the sample of urban women appears to be affected by this problem.[13]

Tables 5 a and b and Tables 6 a and b show the estimates of the wage equations in three different cases: (a) excluding the health variable, (b) including the observed health values, and (c) including the estimated values of the health indicator. The latter were obtained from the regressions in Table 4 and are free from simultaneity and measurement error biases.

As predicted by the theory and suggested by Table 3, health status has a significant and positive effect on productivity. An improvement in health status raises wages in all population groups for both sexes and in both urban and rural areas. The coefficient of the health indicator is positive both with the health variable as exogenous and instrumented (IV). However, both the coefficient and the significance level of the variable health are much greater in the latter case.

The extent to which health impacts productivity varies according to the population group. Improvements in health status have a greater impact on productivity in rural areas, and this effect is greater among rural men than among rural women.[14] Table 7, which shows the impact of one additional healthy day per month, illustrates this finding.[15]

The results for the rest of the variables show that, when health is not controlled for, the coefficients of age and education obtained are upwardly biased. This suggests that when the health variable is omitted, age and education capture part of its effects on productivity.

The negative signs of the quadratic terms of age imply that the impact of age on productivity, though initially positive, declines and, at a certain point, turns negative. The critical age that marks the beginning of the decline in productivity varies from one sample to another. According to the regressions that omit health, in urban areas, maximum productivity is achieved at 49.2 and 46.7

years of age among men and women, respectively. When health is controlled for, the critical age is later: 53.0 and 50.4 years.[16,17]

The inclusion of the instrumented health variable results in an extension of the cycle of productive life for all individuals. This result is explained by the fact that age increases the probability of suffering from some illness or ailment (see Table 4). If health is not controlled for as an explanatory factor, the effect of poor health characteristic of older adults is attributed to age. When health is controlled for, age has a less negative effect on wage level, and the period of productive life is longer.

The effect of one additional year of education depends on the coefficients of the linear and quadratic terms of the education variable and on the individual's years of schooling.[18] Tables 5a and 5b and 6a and 6b evaluate, at the sample mean, the marginal return and its significance. The magnitude of the impact varies from one sample to another. When health is instrumented, the returns to education in urban areas are 7.4% and 5.1% for men and women, respectively, while in rural areas the figures are 5.8% and 10.4%.

When the instrumented health variable is used in the wage equation, it is observed that the returns to education for men are 9.5% and 55.2% higher in urban and rural areas, respectively, than if the observed health variable is used. In the case of women, the proportion of overestimation is 15.7% and 2.9% in urban and rural areas, respectively. This upward bias is explained by an expected positive correlation between the two forms of human capital: education and health (Schultz, 1996). In the absence of the latter, the education variable captures part of the impact of the omitted health variable.

The theory suggests several justifications for this type of correlation. In addition to the existence of individual traits and heterogeneity, the rational behavior of investment in human capital offers other arguments. One is that intertemporal preferences (of the parents) affect in-

---

[12] The endogeneity discussed in footnote 7 might also be important.

[13] Only in this sample did the logarithm of the likelihood function decrease appreciably after correcting for hetereoskedasticity (from -16,107 to -16,069) and significant coefficients were obtained in the explanatory regression of the quadratic error term. As noted in section 3, the heteroskedasticity model included education and number of health facilities per capita as explanatory variables in this regression.

[14] As noted earlier, these results are robust to changes in the health indicator, as long as the indicator shows a marginally decreasing impact for increased days of illness.

[15] Given that $H = 1/(1 + D)$, then $\partial W / \partial D = (\partial W / \partial H) \times (\partial H / \partial D) = -\alpha_H / (1 + D)^2$, where $-\alpha_H$ is the coefficient of the indicator H in the wage equation and D is evaluated at the sample means.

---

[16] Given that the estimated function describes the relationship between health and productivity as an inverted U, the age of maximum productivity (the apex of the parabola) is calculated as $E^* = -a_{E1} / [2 H a_{E2}]$, where a_{E1} and a_{E2} are the coefficients of the linear and quadratic terms of age, respectively. In the case of urban men, for example, productivity reaches its maximum at 53.0 years = $-0.051 / [2 H - 0.00048]$.

[17] For women who live in rural areas, the increase in the critical age is much greater, rising from 37.4 to 62.0 years of age when health is controlled for. In the case of rural men, productivity increases with age.

[18] Given equation (1), one more year of education yields $\Delta \ln(W) = \Delta\% W = \alpha S1 + 2\alpha S2 \, S$, where $\alpha S1$ and $\alpha S2$ represent the coefficients of the linar and quadratic terms of the years of education. Specifically, for urban males, the return ($\Delta\% W$) is equal to 0.074 = 0.094 + 2 (–0.00101) (9.13), where 9.13 is the sample mean of the years of education.

TABLE 5A. Salary equation: males (OLS corrected by Heckman two-stage estimation).[a]

Variables	Without health	Urban areas Health exogenous	Health [IV]
1. Constant	−1.374***	−1.421***	−2.103***
	[−8.50]	[−8.77]	[−8.79]
Individual characteristics			
2. Age	0.052***	0.051***	0.051***
	[7.12]	[6.94]	[6.96]
3. Age squared [× 10⁻²]	−0.053***	−0.051***	−0.048***
	[−5.98]	[−5.77]	[−5.39]
Human capital variables			
4. Years of schooling	0.108***	0.107***	0.094***
	[10.14]	[10.07]	[8.40]
5. Years of schooling squared [× 10⁻²]	−0.143**	−0.140**	−0.101
	[−2.07]	[−2.02]	[−1.45]
6. Health indicator	−	0.090***	0.933***
		[4.19]	[4.13]
Local market variables			
7. Residence in Lima	0.265***	0.265***	0.276***
	[13.91]	[13.90]	[14.32]
8. Unemployment rate [at district level]	0.387*	0.398*	0.486**
	[1.65]	[1.70]	[2.06]
9. Selection term	−0.184***	−0.196***	−0.193***
	[−3.36]	[−3.57]	[−3.53]
Rate of return to education	8.1%	8.0%	7.4%
Return to health	−	0.5%	4.7%
Age of maximum productivity	49.2	49.7	53.0
Joint test of significance [2]–[3]	197.1***	202.1***	181.6***
Joint test of significance [4]–[6]	1,175.3***	1,192.8***	1,192.7***
Joint test of significance [4]–[5]	1,175.3***	1,165.6***	621.6***
Joint test of significance [7]–[8]	233.8***	236.3***	247.9***
Hausman Test	−	−	184.1***
Log likelihood	−18,478	−18,469	−18,469
Chi-square	295.5***	261.1***	261.0***
Adjusted R²	0.126	0.127	0.127
Number of observations	14,321	14,321	14,321

[a] Dependent variable: ln[W], natural logarithm of hourly wage.
[t-statistics in brackets]
(*) Statistically significant at 10% confidence level; (**) Statistically significant at 5% confidence level; (***) Statistically significant at 1% confidence level.

vestment in the education and health of children. In addition, credit restrictions may reduce investment in health and education. Finally, certain personal characteristics—such as intellectual ability—that have an effect on productivity could create incentives for greater investment in human capital in general.[19]

The impact of residing in Lima is always positive and insensitive to the inclusion of health status, whether ob-

served or instrumented. For men, participation in the Lima labor market implies a 28% higher wage and for women, 37% higher. The inclusion of local unemployment (measured at the district level) should control for inter-district differences in labor markets. Except for urban women, positive and significant coefficients are obtained. It could be hypothesized that individuals who are employed achieve higher wage rates in areas with high unemployment. The explanation could be that the expected wage rate in areas with high unemployment is higher than in areas with less unemployment.

The correction term of the selection bias (λ) is significant and negative in the case of urban men. This is an indication that the non-observable characteristics that

[19] The preferences or tastes of households and individual heterogeneity could prompt a decision to invest in education and/or health. Given the individual characteristics of the members of the household, it is possible that the household may make certain decisions in order to compensate for or reinforce the innate endowments (e.g., aspects of health, genetic ability) of its members.

TABLE 5B. Wage equation: males (OLS corrected by Heckman two-stage estimation).[a]

Variables	Rural areas		
	Without health	Health exogenous	Health [IV]
1. Constant	−1.496***	−1.551***	−3.944***
	[−6.03]	[−6.21]	[−9.17]
Individual characteristics			
2. Age	0.029**	0.028**	0.015
	[2.57]	[2.52]	[1.36]
3. Age squared [× 10⁻²]	−0.038***	−0.037***	−0.006
	[−3.05]	[−2.97]	[−0.46]
Human capital variables			
4. Years of schooling	0.024	0.022	−0.057***
	[1.25]	[1.17]	[−2.60]
5. Years of schooling squared [× 10⁻²]	0.537***	0.545***	0.938***
	[3.79]	[3.85]	[6.16]
6. Health indicator	–	0.086*	3.464***
		[1.77]	[6.95]
Local market variables			
7. Residence in Lima	–	–	–
8. Unemployment rate [at district level]	1.180**	1.163**	0.787
	[2.35]	[2.32]	[1.57]
9. Selection term	0.147	0.143	0.129
	[1.61]	[1.56]	[1.42]
Rate of return to education	9.0%	8.9%	5.8%
Return to health	–	0.4%	14.2%
Age of maximum productivity	37.4	37.6	125.6
Joint test of significance [2]–[3]	17.9***	16.2***	15.8***
Joint test of significance [4]–[6]	291.5***	294.8***	343.1***
Joint test of significance [4]–[5]	291.5***	288.6***	150.5***
Joint test of significance [7]–[8]	10.2***	9.8***	5.6*
Hausman Test	–	–	122.1***
Log likelihood	−7,164	−7,162	−7,139
Chi-square	76.6***	66.1***	73.2***
Adjusted R²	0.093	0.093	0.102
Number of observations	4,445	4,445	4,445

[a] Dependent variable: ln[W], natural logarithm of hourly wage.

[t-statistics in brackets]

(*) Statistically significant at 10% confidence level; (**) Statistically significant at 5% confidence level; (***) Statistically significant at 1% confidence level.

determine the probability of labor participation are negatively associated with the wage level in the market and that they are not captured by the explanatory variables in the wage equation.

The interaction effect of health and education was also analyzed. Annex IV shows the results. After instrumenting the interaction term Health × Education, this term was introduced into the wage equation, which revealed that, for men, a positive interaction between the two forms of human capital exists. In the sample comprising males, education and health complement each other. The rate of return to education is higher when the individual is healthy, and health leads to greater productivity when

the individual is better educated. This interpretation would reject the argument that health status is more important when the individual is engaged in physical labor as opposed to intellectual work.

Finally, inclusion of the interaction term of the instrumented health indicator and age shows that productivity is more sensitive to changes in health status especially for older persons. Policies aimed at improving health status in the older adult population would have effects on the relative increase in wages for this population group. A positive coefficient for the crossed term of the health indicator and age is obtained in all the samples, and in the case of rural men and urban women, the coefficients

TABLE 6A. Wage equation: females (OLS corrected by Heckman two-stage estimation).[a]

Variables	Urban areas		
	Without health	Health exogenous	Health [IV]
1. Constant	−1.752***	−1.784***	−2.577***
	[−10.44]	[−10.61]	[−9.81]
Individual characteristics			
2. Age	0.074***	0.073***	0.074***
	[10.26]	[10.18]	[10.26]
3. Age squared [× 10⁻²]	−0.079***	−0.078***	−0.073***
	[−8.77]	[−8.64]	[−8.03]
Human capital variables			
4. Years of schooling	0.105***	0.104***	0.091***
	[10.45]	[10.34]	[8.53]
5. Years of schooling squared [× 10⁻²]	−0.279***	−0.275***	−0.243***
	[−3.96]	[−3.90]	[−3.43]
6. Health indicator	–	0.064***	1.060***
		[2.60]	[4.08]
Local market variables			
7. Residence in Lima	0.383***	0.381***	0.374***
	[15.45]	[15.37]	[15.05]
8. Unemployment rate [at district level]	−0.468	−0.435	−0.125
	[−1.43]	[−1.33]	[−0.37]
9. Selection term	0.002	−0.007	−0.011
	[0.04]	[−0.12]	[−0.19]
Rate of return to education	5.9%	5.9%	5.1%
Return to health	–	0.2%	3.4%
Age of maximum productivity	46.7	47.0	50.4
Joint test of significance [2]–[3]	221.4***	225.7***	206.6***
Joint test of significance [4]–[6]	630.2***	637.3***	647.9***
Joint test of significance [4]–[5]	630.2***	620.4***	268.8***
Joint test of significance [7]–[8]	239.8***	237.7***	227.9***
Hausman Test	–	–	229.3***
Log likelihood	−13,040	−13,036	−13,031
Chi-square	174.3***	153.5***	154.8***
Adjusted R²	0.112	0.113	0.114
Number of observations	9,598	9,598	9,598

[a] Dependent variable: ln[W], natural logarithm of hourly wage.

[*t*-statistics in brackets]

(*) Statistically significant at 10% confidence level; (**) Statistically significant at 5% confidence level; (***) Statistically significant at 1% confidence level.

are significant. Moreover, as noted above, when the interaction between health and education was introduced into the wage equation, it was found that it was significant in the case of men and that the two forms of human capital complement each other.

Higher quality of available housing infrastructure has a favorable effect on wages through better health conditions. This relationship is evaluated by means of simulations that are illustrated in Annex IV. The results suggest that the wages of urban women and rural men are most susceptible to these changes, although the differences are not of great magnitude. For example, an increase of 50% in hours of water supply, quality of flooring, and sewer-age system at the community level produces an increase of 3.5% and 1.8% in women's wages in urban and rural areas, respectively. In the case of men, the increases are 2.1% and 2.3%.

CONCLUSIONS

This study considers health as one of the determinants of human capital that has an influence on wage level, and it shows that public policies that serve to improve the health status of individuals can also raise their wages and consequently improve living standards in their households.

TABLE 6B. Wage equation: Females (OLS corrected by Heckman two-stage estimation).[a]

Variables	Rural areas		
	Without health	Health exogenous	Health [IV]
1. Constant	−2.418***	−2.487***	−4.267***
	−6.78	[−6.95]	[−7.25]
Individual characteristics			
2. Age	0.052***	0.051***	0.054***
	[3.43]	[3.32]	[3.51]
3. Age squared [× 10⁻²]	−0.058***	−0.055***	−0.043**
	[−3.27]	[−3.10]	[−2.40]
Human capital variables			
4. Years of schooling	0.124***	0.124***	0.116***
	[4.78]	[4.78]	[4.44]
5. Years of schooling squared [× 10⁻²]	−0.086	−0.093	−0.130
	[−0.42]	[−0.45]	[−0.63]
6. Health indicator	–	0.146*	2.247***
		[1.93]	[3.94]
Local market variables			
7. Residence in Lima	–	–	–
8. Unemployment rate [at district level]	3.694***	3.646***	3.384***
	[4.52]	[4.47]	[4.14]
9. Selection term	0.087	0.075	0.082
	[1.08]	[0.94]	[1.02]
Rate of return to education	*11.7%*	*11.6%*	*10.4%*
Return to health	*–*	*0.4%*	*6.2%*
Age of maximum productivity	*45.3*	*46.2*	*62.0*
Joint test of significance [2]–[3]	*12.0****	*11.7****	*23.4****
Joint test of significance [4]–[6]	*171.5****	*175.6****	*188.4****
Joint test of significance [4]–[5]	*171.5****	*168.7****	*114.4****
Joint test of significance [7]–[8]	*23.5****	*22.5****	*19.8****
Hausman Test	*–*	*–*	*182.5****
Log likelihood	*−3,254*	*−3,252*	*−3,246*
Chi-square	*41.5****	*36.2****	*38.1****
Adjusted R²	*0.113*	*0.114*	*0.120*
Number of observations	*1,908*	*1,908*	*1,908*

[a] Dependent variable: ln[W], natural logarithm of hourly wage.

[t-statistics in brackets]

(*) Statistically significant at 10% confidence level; (**) Statistically significant at 5% confidence level; (***) Statistically significant at 1% confidence level.

TABLE 7. Productivity returns to health (percentages).

Population group	Rate of return to health (%)[a]
Urban males	4.7
Urban females	3.4
Rural males	14.2
Rural females	6.2

[a]Effect on wage rate of one additional day of good health in 30 days.

The technique of instrumental variables makes it possible to reduce the measurement errors associated with the self-reported health information available in the household survey, and it also takes into account the endogeneity of the health variable. One of the main findings is that, when the observed health variable is used, the returns to education in urban areas appear to be overestimated. It also was found that one additional healthy day has a greater impact on wages among men (4.7% and 10.4% for men in rural and urban areas, respectively) than among women (3.4% and 6.2%).

Results of Peru's 1995 Household Survey show that the reported morbidity rate and number of days ill are negatively associated with individual wages and level of household income. It also shows that individuals with more years of education report higher rates of illness and receive more health care.

Significant and positive effects of health were estimated in the wage equation. The results are the same regardless of whether the dummy variable "reported morbidity rate" or "days ill" is used as a health indicator. The productivity of rural men and women was most sensitive to health status. Empirically, if the simultaneity and measurement error had not been corrected, they would have biased the health coefficients downward.

In all the samples, the effects of age and education decreased when health was controlled for. As predicted by the theory, when the health variable is omitted from the wage equation, the estimates for the education variable are overestimated, especially in the case of rural men and urban women.

When the impact of public health care services was studied, health status in rural areas was found to be sensitive to access to such services and the health of rural men appeared to benefit the most from increased access. However, there is evidence that the returns to health are slightly underestimated if the interaction terms are omitted. An omitted positive interaction downwardly biases the health coefficient, while a negative interaction produces an upward bias.

Wealthier individuals—excluding rural men and controlling for age, education, variables of housing and health infrastructure, regional variables, and food prices—have better health status. However, the health status of individuals was found to be negatively influenced by living conditions and by the labor market in the districts in which they reside. Hence, the poverty indicator and district unemployment rate variables have a negative effect on individual health status.

In rural areas, housing infrastructure, the community environment, and availability of health infrastructure were significant in explaining health status. This finding is important in that it may facilitate the identification of public policy measures that lead to improved health status for individuals and, consequently, higher wages. The results of the simulations indicate that the hourly wages of urban men and rural women are positively sensitive to investment in housing infrastructure, which generates positive effects on their health status and thus on the level of their wages. It would, therefore, appear that public investment can be targeted so as to improve the level of equity in the labor market.

One of the problems encountered in this study was the scant availability of information on other policy variables that might be incorporated into the health equation. Peru's 1995 NHS includes only information on morbidity rate and reported number of days ill. Some variables that might, in theory, explain health status—such as number of doctors and/or nurses per 10,000 population, number of beds per district, and level of coverage of the Social Security Institute per district—were not among the expected coefficients in accordance with the theory. It is impossible to discern whether this was due to poor quality of information, insufficient disaggregation, serious measurement problems, or the simple fact that they do not have an impact on health status.

Number of days disabled by illness was not reported in the survey. To the author's knowledge, neither is anthropometric information for adults available in any of Peru's household surveys to date. Future studies should attempt to verify the trend of returns to health with the inclusion of these other indicators, as well as information from other variables derived from other sources of information, especially those associated with policy instruments—for example, indicators of the availability of the health and feeding programs that they are of great importance in the country's budget and whose evaluation in terms of effects on the health of individuals would make it possible to evaluate their indirect impacts on wage rates. Such research could be enormously useful in the design of new schemes for targeting social expenditure.

REFERENCES

Becker SG. A theory of the allocation of time. *Economic Journal* 1965;LXXX (200):493–517.

Barrera A. The role of maternal schooling and its interaction with public health programs in child health production. *Journal of Development Economics* 1990;32:69–91.

Behrman J, Deolalikar A. Health and nutrition. In: Chenery H and Srinivasan TN (eds.). *Handbook of Development Economics*. New York: North Holland; 1988. pp. 631–711.

Behrman JR. Macroeconomic adjustment, household food consumption, nutrient intakes, and health status. In: *Macroeconomic Reforms, Poverty and Nutrition: Analytical Methodologies*. New York: Cornell Food and Nutrition Policy Program; 1990.

Behrman J. The economic rationale for investing in nutrition in developing countries. *World Development* 1993;21(11): 749–771.

Deolalikar A. Nutrition and labor productivity in agriculture: estimates for rural south India. *The Review of Economics and Statistics* 1988;70(3):406–413.

Haddad L, Kennedy E, Sullivan J. Choice of indicators for food security and nutrition monitoring. *Food Policy* 1994;19 (3):329–343.

Heckman J. Sample selection bias as a specification error. *Econometrica* 1979;47(1):143–161.

Lee L-F. Generalized econometric models with selectivity. *Econometrica*. 1983;51(2):507–512.

Lee, L-F. Some approaches to the correction of selectivity bias. *Review of Economic Studies* 49:355–372.

Maddala GS. *Limited Dependent and Qualitative Variables in Econometrics*. Cambridge: Cambridge University Press; 1983. (Econometric Society Monographs 3).

Mincer J. On-the-job training: costs, returns and some implications. *Journal of Political Economy* 1962;70(5):50–79.

Pitt MM, Rosenzweig M. Health and nutrient consumption across and within farm households. *The Review of Economics and Statistics* 1985;67(2):212–223.

Pitt MM, Rosenzweig MR, Gibbons DM. The determinants and consequences of the placement of government programs in Indonesia. In: van de Walle D, Nead K (Eds). *Public Spending and the Poor: Theory and Evidence*. Baltimore and London: World Bank; 1995.

Pitt MM, Rosenzweig M, Hassan MN. Productivity, health and inequality in the intrahousehold distribution of food in low-income countries. *The American Economic Review* 1990;80(5): 1139–1156.

Rosenzweig MR, Schultz TP. Market opportunities, genetic endowments and intrafamily resource distribution: child survival in rural India. *The American Economic Review* 1982;72(4):803–815.

Rosenzweig MR, Schultz TP. Estimating a household production function: heterogeneity, the demand for health inputs, and their effects on birth weight. *Journal of Political Economy* 1983;91(5): 723–746.

Rosenzweig RM, Wolpin KI. Evaluating the effects of optimally distributed public programs: child health and family planning interventions. *The American Economic Review* 1986;76(3):470–482.

Sahn DE, Alderman H. The effects of variables of human capital on wages, and the determinants of labor supply in a developing country. *Journal of Development Economics* 1988;29(2):157–183.

Schultz TP. Wage rentals for reproducible variables of human capital: evidence from two West African countries. 1996. (mimeograph).

Schultz TP, Tansel A. Wage and labor supply effects of illness in Côte d'Ivoire and Ghana: instrumental variable estimates for days disabled. *Journal of Development Economics* 1997;53(2):251–286.

Strauss J, Gertler P, Rahman O, Fox K. Gender and life-cycle differentials in the patterns and determinants of adult health. *The Journal of Human Resources* 1993;28(4):791–837.

Thomas D, Strauss J. Health and wages: evidence on men and women in urban Brazil. *Journal of Econometrics* 1997;77(1):159–186.

Sen A. The political economy of targeting. In: van de Walle D, Nead K (Eds). *Public Spending and the Poor: Theory and Evidence.* Baltimore and London: World Bank; 1995.

Strauss J. Does better nutrition raise farm productivity? *Journal of Political Economy* 1986;94(2):297–320.

Wolfe B, Behrman J. Is income overrated in determining adequate nutrition? *Economic Development and Cultural Change* 1983;31(3): 525–549.

Wolfe B, Behrman J. Determinants of women's health status and health-care utilization in a developing country: a latent variable approach. *Review of Economics and Statistics* 1984;56(4):703–720.

ANNEX I. DEFINITIONS AND SAMPLE MOMENTS OF THE VARIABLES.

Variable	Definition	Mean[†]	Standard deviation[†]
Dependent Variables			
Reported days ill	Number of days of illness during the 15 days preceding the interview	2.21	4.49
Reported illness rate	Reported ailment or illness in the 15 days preceding the interview = 1, otherwise = 0	0.27	0.44
Ln(Wage)	Natural logarithm of the individual's hourly wage in new soles (Peruvian currency) calculated on the basis of hours worked per week and monthly salaries, weekly wages, and half-year earnings	0.34	1.15
Independent Variables			
Age	Years of age (not including any fractions of years)	23.22	82.92
Years of schooling	Years of schooling (calculated on the basis of grades passed)	8.07	4.08
Automobile	Dichotomous: Owns an automobile = 1; otherwise = 0.	0.10	0.31
Other vehicle	Dichotomous: Household has any vehicle other than an automobile = 1; otherwise = 0	0.32	0.47
Non-labor income	Income in new soles (labor and non-labor) received by the household as a whole in the preceding month, excluding labor income of the individual under observation, divided by family size.	6.23	57.37
Residence in the coastal region	Dichotomous: Resides in the coastal region = 1; otherwise = 0.	0.44	0.50
Residence in Lima	Dichotomous: Resides in Lima = 1; otherwise = 0.	0.14	0.35
Hours of water supply	Hours of drinking water supply from the public system during the last week	76.22	98.78
Adequate sewerage system	Dichotomous: Access to the public sewerage system in the household = 1; otherwise = 0	0.56	0.50
Non-dirt floor	District rate of households without dirt floors	0.60	0.25
Health care facilities per capita	Number of hospitals, health posts or centers operated by the Ministry of Health, Peruvian Social Security Institute, local government, or other state agency in the district, per 10,000 population	4.06	8.72
Unemployment rate	District rate of unemployment	7.76	3.13
Poverty rate	Provincial rate of unmet needs calculated by FONCODES	2.22	2.22
Head of household	Dichotomous: The individual is the head of household = 1; otherwise = 0.	0.35	0.48
Price of rice	Price in new soles of a kilogram of ordinary rice in the department as of November 1995	1.27	0.15
Price of milk	Price in new soles of a large can of evaporated milk in the department as of November 1995	1.57	0.11
Price of tomatoes	Price in new soles of a kilogram of tomatoes in the department as of November 1995	1.12	0.33
Residence in urban area	Dichotomous: Resides in urban or semi-urban area = 1 (based on INEI classification included in the survey); otherwise = 0.	0.78	0.42

[†] Calculated for the sample aged over 17 to under 70 years of age.

ANNEX II. LABOR PARTICIPATION EQUATION BY SEX AND REGION: PROBIT REGRESSION.[a]

Independent variables	Males		Females	
	Urban	Rural	Urban	Rural
1. Constant	−3.251***	−1.847***	−2.067***	−1.876***
	[−11.69]	[−4.02]	[−9.26]	[−4.89]
Individual characteristics	*1,735.9****	*101.5****	*1,021.5****	*109.1****
2. Age [10⁻²]	0.213***	0.107***	0.131***	0.088***
	[38.60]	[10.07]	31.21	[10.39]
3. Age squared [× 10⁻⁴]	−0.267***	−0.123***	−0.171***	−0.103***
	[−41.01]	[−9.80]	−31.96	[−9.98]
Human capital variables	*173.5****	*22.2****	*2.5*	*79.7****
4. Years of schooling [10⁻²]	0.133***	0.067***	0.014	0.044***
	[9.48]	2.81	[1.57]	[2.74]
5. Years of schooling squared [× 10⁻²]	−1.017***	−0.637***	−0.089	0.050
	[−11.69]	[−3.76]	[−1.41]	[0.40]
Household characteristics				
6. Head of household [X_L]	0.753***	1.369***	0.794***	1.763***
	[22.93]	[22.65]	[24.70]	[24.10]
Household assets	*135.6****	*4.7*	*22.1****	*13.2****
7. Non-labor income	−0.126***	−0.001	−0.041***	−0.242***
	[−11.42]	−0.01	[−3.74]	[−3.00]
8. Automobile [X_L]	0.006	−0.242**	−0.005	−0.092
	[0.16]	−2.15	[−0.17]	[−0.91]
9. Other vehicle [X_L]	0.044*	−0.006	0.053***	0.081*
	[1.84]	[−0.12]	[2.75]	[1.75]
Housing infrastructure	*14.8****	*11.4****	*11.7****	*49.2****
10. Hours of water supply [× 10⁻⁴]	1.134	6.625***	−0.577	7.488***
	[0.90]	[2.64]	−0.59	[4.28]
11. Adequate sewerage system	−0.104***	−0.236**	0.074***	0.218***
	[−3.74]	[−2.47]	[3.40]	[2.68]
12. Non-dirt floor	−0.022	−0.007	−0.011	0.320***
	[−0.30]	[−0.08]	[−0.19]	[4.15]
Regional variables	*111.2****	–	*6.3***	–
13. Residence in coastal region	0.074*	0.098	−0.076**	0.062
	[1.79]	[1.41]	[−2.28]	[1.11]
14. Residence in Lima	0.346***	–	0.089**	–
	[6.93]		[2.27]	
Community variables	*10.3****	*18.0****	*38.6****	*21.6****
15. Poverty indicator	−0.141	−1.035	0.578	6.691**
	[−0.27]	[−0.26]	[1.31]	[2.02]
16. Unemployment rate	−1.499***	−2.966***	−2.354***	−2.024***
	[−3.17]	[−4.15]	[−6.15]	[−3.42]
Health infrastructure	*2.0*	*3.1*	*4.1*	–
17. Number of health care facilities per capita	−0.319	−0.220	0.522	−0.251***
	[−0.58]	[−0.96]	[1.38]	[−3.86]
18. Number of health care facilities per capita squared	0.385	0.092	−0.569	0.018***
	[0.72]	[0.47]	[−1.55]	[3.11]
Food prices	*14.8****	*18.1****	*80.6****	*33.5****
19. Price of rice	−0.348***	−0.270	0.060	−0.154
	[−3.43]	[−1.59]	[0.74]	[−1.10]
20. Price of tomatoes	0.002	−0.128	0.033	0.040
	[0.04]	[−1.55]	[1.00]	[0.59]
21. Price of milk	0.205	0.366	−0.203*	−0.393**
	[1.55]	[1.60]	[−1.90]	[−1.99]
Joint test of significance [13]–[16]	*120.8****	*18.9****	*74.8****	*34.7****
Ln (Likelihood function)	*−7,908*	*−2,003*	*−13,201*	*−3,107*
Chi-square	*4,791****	*1,798.2****	*1,853****	*1,029.2****
X² [X_L] (identification variables)	*529.7****	*524.8****	*615.4****	*584.5****
Percentage accuracy	*81.9%*	*84.1%*	*61.0%*	*73.9%*
Number of observations	*18,787*	*5,633*	*20,465*	*5,671*

[a] Dependent variable: L = 1, if the individual works; otherwise, I = 0.

[t-statistics in brackets] and joint significance tests italicized

(*) Statistically significant at 10% confidence level; (**) Statistically significant at 5% confidence level; (***) Statistically significant at 1% confidence level.

ANNEX III. POLICY INSTRUMENT SIMULATIONS BY SEX AND REGION.

Simulation 1				
Policy	Urban males	Rural males	Urban females	Rural females
Mean of hours of water supply (by district) * 1.1	0%	0.1%	0%	0.1%
Mean of adequate drainage system (by district) * 1.1	0.1%	0%	0%	−0.1%
Mean of quality of flooring (by district) * 1.1	0.4%	0.3%	0.7%	0.3%
Percentage increase in hourly wage due to a 50% improvement in housing infrastructure at the district level	**0.4%**	**0.4%**	**0.7%**	**0.3%**

Simulation 2				
Policy	Urban males	Rural males	Urban females	Rural females
Mean of hours of water supply (by district) * 1.3	0.1%	0.4%	0.0%	0.3%
Mean of adequate drainage system (by district) * 1.3	0.0%	0.1%	0.1%	−0.2%
Mean of quality of flooring (by district) * 1.3	1.2%	0.9%	2.0%	1.0%
Percentage increase in hourly wage due to a 50% improvement in housing infrastructure at the district level	**1.3%**	**1.4%**	**2.1%**	**1.1%**

Simulation 3				
Policy	Urban males	Rural males	Urban females	Rural females
Mean of hours of water supply (by district) * 1.5	0.1%	0.7%	0.0%	0.4%
Mean of adequate sewerage system (by district) * 1.5	0.0%	0.1%	0.2%	−0.3%
Mean of quality of flooring (by district) * 1.5	2.0%	1.5%	3.3%	1.7%
Percentage increase in hourly wage due to a 50% improvement in housing infrastructure at the district level	**2.1%**	**2.3%**	**3.5%**	**1.8%**

ANNEX IV. WAGE EQUATIONS BY SEX AND REGION.

A. Wage Equation by Sex and Region, Including the Interaction Term of Health (IV) x Years of Schooling, Two-stage Estimation.[a]

Variables	Males		Females	
	Urban	Rural	Urban	Rural
1. Constant	−1.291**	−1.237*	−2.744***	−4.575***
	[−2.48]	[−1.65]	[−5.12]	[−5.82]
Individual characteristics				
2. Age	0.053***	0.056***	0.072***	0.047**
	[7.12]	[3.85]	[7.51]	[2.47]
3. Age squared [$\times 10^{-2}$]	−0.050***	−0.060***	−0.071***	−0.034
	[−5.53]	[−3.30]	[−5.84]	[−1.46]
Human capital variables				
4. Years of schooling	0.001	−0.635***	0.117	0.221
	[0.02]	[−4.76]	[1.59]	[1.23]
5. Years of schooling squared [$\times 10^{-2}$]	−0.280**	−0.715*	−0.177	0.153
	[−2.27]	[−1.76]	[−0.89]	[0.29]
6. Health [IV]	−0.261	−1.462	1.379	2.864**
	[−0.36]	[−1.19]	[1.48]	[2.41]
7. Health × Years of Schooling [IV]	0.154*	1.011***	−0.049	−0.182
	[1.76]	[4.39]	[−0.36]	[−0.59]
Local labor market variables				
8. Residence in Lima	0.278***	–	0.375***	–
	[14.40]		[15.00]	
9. Unemployment rate	0.526**	−0.211	−0.112	3.456***
	[2.22]	[−0.38]	[−0.33]	[4.18]
10. Selection term	−0.205***	0.139	−0.011	0.084
	[−3.71]	[1.53]	[−0.18]	[1.05]
Impact of health	*1.193***	*4.749***	*0.972***	*2.065***
	[4.4]	*[8.2]*	*[2.7]*	*[3.2]*
Rate of return to education	*7.4%***	*5.8%***	*5.1%***	*10.6%***
	[18.2]	*[8.1]*	*[12.0]*	*[9.2]*
Rate of return to health	6.0%	19.5%	3.1%	5.7%
Joint significance test [2]–[3]	182.6***	22.1***	163.6***	22.1***
Joint significance test [4]–[7]	1,194.4***	363.7***	648.0***	188.8***
Joint significance test [4]–[5]	10.1***	42.7***	24.9***	3.6
Joint significance test [8]–[10]	250.7***	2.4	226.1***	20.1***
Ln (Likelihood function)	−18,467	−7,129	−13,030	−3,245
Chi-square	232.4***	66.8***	137.6***	33.3***
Adjusted R²	0.127	0.106	0.114	0.119
Number of observations	14,321	4,445	9,598	1,908

[a] Dependent variable: ln(W), natural logarithm of hourly wage.
[t-statistic in brackets]
(*) Statistically significant at 10% confidence level; (**) Statistically significant at 5% confidence level; (***) Statistically significant at 1% confidence level.

B. Wage Equation by Sex and Region, Including the Interaction Term of Health (IV) x Age, Two-stage Estimation.[a]

Variables	Males		Females	
	Urban	Rural	Urban	Rural
1. Constant	−2.025***	−0.145	0.244	−3.877**
	[−2.66]	[−0.11]	[0.31]	[−2.36]
Individual characteristics				
2. Age	0.049*	−0.114**	−0.030	0.040
	[1.88]	[−2.47]	[−1.05]	[0.72]
3. Age squared [×10⁻²]	−0.047***	0.052**	−0.023	−0.036
	[−3.50]	[2.16]	[−1.44]	[−1.10]
Human capital variables				
4. Years of schooling	0.093***	−0.092***	0.076***	0.113***
	[8.07]	[−3.67]	[6.70]	[4.13]
5. Years of schooling squared [×10⁻²]	−0.099	1.161***	−0.177**	−0.110
	[−1.37]	[6.81]	[−2.41]	[−0.50]
6. Health [IV]	0.857	−0.296	−1.748**	1.841
	[1.16]	[−0.21]	[−2.23]	[1.08]
7. Health × Age [IV]	0.002	0.115***	0.092***	0.012
	[0.11]	[2.88]	[3.79]	[0.25]
Local labor market variables				
8. Residence in Lima	0.275***	–	0.359***	–
	[14.24]		[14.26]	
9. Unemployment rate	0.493**	0.689	0.188	3.387***
	[2.02]	[1.37]	[0.54]	[4.15]
10. Selection term	−0.194***	0.136	−0.031	0.083
	[−3.51]	[1.50]	[−0.52]	[1.04]
Impact of health	*0.940***	*3.952***	*1.500***	*2.285***
	[4.0]	*[7.5]*	*[5.3]*	*[3.9]*
Rate of return to education	*7.4%***	*5.0%***	*4.7%***	*10.4%***
	[18.4]	*[6.6]*	*[11.5]*	*[9.1]*
Rate of return to health	*4.7%*	*16.2%*	*4.8%*	*6.4%*
Joint significance test [2]–[3]	*21.2***	*6.3**	*49.8***	*2.2*
Joint significance test [4]–[7]	*1,192.6***	*352.0***	*663.0***	*188.5***
Joint significance test [4]–[5]	*615.2***	*182.5***	*156.3***	*114.4***
Joint significance test [8]–[10]	*247.8***	*5.2*	*208.8***	*19.9***
Ln (Likelihood function)	*−18,468*	*−7,134*	*−13,023*	*−3,245*
Chi-square	*232.0***	*65.2***	*139.4***	*33.3***
Adjusted R²	*0.127*	*0.104*	*0.115*	*0.119*
Number of observations	*14,321*	*4,445*	*9,598*	*1,908*

[a] Dependent variable: ln(W), natural logarithm of hourly wage.
[t-statistic in brackets]
(*) Statistically significant at 10% confidence level; (**) Statistically significant at 5% confidence level; (***) Statistically significant at 1% confidence level.

ANNEX V. HEALTH AND SALARY EQUATIONS BY SEX AND REGION.

TABLE Va. Health Equation by Sex and Region: Censured Tobit.[a]

Variables	Males		Females	
	Urban	Rural	Urban	Rural
1. Constant	−29.091***	−4.158	−22.100***	−11.736**
	[−5.46]	[−0.67]	[−5.60]	[−2.21]
Individual characteristics				
2. Age	−0.017	−0.146	0.149**	0.202*
	[−0.18]	[−1.14]	[2.08]	[1.76]
3. Age squared [×10⁻²]	0.274**	0.376**	0.085	0.021
	[2.30]	[2.44]	[0.97]	[0.16]
Human capital variables				
4. Years of schooling	−1.398***	−1.431***	−0.619***	−0.229
	[−5.19]	[−4.87]	[−3.94]	[−1.03]
5. Years of schooling squared [×10⁻²]	0.046***	0.070***	0.016	−0.008
	[2.66]	[3.19]	[1.46]	[−0.45]
Household assets				
7. Non-labor income	−0.262	0.439	−0.507**	1.221
	[−1.04]	[0.86]	[−2.47]	[1.39]
Housing infrastructure				
10. Hours of water supply [×10⁻²]	−0.104	−0.266	0.080	−0.577**
	[−0.46]	[−0.83]	[0.47]	[−2.05]
11. Adequate sewerage system	0.340	−1.329	−0.105	2.705**
	[0.66]	[−0.93]	[−0.27]	[2.32]
12. Non-dirt floor	−4.152***	−0.954	−4.262***	−2.112*
	[−2.96]	[−0.77]	[−4.14]	[−1.95]
Regional variables				
13. Residence in coastal region	1.864**	−1.467	1.903***	−2.934***
	[2.30]	[−1.58]	[3.19]	[−3.72]
14. Residence in Lima	−2.729***	−	−2.557***	−
	[−2.93]		[−3.69]	
Community variables				
15. Poverty indicator (at district level)	0.138	0.921*	0.103	0.012
	[1.50]	[1.74]	[1.41]	[0.03]
16. Unemployment rate (at district level)	0.174*	0.162*	0.198***	0.213***
	[1.90]	[1.66]	[2.94]	[2.63]
Health infrastructure				
17. Number of health care facilities per capita [×10⁻²]	0.053	−0.023**	0.127*	−0.011
	[0.58]	[−2.18]	[1.91]	[−1.26]
18. Number of health care facilities per capita squared [×10⁻²]	4.040	0.221**	−11.254*	0.160**
	[−0.46]	[2.38]	[−1.76]	[2.13]
Food prices				
19. Price of rice	15.590***	5.295**	10.761***	5.033**
	[7.99]	[2.30]	[7.53]	[2.57]
20. Price of tomatoes	4.266***	0.737	2.980***	1.115
	[5.33]	[0.67]	[5.02]	[1.15]
21. Price of milk	−5.430**	−8.001***	−4.983***	−6.033**
	[−2.20]	[−2.63]	[−2.68]	[−2.21]
∂H/∂ [Facilities]	4.045	−0.653**	3.852*	−0.402
	[0.35]	[4.72]	[3.70]	[1.53]
Joint test of significance [2]–[3]	135.6***	53.3***	236.0***	104.1***
Joint test of significance [4]–[5]	102.0***	45.3***	73.0***	16.4***
Joint test of significance [7]–[9]	9.1**	2.6	17.9***	11.9**
Joint test of significance [10]–[11]	8.9**	−	14.7***	−
Joint test of significance [12]–[13]	6.3**	4.5	11.3***	7.6**
Joint test of significance [14]–[15]	1.2	5.7*	4.8*	9.7***
Joint test of significance [16]–[18]	73.8***	10.4**	69.1***	9.8**
Ln (Likelihood function)	−23,367	−8,231	−33,104	−10,013
Chi-square	481.9***	214.0***	693.1***	288.0***
Prob [H*<1]	22.7%	29.1%	32.7%	38.0%
Number of observations	18,787	5,633	20,435	5,671

[a]Dependent variable: number of days ill.

[*t*–statistic in brackets]

TABLE Vb. Health Equation by Sex and Region: Probit Regression.[a]

Variables	Males		Females	
	Urban	Rural	Urban	Rural
1. Constant	−1.790***	−0.399	−1.449***	−0.621*
	[−7.04]	[−1.06]	[−6.33]	[−1.71]
Individual characteristics				
2. Age [×10⁻²]	0.472	−0.188	0.996**	1.306*
	[1.01]	[−0.24]	[2.38]	[1.65]
3. Age squared [×10⁻⁴]	0.808	1.666*	0.447	0.399
	[1.40]	[1.75]	[0.86]	[0.42]
Human capital variables				
4. Years of schooling	−0.034***	−0.060***	−0.027***	0.004
	[−2.58]	[−3.32]	[−2.91]	[0.26]
5. Years of schooling squared [×10⁻²]	0.067	0.294**	0.045	−0.185
	[0.79]	[2.18]	[0.69]	[−1.49]
Household assets				
7. Non-labor income	−0.016	0.014	−0.043***	0.145**
	[−1.34]	[0.42]	[−3.57]	[2.09]
Housing infrastructure				
10. Hours of water supply [×10⁻⁴]	−1.359	−3.668*	0.116	−3.196*
	[−1.24]	[−1.84]	[0.12]	[−1.69]
11. Adequate drainage system	−0.006	−0.047	−0.015	0.127
	[−0.26]	[−0.55]	[−0.68]	[1.57]
12. Non-dirt floor	−0.246***	−0.086	−0.295***	−0.140*
	[−3.67]	[−1.13]	[−4.91]	[−1.89]
Regional variables				
13. Residence in coastal region	0.113***	−0.136**	0.102***	−0.267***
	[2.91]	[−2.40]	[2.94]	[−4.95]
14. Residence in Lima	−0.164***	–	−0.188***	–
	[−3.69]		[−4.66]	
Community variables				
15. Poverty indicator [×10⁻²]	0.921**	7.260**	0.785*	1.609
	[2.07]	[2.25]	[1.79]	[0.51]
16. Unemployment rate [×10⁻²]	1.021**	1.096*	1.515***	1.520***
	[2.33]	[1.84]	[3.86]	[2.72]
Health infrastructure				
17. Number of health care facilities per capita	0.301	−0.146**	0.856**	−0.109*
	[0.68]	[−2.28]	[2.24]	[−1.82]
18. Number of health care facilities per capita squared	−0.206	0.015*	−0.749**	0.016***
	[−0.49]	[2.63]	[−2.04]	[3.00]
Food prices				
19. Price of rice	0.872***	0.412***	0.765***	0.366***
	[9.39]	[2.94]	[9.20]	[2.73]
20. Price of tomatoes	0.261***	0.101	0.219***	0.115*
	[6.85]	[1.50]	[6.37]	[1.74]
21. Price of milk	−0.259**	−0.629***	−0.303***	−0.567***
	[−2.19]	[−3.36]	[−2.79]	[−2.99]
∂H/∂ [Facilities]	0.285	0.795**	−0.142**	−0.104*
	[0.49]	[5.10]	[5.14]	[3.18]
Joint test of significance [2]–[3]	176.3***	68.9***	270.4***	120.5***
Joint test of significance [4]–[5]	46.8***	21.6***	56.8***	12.4***
Joint test of significance [7]–[9]	16.5***	5.7	7.1**	8.1**
Joint test of significance [10]–[11]	14.1***	–	21.8***	–
Joint test of significance [12]–[13]	10.5***	6.6**	19.1***	7.5**
Joint test of significance [14]–[15]	2.8	–	7.1**	–
Joint test of significance [16]–[18]	104.4***	17.9***	101.2***	15.0***
Ln (Likelihood function)	−9,492	−3,176	−12,116	−3,492
Chi-square	501.0***	219.0***	773.1***	327.8***
Percentage accuracy	78.6%	73.4%	70.0%	70.0%
Number of observations	18,787	5,633	20,435	5,671

[a]Dependent variable: reported illness rate.
[t-statistic in brackets]

TABLE Vc.   Salary Equation: Use of Number of Days III (OLS corrected by Heckman two-stage estimation).[a]

Variables	Males		Females	
	Urban	Rural	Urban	Rural
1. Constant	−1.164***	−0.091	−1.561***	−2.034***
	[−6.54]	[−0.27]	[−8.56]	[−5.42]
Individual characteristics				
2. Age	0.051***	0.004	0.073***	0.051***
	[6.87]	[0.32]	[10.14]	[3.35]
3. Age squared [$\times 10^{-2}$]	−0.049***	0.007	−0.074***	−0.043**
	[−5.38]	[0.49]	[−8.02]	[−2.35]
Human capital variables				
4. Years of schooling	0.088***	−0.109***	0.091***	0.103***
	[6.92]	[−3.86]	[8.02]	[3.84]
5. Years of schooling squared [$\times 10^{-2}$]	−0.067	1.242***	−0.231***	−0.026
	[−0.90]	[6.88]	[−3.18]	[−0.12]
6. Health indicator	−0.045***	−0.269***	−0.053***	−0.142***
	[−2.80]	[−6.25]	[−2.69]	[−3.19]
Local labor market variables				
7. Residence in Lima	0.274***	–	0.383***	–
	[14.17]		[15.44]	
8. Unemployment rate (at district level)	0.455*	1.246**	−0.211	3.722***
	[1.93]	[2.50]	[−0.62]	[4.57]
9. Selection term	−0.187***	0.117	−0.005	0.084
	[−3.41]	[1.28]	[−0.09]	[1.05]
Rate of return to education	7.5%	4.3%	5.3%	10.%
Age of maximum productivity	52.1	–	49.4	59.6
Joint test of significance [2]–[3]	159.5***	12.7***	184.0***	37.2***
Joint test of significance [4]–[6]	1,183.5***	333.4***	637.9***	182.6***
Joint test of significance [4]–[5]	429.0***	151.3***	232.5***	104.2***
Joint test of significance [7]–[8]	199.0***	–	238.7***	–
Hausman Test	127.9***	13.3***	405.5***	27.3***
Ln (Likelihood function)	−18,474	−7,144	−13,036	−3,248
Chi-square	259.7***	71.8***	153.5***	19.6***
Adjusted R^2	0.127	0.100	0.113	0.117
Number of observations	14,321	4,445	9,598	1,908

[a] Dependent variable: ln[W], natural logarithm of hourly wage.
[t-statistics in brackets]

TABLE Vd.   Salary Equation: Including Reported Illness Rate (OLS Corrected by Heckman Two-stage Estimation).[a]

Variables	Males		Females	
	Urban	Rural	Urban	Rural
1. Constant	−1.378***	−1.473***	−1.753***	−2.357***
	[−8.53]	[−5.79]	−[10.23]	[−6.34]
Individual characteristics				
2. Age	0.052***	0.028**	0.074***	0.049***
	[7.14]	[2.41]	[10.00]	[2.91]
3. Age squared [× 10⁻²]	−0.053***	−0.037***	−0.079***	−0.052**
	[−6.01]	[−2.83]	[−8.46]	[−2.55]
Human capital variables				
4. Years of schooling	0.108***	0.022	0.105***	0.124***
	[10.18]	[1.14]	[10.22]	[4.74]
5. Years of schooling squared [× 10⁻²]	−0.146**	0.548***	−0.280***	−0.080
	[−2.11]	[3.80]	[−3.90]	[−0.39]
6. Health indicator	0.296	−0.057	0.001	−0.078
	[1.12]	[−0.41]	[0.01]	[−0.58]
Local labor market variables				
7. Residence in Lima	0.266***	–	0.383***	–
	[13.91]		[15.44]	
8. Unemployment rate (at district level)	0.384	1.183**	−0.469	3.703***
	[1.64]	[2.36]	[−1.42]	[4.53]
9. Selection term	−0.185***	0.145	0.002	0.086
	[−3.38]	[1.59]	[0.04]	[1.08]
Rate of return to education	*8.1%*	*8.9%*	*5.9%*	*11.7%*
Age of maximum productivity	*49.1*	*37.3*	*46.7*	*46.8*
Joint test of significance [2]–[3]	*195.4*** *	*14.7*** *	*220.2*** *	*10.8*** *
Joint test of significance [4]–[6]	*1,176.5*** *	*291.7*** *	*630.2*** *	*171.8*** *
Joint test of significance [4]–[5]	*1,176.5*** *	*290.6*** *	*610.8*** *	*170.7*** *
Joint test of significance [7]–[8]	*238.6*** *	*–*	*238.5*** *	*–*
Hausman Test	*176.0*** *	*0.0*	*272.4*** *	*42.4*** *
Ln (Likelihood function)	*−18,477*	*−7,163*	*−13,039*	*−3,253*
Chi-square	*258.8*** *	*65.4*** *	*152.5*** *	*35.6*** *
Adjusted R²	*0.126*	*0.092*	*0.112*	*0.113*
Number of observations	*14,321*	*4,445*	*9,598*	*1,908*

[a] Dependent variable: ln[W], natural logarithm of hourly wage.
[t-statistics in brackets]

ANNEX VI. HEALTH AND PRODUCTIVITY STATISTICS.

TABLE VIa. Reported Illness Rates (%), by Age.

| | Reported illness rates (%) | |
Age groups	Illness rate	Distribution of the ill population
[0–10]	35.2	32.3
[11–20]	22.8	17.8
[21–30]	21.3	12.0
[31–40]	26.2	11.3
[41–50]	30.9	9.0
[51–60]	36.2	7.3
[61–70]	44.1	5.8
[70–]	50.3	4.5
Total	–	100.0

Source: National Household Survey, Peru, 1995.
Table prepared by the author.

TABLE VIb. Illness rate by per capita income.

| Per capita income quintiles | Reported illness rate (%) | |
	Males	Females
1	25.4	32.0
2	23.0	33.0
3	22.8	29.1
4	21.7	29.9
5	18.3	22.8
Total	22.2	29.4

Source: National Household Survey, Peru, 1995.
Table prepared by the author.

TABLES VIc. Reported illness rate.

1. By age and sex

| Age | Sex (%) | | Total (%) |
	Males	Females	
[18–24]	17.7	21.5	19.7
[25–34]	20.1	27.3	23.8
[35–44]	22.7	32.3	27.7
[45–59]	28.4	38.8	33.7
[60–70]	37.9	47.7	42.9
Total	23.2	30.8	27.2

Source: National Household Survey, Peru, 1995.
Table prepared by the author.

2. By age and years of schooling

| Age | Years of schooling (%) | | | | Total (%) |
	[0]	[1–6]	[7–12]	[13–]	
[18–24]	29.0	22.8	19.0	17.1	19.7
[25–34]	34.3	27.8	22.7	20.7	23.9
[35–44]	38.8	30.7	26.6	21.7	27.7
[45–59]	45.3	34.8	29.2	24.7	33.8
[60–70]	51.5	43.2	35.8	31.4	42.9
Total	43.1	31.6	23.3	21.2	27.2

Source: National Household Survey, Peru, 1995.
Table prepared by the author.

TABLES VId. Reported number of days ill.

1. By age and sex

| Age | Sex | | Total |
	Males	Females	
[18–24]	9.7	8.9	9.2
[25–34]	8.8	9.1	9.0
[35–44]	9.5	9.8	9.7
[45–59]	10.2	10.1	10.2
[60–70]	12.4	11.8	12.0
Total	9.9	9.8	9.9

Source: National Household Survey, Peru, 1995.
Table prepared by the author.

2. By age and years of schooling

| Age | Years of schooling | | | | Total |
	[0]	[1–6]	[7–12]	[13–]	
[18–24]	17.8	9.7	8.4	9.2	9.2
[25–34]	14.0	9.0	8.4	8.7	9.0
[35–44]	12.4	9.8	8.6	9.4	9.6
[45–59]	10.7	9.6	11.3	9.0	10.2
[60–70]	11.6	12.7	11.6	10.3	12.0
Total	12.0	10.1	9.0	9.1	9.8

Source: National Household Survey, Peru, 1995.
Table prepared by the author.

3. By years of schooling and area of residence

| Schooling (years) | Area | | Total |
	Urban	Rural	
[0]	11.9	12.1	12.0
[1–6]	10.4	9.4	10.1
[7–12]	9.0	8.8	9.0
[13–]	9.2	8.5	9.1
Total	12.5	11.8	9.8

Source: National Household Survey, Peru, 1995.
Table prepared by the author.

4. By years of schooling and sex

| Schooling (years) | Sex | | Total |
	Males	Females	
[0]	15.5	10.9	12.0
[1–6]	10.5	9.8	10.1
[7–12]	9.0	9.0	9.0
[13–]	8.3	9.9	9.1
Total	9.9	9.8	9.8

Source: National Household Survey, 1995.
Table prepared by the author.

TABLE VIe. Health care by income deciles (percentages).

Deciles of per capita income	Health services received by individuals who reported illness (%)
1	34.0
2	36.1
3	36.8
4	37.9
5	41.2
6	41.7
7	45.3
8	45.9
9	50.0
10	51.3
Total	41.4

Source: National Household Survey, Peru, 1995.
Table prepared by the author.

TABLE VIf. Household poverty rate by region (percentages).

Region	Poverty rate (%)			
	Non-poor	Poor	Extremely poor	Total (%)
Northern coast	63.9	21.7	14.4	100.0
Central coast	68.5	22.1	9.5	100.0
Southern coast	69.3	19.8	11.0	100.0
Northern highlands	53.5	25.6	20.9	100.0
Central highlands	61.9	20.2	17.8	100.0
Southern highlands	65.0	19.6	15.5	100.0
Jungle	61.0	20.1	18.9	100.0
Metropolitan Lima	78.8	17.4	3.8	100.0
Total	67.6	20.0	12.6	100.0

Source: National Household Survey, Peru, 1995.
Table prepared by the author.

Part III

Investment in Health and Poverty Reduction

HEALTH SYSTEM INEQUALITIES AND INEQUITIES IN LATIN AMERICA AND THE CARIBBEAN: FINDINGS AND POLICY IMPLICATIONS

Rubén M. Suárez-Berenguela[1]

BACKGROUND

This paper summarizes the results of studies on health system inequalities, inequities, and poverty carried out within the framework of the World Bank's EquiLAC Project and the PAHO/UNDP-sponsored Investments in Health Equity and Poverty Project (IHEP). Development of the EquiLAC and IHEP projects involved adopting an analytical framework and producing background and demonstration papers, regional overviews, and country case studies. The analytical framework adopted was an extension of the framework used in a comparative study on equity in the finance and delivery of health care systems in 10 developed countries—the ECuity Project—which was sponsored by the Commission of the European Communities (van Doorslaer et al., 1993).

The background papers include a review of state-of-the-art concepts and methods for assessing health system inequalities and inequities in developed and developing countries (van Doorslaer and Wagstaff, 1997) and of concepts and issues related to the analysis of poverty and health inequalities (Whitehead, 1999). Two demonstration papers use data from a 1988 Jamaican Living Standard Measurement Survey (LSMS) to show the ap-

plications of some of these concepts and methods. One paper focuses on concepts and methods for measuring health status inequalities (van Doorslaer and Wagstaff, 1998a), and another deals with measuring inequities in the delivery of health care (van Doorslaer and Wagstaff, 1998b). The regional overviews include a paper on health systems and health sector reform policies in Latin American and Caribbean countries (Bengoa et al., 1998) and a paper that proposes a taxonomy of national health systems of countries of the Latin America and Caribbean region (Suárez, 1998a).

The EquiLAC and IHEP projects sponsored eight case studies covering different aspects of health system inequalities, inequities, and poverty in six countries. The EquiLAC case studies focused on measuring health system inequalities in Brazil, Ecuador, Jamaica, and Mexico. The IHEP case studies focused on assessing the nature of health system inequalities affecting the poor (the lowest 20% of the income distribution) in Brazil, Ecuador, Guatemala, Jamaica, and Peru. These countries account for more than two-thirds of the Latin America and Caribbean region's population, GDP, and overall health expenditures.

All the case studies shared similar terms of reference and were based on intensive use of micro-data, or household-level data; health status; health service utilization; income and expenditures; and other socioeconomic characteristics of individuals and populations. The country case study reports include a description of the institutional structure and organization of national health systems, as well as a summary of national health expenditure accounts (flows of expenditure and sources of finance). They also include the results of the measurement and analysis of health care system inequalities and inequities: health status inequalities, inequalities and inequities in access to or utilization of health care services, and inequalities and inequities in the financing of national

[1] Economic Adviser, Consultant to the World Bank's "Equity in Health in LAC" (EquiLAC) project and to the Pan American Health Organization (PAHO)–United Nations Development Program (UNDP) project on "Investments in Health Equity and Poverty" (IHEP). My thanks to Noberto Dachs, Edward Greene, David Gwatkin, Amparo Gordillo, Cesar Vieira, and Jose Vicente Zevallos for their helpful comments on the earlier drafts. Also, I thank for their comments Arnab Acharya, George Alleyne, Ichiro Kawachi, Elsie Le Franc, William Savedoff, Michael Ward, Adam Wagstaff, and other participants at the International High-Level Meeting of Experts in Economics, Social Development, and Health on the "Impact of the Investments in Health on the Economic Growth, Household Productivity, and Poverty Reduction," organized by PAHO, at which partial results of the EquiLAC and IHEP projects were presented (5–6 October 1999). The usual disclaimer applies.

health systems. Most of the data were obtained from the most recent national household surveys, mainly Living Standards Measurement Study (LSMS) and national Household Income-Expenditure Surveys (HIES).

Most of the country case studies were carried out by local multidisciplinary research teams between June 1998 and January 1999. The Mexico case study began in November 1998, and a first draft of the report was completed in June 1999; preliminary findings of that report are included here. The team coordinators for the country case studies were Antonio Campino for Brazil, Enrique Lasprilla for Ecuador, Edgard Barillas for Guatemala, Karlt Theodore and Althea Lafoucade for Jamaica, Eduardo Gonzales and Susan Parker for Mexico, and Margarita Petrera and Luis Cordero for Peru. A list of country reports and members of national teams is included in this chapter's Annex.

LIVING CONDITIONS, INCOME INEQUALITIES, AND POVERTY: RESULTS

The countries included in the EquiLAC and IHEP studies differ widely in terms of population size and living conditions as assessed by the level of per capita income, income inequalities, and poverty. Despite this heterogeneity, however, these countries share some characteristics—a relatively high degree of income inequality, as compared with other countries in the world, and a large proportion of their population living in poverty.

Table 1 summarizes the indicators of the socioeconomic characteristics of these countries. In 1998, these countries' population ranged from 2.5 million in Jamaica, to 94 million in Mexico, and 165 million in Brazil. Ecuador and Guatemala had a total population of around 12 million each, and Peru's population was twice that size. All the countries included in the study can be classified as middle-income countries (per capita income above US$ 400). Per capita income in these countries, expressed in United States dollars (US$) adjusted for purchasing power parity (PPP), ranged from less than US$3,500 in Jamaica to around US$4,000 in Guatemala, US$4,500 in Ecuador and Peru, US$6,200 in Brazil, and more than US$8,000 in Mexico.

The countries included in the study can be characterized as countries with a relatively high degree of income inequality and a high percentage of their population living in poverty. The average Gini coefficient for countries of the Latin American and Caribbean region is 0.50. The Gini coefficients for these countries range from 0.41 to 0.60, which is above the average of 0.32 for developed countries. Moreover, the lowest degree of income inequality in the region, around 0.41 for Jamaica and Uruguay,

is similar to the average value of the Gini coefficient for East Asian countries.[2]

The relationship between the level of per capita income and the degree of income inequality and poverty is weak. Brazil, with almost twice the level of income as Jamaica, is the country with the greatest degree of income inequality; Jamaica has the lowest degree of income inequality. The Gini coefficient for Brazil is 0.60, and the ratio of the share of income going to the top and bottom quintiles of the income distribution is 26. Jamaica has a Gini coefficient of 0.41 and an income share ratio of top to bottom quintiles of 8. However, in spite of the high degree of income inequality, Brazil is the country with the lowest percentage of the population living in poverty—around 28%—because of its level of income per capita. For the rest of the countries included in the case studies, the Gini coefficient ranged from 0.46 (Peru) to 0.54 (Mexico), with large variations in the income share ratio of top to bottom quintiles (see Table 1). The population living in poverty—defined as those whose income is below the cost of a market basket of commodities providing a minimum intake or consumption of calories and proteins—ranged from less than one-third of the population in Brazil to more than three-fourths of the population in Guatemala. For the rest of the countries, the percentage of the population living in poverty fluctuated between 34% in Jamaica, 38.6% in Mexico, 49% in Peru, and 54.7% in Ecuador.

NATIONAL HEALTH SYSTEMS: A TAXONOMY

The national health care systems of Latin American and Caribbean countries are very diverse. History, ideology, and economic conditions have shaped and constantly modified the structure of national health systems. National health systems differ in terms of their organizational structure or institutional configuration, the principles guiding the role of government, and the role of the public and private sectors in the provision (financing and/or delivery) of health care services.

To analyze how national health systems performed in terms of equity, the systems were broadly classified into three categories: national health service systems (NHS),

---

[2] The Gini coefficient is an index for measuring income distribution inequality. The values of the coefficient range from 0 to 1. The value of the coefficient is close to 0 for a low degree of income distribution inequality and close to 1 for a high degree of income inequality. Data on regional averages of income distribution Gini coefficients are based on data from Denninger and Squire (1996) and are taken from the Inter-American Development Bank (1999). Gini coefficients for the countries presented in Table 1 were taken from the World Bank (1999) and the Inter-American Development Bank (1999).

TABLE 1. Summary indicators of countries participating in the EquiLAC and IHEP projects.

Country	Population (millions) 1998	Per capita income, 1998 PPP*	Gini coefficient	Ratio 20/20	% of population below PL-C[†]
Brazil	165.2	6,160	0.60	26	27.2
Ecuador	12.2	4,630	0.47	10	54.7
Guatemala	11.6	4,070	0.60	30	75.2
Jamaica	2.5	3,210	0.41	8	34.2
Mexico	95.8	8,190	0.54	16	38.6
Peru	24.7	4,410	0.46	12	49.0

Source: World Bank, *Social Indicators of Development*, database, 1999 (CD-ROM). PAHO Health Status Indicators, 1999.
*PPP = purchasing power parity, international dollars.
[†]PL-C = consumption-based poverty line.

national health insurance systems (NHIS), and highly fragmented or mixed national health systems (MNHS).[3] The systems were then ranked according to the relative importance of the government's role, from more statutory (mostly public) to less statutory (mostly private, market-oriented) national health systems.

The national health systems of countries included in the case studies range from a predominantly public national health services system (NHS) in Jamaica to a highly fragmented, market-oriented (predominantly private) mixed health system in Guatemala. In between, are Mexico, with a national social insurance system (NHIS), and Brazil, Ecuador, and Peru, with mixed national health systems (MNHS) characterized by various degrees of participation by public sector institutions (ministry of health and social security) in the provision of health care.

Countries with NHS were defined as those in which a central government institution plays a major role in the provision of health care services. Social health insurance institutions are nonexistent or play a minor role in the financing of the systems. The presence of private providers and the magnitude of private expenditures varies across the countries. To differentiate countries with effective restriction of the private market of health services and health insurance, NHS were further subdivided into nonmarket and open-market systems. Cuba is the only country with a nonmarket NHS system, as it is the only country in the Region where market transactions of health care services and health insurance are not allowed.

Countries defined as NHIS were those in which one or more social insurance institutions play a major role in providing (delivery and/or financing) health care services. Statutory social insurance systems cover about 50% or more of the total population. Health care expenditures through social insurance schemes are the main compo-

nent of public expenditures on health. The presence and relative importance of private sector institutions involved in managing social insurance funds and providing health care and health insurance services (including prepaid health plans) varies greatly across these countries. Table A1 in the Annex further differentiates NHIS according to their public or private nature and whether the health insurance system is organized into a single national system or multiple provincial or occupational-based systems.

Countries with MNHS were characterized as those in which public sector institutions play a relatively minor role in the provision of health care services. Resources of central government institutions involved in the delivery of health care services are limited (less than US$20 per capita). The coverage of mandatory social health-insurance systems is limited to fewer than one-third of the total population. The magnitude of private out-of-pocket expenditures on health services is relatively large, and the presence and relative importance of private insurance and prepaid health plans varies greatly according to the country's income per capita.

The broad classification categories presented above are similar to those used to classify national health systems of developed countries, based on the predominance of actual or planned methods of financing (Organization of Economic Cooperation and Development [OECD], 1987; van Doorslaer et al., 1993; WHO, 1997). However, within the framework of the OECD and WHO classification, most national health systems of Latin American and Caribbean countries would be classified as MNHS. Despite this, national health systems in Latin American and Caribbean countries are rather heterogeneous, with a relatively weak predominance of a "main" institution or source of finance characterizing most national health systems. None of the systems provides the universal and comprehensive coverage of health care services achieved by European national health systems.

---

[3] This section of the chapter is based on the background papers on health systems in Latin America and the Caribbean prepared by Bengoa et al. (1998) and Suárez (1998b).

Table 2 illustrates the characteristics of national health systems in terms of selected indicators. It includes the type of national health system, the number of public and private institutional providers of health care services, the level and public-private composition of national health care expenditures (total, per capita, and as a percentage of GDP), and the percentage of the population covered by the national social insurance systems.

The national health care systems of these countries can be characterized as open-market systems. The number of for-profit institutional providers of health care and their market share are relatively large compared with national health systems in developed countries. There are a significant number of private providers of health care and a relatively large private sector in the provision of health care services. Private expenditure on health—i.e., direct out-of-pocket expenditures and voluntary contributions to privately managed prepaid health plans and health insurance schemes—is the largest component of national health care expenditures. It represents around 53% in Mexico and 66% in Brazil. In Ecuador, Jamaica, and Peru, the public-private mix is around 50/50. In developed countries, excluding the United States, most institutional providers are public and not-for-profit institutions; the coverage of the systems is universal; and public expenditure and financing represent more than 70% of national expenditures on health.

In Brazil, whose system is classified as an MNHS, the public component of the Unified National Health System (Sistema Único de Saúde, SUS) has been financed through consolidation of the funds of public-sector institutions since 1989. Resources from the social insurance fund, managed by a decentralized government institution (INAMPS), were transferred to a national health fund. The management of the national health fund is being decentralized and administered by local (municipal) governments. In addition, there are a large number of decentralized public sector institutions (62) involved in providing specialized health care services or managing specific public health programs. These institutions have their own budgets but also receive transfers from the central government. In Brazil it is estimated that there are a total of 6,124 institutional care providers (hospitals and clinics). Of a total of 2,874 private hospitals, more than

TABLE 2. National health systems in Latin America and the Caribbean, selected indicators.

	Brazil	Ecuador	Jamaica	Mexico	Peru	Guatemala
Type of system	MNHS	MNHS	NHS	NHIS	MNHS	MNHS
Total national health expenditure (NHE) (millions US$, PPP)	74,410	3,010	470	38,160	5,190	1,080
NHE (% GDP)	7	5	5	5	5	3
NHE per capita (per capita US$, PPP)	456	251	186	406	216	103
Number of health sector institutions						
Public sector						
General budget	1 (24)	21	1	16 (31)	n.a.	n.a.
Own budget	62			2		
Of which						
Social security	4	1	(1)	4	1	1
Coverage of SI	n.a.	19%	n.a.	60%	30%	16%
Total institutional providers	6,124	299	31	3,033	n.a.	n.a
Of which						
Private sector						
hospital	2,874	132	7	2,096	n.a.	n.a.
Not-for-profit hospital	1,197	4	0	16	n.a.	n.a.
NHE composition						
Public (%)	34	52	49	47	51	45
Private (%)	66	48	51	53	49	55
Total (%)	100	100	100	100	100	100

Numbers in parentheses in Brazil and Mexico indicate the number of local governments; for Jamaica the number indicates the existence of a National Insurance Board that deals with health care insurance issues.

n.a. = not available.

Source: Developed by the author based on information from PAHO (1998, 1999), Suárez (1998a), World Bank (1999), and the country case study reports.

half are for-profit institutions. Direct out-of-pocket expenditures account for 40% of total national health expenditures. Contributions to privately managed prepaid health plans or private health insurance schemes represented 26% of national health care expenditures. It is estimated that around 30 million Brazilians (20% of the population) are enrolled in private health insurance or prepaid plans.

In Jamaica, which is classified as an NHS country, the Ministry of Health operates an extensive network of health posts, clinics, and hospitals. There are a limited number of private institutional care providers (private hospitals and clinics) and an incipient health insurance market. Seven of the thirty-one institutional providers are private for-profit hospitals. User fees are charged at many public facilities. There is a tendency for health professionals from the Ministry of Health to supplement low government salaries through private practice, often in government facilities, for which they pay a nominal fee to the government. Private practice by Ministry physicians and other health sector workers is widespread.

Mexico's system is classified as an NHIS. More than 60% of the population (around 54 million persons) is covered by a national health insurance system: the Mexican Social Security Institute (Instituto Mexicano de Seguridad Social; IMSS) for private sector workers and the Social Security and Services Institute for Government Employees (Instituto de Seguridad y Servicios Sociales de los Trabajadores del Estado; ISSSTE) for government employees. These two institutions own and manage a large network of health facilities. Participation of the Ministry of Health in the provision of curative services and in expenditure on health care delivery is relatively minor. There are many private providers of institutional and individual health care. Private hospitals account for around two-thirds of the total number of institutional providers, mostly for-profit institutions. The proportion of the population using private health care services is larger in the lowest and highest income quintiles than in the middle quintiles of the income distribution.

The national health systems of Ecuador, Guatemala, and Peru are classified as MNHS. In these countries the national health insurance fund is financed by compulsory employee-employer contributions to a national social insurance scheme, which is managed by decentralized public sector institutions. Coverage of the social insurance system is limited to fewer than 20% of the population. Ministry of Health budgets are relatively small—about half the amount of the budget managed by the social insurance institutions. Direct out-of-pocket payments are the main source of financing for national health expenditures. Coverage of and expenditures on private health plans and health insurance schemes are negligible.

The national health systems of these countries were ranked from more statutory (mostly public) to less statutory (mostly private, market-oriented): Jamaica (NHS) and Mexico (NHIS) thus form a first group, Brazil and Peru are a second group, and Ecuador and Guatemala are a third group. All the countries in the second and third groups have MNHS. This ranking is based on the institutional configuration of the systems and the relative importance of public sector institutions, the coverage of the population, and the relative importance of the resources managed by the systems. The relationship between the type of system and the degree of health inequalities is explored in the following section.

MEASURING HEALTH SYSTEM INEQUALITIES AND INEQUITIES

Concepts

Illness and medical care concentration curves, concepts of vertical and horizontal equity, and inequality and inequity indices were used to describe and measure the extent of health system inequalities and inequities: health status inequalities, inequities and inequalities in access/utilization of health care services, and inequities in financing.

Assessment of the inequalities in the health status of the population was based on the concept of illness concentration curves and an inequality index proposed by Wagstaff, van Doorslaer, and Paci (1989). The illness concentration curve (similar to Lorenz curves) plots the cumulative proportion of the population ranked by socioeconomic status (SES) against the cumulative proportion of ill health. Ill health or health status of the population was assessed in terms of the observed distribution of self-reported health status–related variables from survey questionnaires (LSMS). Depending on the country and year, surveys included questions on self-assessed health status (SAH) or on self-reported symptoms of illness or accident (SIA), and, in a few cases, questions on the number of restricted activity days (RAD) or days of impairment due to illness or accident. A direct standardization procedure was used to isolate the inequalities in health status and health needs arising from differences in the age and sex composition of different socioeconomic or income groups. The standardized illness concentration curve describes what have been called avoidable inequalities (Whitehead, 1998)—health inequalities attributable to differences in socioeconomic status. A health status inequality index (I^*) is defined as twice the area between the unstandardized and standardized illness concentration curves. The value of the inequality index is negative (<0) if there are avoidable inequalities favoring the rich; it is positive (>0) if inequalities favor the poor. A value of the inequality index close to zero indicates that existing inequalities are due to differences in the demographic characteristics of different socioeconomic groups rather than to differences in socioeconomic characteristics.

Inequalities in the delivery or access to health care services were assessed by the distribution of the utilization of health care services—curative, preventive, chronic care, or hospitalization—by socioeconomic groups. It was described by medical care concentration curves and health care and was measured by a medical care use concentration index (similar to Lorenz curves and Gini coefficient, respectively). A summary of the concepts for measuring health status inequalities is presented in Box 1.

Concepts of vertical and horizontal equity similar to those developed in the literature on public finance were used to assess inequities in the delivery and financing of health care systems.[4] The concept of horizontal equity applied to the delivery or utilization of health care services refers to the principle or requirement that persons with equal health needs be treated equally. The concept of vertical equity implies that persons with unequal health needs should be treated differently. The EquiLAC studies focus on assessing the horizontal equity principle: the extent to which persons in equal need have similar access/utilization of health care services.

Inequities in access to health care services were assessed by comparing observed patterns of utilization of health care services with estimates of the distribution of health care needs for those services. The "need for health care services" was derived by estimating what utilization of health care services would have been, by income group, once differences in utilization due to differences in age, sex, and differences in SAH, SIA, etc., were taken into account (standardized distribution of the utilization of health care). Several regression models and techniques were used to derive the (standardized) distribution of need for health care services. Differences between estimated "health care needs" and observed utilization of health care services were used to derive the index of (horizontal) inequity in access (*Hiwv*). The inequity in access is positive in the case of pro-rich inequity and negative in the case of pro-poor inequity. A comprehensive presentation of alternative concepts, methods, and statistical and econometric techniques for measuring health status inequalities and inequalities and inequities in delivery is contained in the background and demonstration papers prepared for the EquiLAC project (van Doorslaer and Wagstaff, 1997; 1998a; 1998b). A summary of the concepts for measuring inequalities and inequities in access/delivery of health care services is presented in Box 2.

Equity in the financing of national health systems was assessed in terms of the progressivity, regressivity, or proportionality or neutrality of the sources of revenue to finance government expenditures on health. The concepts of vertical and horizontal equity, combined with the benefit principle or the ability-to-pay principle, provide the framework for different approaches commonly used in assessing the equity of a tax system. The benefit principle states that individuals should be taxed according to the benefits they receive from the expenditure that is financed by tax revenue. The ability-to-pay principle states that individuals should be taxed according to their abilities to bear the tax burden. Under the benefit principle the concepts of horizontal and vertical equity will imply that individuals receiving the same (different) benefits will be identically (differentially) taxed. The concepts of horizontal and vertical equity imply that individuals with the same (different) ability to pay should be taxed similarly (differentially).

The EquiLAC studies assessed the equity in financing considering the ability to pay principle: the extent to which payments for health care services or contributions to the financing of national health care systems should be commensurate with the individual's or the family's ability to pay.[5] To assess the distribution of the benefits of government expenditures on health, the country case studies focused on a partial benefit incidence analysis, which measured the distribution of government expenditure on health care services by income groups. The concepts and methods used were similar to those used in the analytical and empirical work on fiscal incidence analysis sponsored by the World Bank and the International Monetary Fund (Selowsky, 1979; May, 1996; International Monetary Fund, 1998). Concerns about policy relevance and methods used in assessing the full fiscal incidence, coupled with limited availability of empirical studies and micro-level data, prevented us from asking investigators to conduct a full fiscal incidence analysis of government expenditure on health similar to the one conducted for the OECD countries.[6]

---

[4]A summary presentation of concepts and issues of equity and taxation can be found in an article by Zee H. in the IMF Tax Policy Handbook (Shome, 1995). Application of the concepts of vertical and horizontal equity to measure health system inequities is presented by Kakwani *et al.* (1997).

[5]Several methodological issues remain to be resolved, including the definition of income to be used, whether the ability to pay should be measured in relative or absolute terms, the degree of progressivity, and others.

[6]The case was made that an analysis of the distributive impact of government expenditures on health was a more relevant policy issue than the fiscal incidence of the sources of revenue. A common argument was that optimal revenue (tax) collection policies are based on efficiency rather than on equity considerations. Sector policies should focus on maximizing the distributive impact of government expenditures if equity is the main policy objective.

Box 1: Illness Concentration Curve, Standardization Methods, Inequality Index, and Measuring Avoidable Inequalities

The **illness concentration curve** $L(s)$ plots the cumulative proportion of the population ranked by socioeconomic status (SES), beginning with the least advantaged, against the cumulative proportion of illness, perception of illness, or another health status variable. If illness is equally distributed across all socioeconomic groups, the illness concentration curve will coincide with the diagonal line, the perfect equality line. If the illness concentration curve lies above (below) the diagonal, inequalities in illness favor the more (less) advantaged member of society. Health inequality is measured by a concentration index C, the value of which is twice the area between the illness concentration curve and the equality line. If the illness concentration curve coincides with the diagonal, the difference is zero ($C = 0$). If all illness is concentrated among the least advantaged, the illness concentration curve will be bowed out, above the equality line, and the concentration index C will be negative with values tending to -1. If illness is concentrated among the most advantaged, the illness concentration curve will be bowed in, below the equality line, and the value of C will tend to $+1$.

Direct and indirect **standardization** procedures were used to take into account the confounding effects of demographic factors on inequalities—i.e., differences in illness associated with differences in the age-sex structure of different SES groups or individuals. The standardized illness concentration curves describe health inequalities attributable to socioeconomic characteristics (avoidable inequalities). **Direct standardization** involves applying the age-sex-specific average illness rate of each SES group (ranked by social class, groups of persons with similar levels of educational attainment, or income groups) to the age-gender structure of the population. A concentration index ($C+$ or $I+$) is defined as twice the area between $L+(s)$ and the equality line. If the standardized illness concentration curve $[L+(s)]$ is close to diagonal, the corresponding concentration indices will tend to zero ($C+ > 0$). If the demographic characteristics of the least-advantaged groups of the society (the poor) make them more prone to illness, the standardized concentration curves will be bowed out, above the equality line, and the concentration indices will be negative (<0). If the demographic characteristics of the least-disadvantaged group of the society (the rich) make them more prone to illness, the concentration curve will be bowed in, below the equality line, and the value of the concentration index will be positive (>0).

Indirect standardization uses individual-level data. It involves substituting an individual's degree of illness with the degree of illness suffered on average by persons of the same age and gender. The standardized concentration curve is denoted by $L^*(s)$ and is measured by concentration index C^*, defined as twice the area between the standardized concentration curve and the equality line. An alternative **inequality index** (I^*) for measuring avoidable inequalities is defined as the difference between the concentration indices for the unstandardized and standardized illness concentration curves ($I^* = C - C^*$). The value of I^* is negative (<0) if there are avoidable inequalities favoring the rich (pro-rich inequalities) and positive (>0) if there are avoidable inequalities favoring the less-advantaged members of society (pro-poor inequalities).

Further readings: Wagstaff, van Doorslaer, and Paci (1991); Kakwani et al. (1997); van Doorslaer and Wagstaff (1998a).

All case studies used a common analytical framework, shared similar terms of reference, and were based on intensive use of micro-data, or household-level data, from the most recent national household surveys, mainly LSMS, national health surveys (ENSA), and (HIES). A summary of surveys used in the country case studies is presented in Table A2 of the Annex at the end of this chapter. Table 3 summarizes health status and health services variables used in the country studies to measure health status inequalities, inequalities and inequities in access/delivery of health care services, and the distribution of the benefits of government expenditures on health. The table also includes a description of the most common ranking variables used to assess the population's socioeconomic status.

The results obtained from country case studies should be seen as a first systematic attempt to measure health system inequalities in Latin American and Caribbean countries. The qualitative results, particularly those assessing health status inequalities, inequities in the delivery of or access to health care services, and distribution of the benefits of government expenditures on health, are very robust. Cross-country comparison of quantitative results is somewhat more limited. Differences in definition of variables, coverage, reference period, and contents of the surveys, together with some differences in estimation procedure, limit a direct cross-country comparison of all the quantitative results.

Different variables and models were used to assess health status inequalities. All the country case studies reported or acknowledged the existence of large health status inequalities, as measured by difference in mortality and/or incidence or prevalence of diseases and injuries (Zt) by different socioeconomic groups. However,

BOX 2: EQUITY IN DELIVERY/UTILIZATION OF HEALTH SERVICES: INEQUALITY AND INEQUITY INDICES

Equity in the delivery/utilization of health care is defined as a system in which consumption of health care is allocated or distributed according to need rather than socioeconomic status. This egalitarian view is consistent with policy statements in European countries and Canada, with national health care systems providing universal coverage, as well as policy objectives of health sector reform in countries of the Latin America and Caribbean region. The principle of horizontal equity applied to the delivery of health care requires that persons with equal needs should be treated the same; thus, persons with equal needs should have similar patterns of utilization of health care services. The distribution of utilization of health care services is described by a *medical care concentration curve* [$Lm(s)$]. The $Lm(s)$ curve plots the cumulative proportion of utilization of health care services (vertical axis) ranked by socioeconomic group (horizontal axis) similar to the Lorenz curve. **Inequality in the utilization** of health care services is measured by the corresponding concentration index Cm (similar to a Gini concentration coefficient). It is defined as the area between the medical care concentration curve and the equality line (horizontal).

Need for medical care utilization of different socioeconomic groups is estimated by the method of indirect standardization. This method provides estimates of the amount of medical care a person would have received if he/she had been treated in the same way that others with the same characteristics of need were, on average, treated. Distribution of "need" is described by a *need concentration curve* [$Ln(s)$]. The $Ln(s)$ curve plots the cumulative proportion of the population—ranked by SES—against the cumulative proportion of "needed" medical care utilization. The corresponding index of inequality of health needs is denoted by Cn and defined by the area between the need concentration curve and the equality line.

Horizontal inequity is assessed by comparing the distribution of utilization (medical care concentration curve) with the distribution of need (need concentration curve). If the need concentration curve [$Ln(s)$] lies above the medical care concentration curve [$Lm(s)$], there is horizontal inequity favoring the better off (pro-rich inequity). If the $Ln(s)$ lies below $Lm(s)$, there is inequity favoring the worst-off (pro-poor inequities in access/utilization). Inequity in the delivery is measured by an **inequity index** ($Hiwv$) derived by comparing the actual distribution of the utilization of health care across socioeconomic groups with the distribution of need. $Hiwv$ is defined as twice the area between the need and utilization or medical care concentration curves, or, equivalently, as the difference between the concentration index of utilization of health care (Cm) and the concentration index for need (Cn): $Hiwv = Cm - Cn$. If the distribution of utilization of medical care and need coincide, health services are being used according to need, and the inequity index is equal to zero. It indicates proportionality in the distribution of health need and utilization of health care services. A positive value of the inequity index ($Hiwv > 0$) indicates horizontal inequity favoring the rich (pro-rich inequity), and a negative value of the inequity index ($Hiwv < 0$) indicates horizontal inequity favoring the poor (pro-poor inequity).

Further readings: Wagstaff, van Doorslaer, and Paci (1991), van Doorslaer and Wagstaff (1997, 1998b).

the analysis of health status inequalities focuses on the analysis of self-reported health status variables belonging to the subjective, medical, and functional models. Questions on qualitative (very poor, poor, fair, good, or very good) SAH—the subjective model—were included in the questionnaire of one round of the LSMS in Brazil (1996–1997), Jamaica (1989), and Mexico (1994). The country reports from these three countries present the findings on illness concentration curves and the inequality index of SAH variables. All the surveys included questions on self-reported SIA—the medical model. Few surveys (only those in Brazil, Ecuador, and Jamaica) included questions on the days of disability or RAD due to illness or injury—the functional model. Several of the surveys included specific questions on whether the onset of the illness or injury occurred in the preceding four weeks, the number of days suffered from the symptoms of reported illness or injury, and the existence of a chronic health problem.

In all the surveys the general questions about SAH, SIA, and RAD were very similar. However, there were some differences in the reference period and the person answering the surveys. In most surveys (LSMS) the reference period for the general health questions was the four weeks before the interview. The Mexican survey (ENSA), however, used a reference period of only two weeks. Also, whereas in most countries the reporting on SAH and/or SIA was done by the person concerned, in the Mexican case study the woman in the home (mother or wife) answered for all the household members.

The perceived health status questions were aimed at detecting subjective factors that may affect the demand for services rather than the actual health status of individuals. However, it was noted that self-reported health

TABLE 3. Variables used in assessing health system inequalities and inequities, selected countries, summary.

	Countries					
	Brazil	Ecuador	Jamaica	Mexico	Peru	Guatemala
Health status						
Mortality/morbidity indicators (Zt)	x	x	x	x	x	x
SAH	x		x	x		
SIA[a]	x	x	x	x	x	
RAD due to illness or accident	x	x				
Health care services						
Curative	x			x		
Chronic	x					
Preventive	x			x		
Outpatient		x				
Hospitalization		x		x		
Institutional					x	
Noninstitutional (private)					x	
Other			x			x
Benefit incidence analysis (partial)	n.a.			n.a.		
MOH, total		x	x			x
MOH, hospitals and health center/posts					x	
Ranking SES variable(s)	Pcy	Pce	Pce	Pce	Phy	Geo

[a]In general a four-week reference period, with the exception of Mexico, where it was two weeks.
x = variables included in the analysis. n.a. = not applicable.
Definitions of ranking SES variables: Pcy, per capita income; Pce, per capita consumption expenditure (adult) equivalent; Phy, average household income; Geo, geographical, by province or department according to level of poverty.

status variables do not reflect actual health status inequalities as measured by differences in morbidity and mortality by different socioeconomic groups. In addition, concerns were expressed by the investigators involved in the studies about the fact that the inequality index of standardized variables, by eliminating existing differences in the age and sex composition of different socioeconomic groups, would show a lesser degree of inequality.

Estimates of inequalities and inequities in access to and/or delivery of health care services were based on data on health care utilization patterns. General questions on care-seeking behavior by income group were supplemented with detailed information on the type of services and type of providers. However, not all the countries classify health care services in the same way. The Brazil study was based on a differentiation between curative, preventive, and chronic care. Services were classified into outpatient and hospital services in the case of Ecuador. The Mexican case study used curative, preventive, and hospital-type services, whereas in Peru services were classified as institutional (hospitals, health centers, and health posts) and noninstitutional (private). Several surveys included basic and follow-up questions on the type of illness or condition for which health care services were sought. The country case studies went to different lengths and depths in analyzing detailed data on more specific types of services and illness conditions.

The population's socioeconomic status (the ranking variable) was measured by household income, household expenditure, or the percentage of population living in poverty in the place of residence or province/department. It was suggested that, ideally, households should be ranked in terms of expenditure per adult equivalent to correct for differences in household size and composition (numbers of adults and children). The equivalence scales suggested were similar to those proposed by Aronson et al. (1994).[7] However, not all the case studies were able to follow this adjustment procedure. In Ecuador, Jamaica, and Mexico, the distribution of household income was adjusted by using consumption adult equivalence scales (Pce) by quintiles and deciles. The ranking variable used in the Brazil study was per capita income by quintiles; in Peru, per capita household income by deciles and quintiles (Phy) was used. Data on income or expenditures were not available for Guatemala, so the population was grouped by quintiles according to degree of rural poverty in the province or department (Geo).

In addition to income or expenditure variables, some of the case studies explored inequalities with other socioeconomic ranking variables. Urban/rural and indigenous/nonindigenous categories were used in the

---

[7]The rationale for this adjustment procedure is discussed in the demonstration paper by van Doorslaer and Wagstaff (1998b, p. 11).

Ecuador and Guatemala case studies. City size and rural area categories were used in Ecuador and Jamaica, and extremely poor, poor, and nonpoor categories were used in the Guatemala and Peru studies. Gender and age variations were analyzed in the Jamaica, Mexico, and Peru case studies.

Most of the estimates on inequity in the financing of national health care systems were based on results from secondary sources on the fiscal incidence of different sources of government revenues. These results, combined with those relating to the structure of financing of health sector public institutions, were used to assess the proportionality, progressivity, or regressivity of the financing of government expenditures on health. Methods used in assessing fiscal incidence varied significantly across countries, and the authors of the country case studies of the EquiLAC and IHEP projects expressed concerns about the methods and some of the results of those studies. Limited availability of micro-level data on taxes and contributions to social security by different income groups did not allow estimation of an inequity index (Kakwani's index) for financing; instead, only qualitative results are presented.[8]

In general, all the countries reporting estimates of the distribution of the benefits of government expenditures on health followed a similar procedure. Data on government expenditures by different types of services, combined with data on health care utilization patterns (both public and private services), were used to allocate government expenditures to different income groups on a cost-of-services basis (average expenditure by type of services). Differences in allocation procedures will not significantly change the distribution of benefits by different socioeconomic or income groups.[9]

Differences in the definition of variables and estimation methods are major drawbacks for a direct cross-country comparison of the quantitative results of concentration curves and inequality and inequity indices.[10] However, in spite of these differences, there are some common findings with regard to the signs of inequalities and the relative magnitudes of health inequalities that seem to hold across countries. These findings are summarized in the following section.

Findings

The general findings from the country case studies are as follows:

- In all the countries except Jamaica, the studies found significant pro-rich health status inequalities. These pro-rich health status inequalities were constant regardless of the proxy variables used to measure such inequalities: SAH status in Brazil, Jamaica, and Mexico; SIA in Brazil, Ecuador, Mexico, and Peru; and chronic illness in Brazil and Jamaica. Although small pro-poor inequalities were found in Jamaica (SIA) and in Mexico (chronic illness), they were statistically significant only in the case of Mexico (Table A3).

- Inequalities in perceived health status were relatively small compared with the large overall socioeconomic and income inequalities and with inequalities in mortality rates by income groups. The health status inequalities index (I^*) ranged from −0.09 to +0.018, over possible values of −1 to +1. Socioeconomic inequalities measured by Gini coefficients of the income distribution ranged from 0.41 to 0.60, over possible values of 0 to 1.[11]

- All the country case studies found significant pro-rich inequities in access ($Hiwv > 0$). Inequities in access to preventive care (Brazil, Ecuador, and Mexico) were more pronounced than inequities in access to curative care. The average $Hiwv$ of these countries was +0.130 for preventive care and +0.080 for curative care. Jamaica and Peru were the two countries with the largest inequities in access to curative care: inequity indices of +0.170 and +0.111, respectively. A lower degree of inequity in access to chronic care was found in the case of Brazil (+0.06). Inequalities in access/delivery of health care were less pronounced overall than socioeconomic or income inequalities (see Table A4).

- Private expenditures—which are the main source of financing for national health systems, accounting for between 48% and 66% of overall national expenditures on health—were found to be progressive. Private expenditure inequalities are closely related to income inequalities. Private expenditures on health

---

[8]The Kakwani index of inequity measures the changes in the distribution of income resulting from different types of taxes; it is equivalent to the difference in the Gini coefficients of the pretax and the actual income distributions (after taxes).

[9]An alternative method, although more difficult, would have been to allocate the benefits of government expenditures on a "willingness to pay" basis. This method would have better captured differences in the quality of services provided by public and private providers.

[10]These problems with differences in definition of health status and health variables of data sources and estimation procedures are not more severe than the ones encountered in the ECuity study [see van Doorslaer *et al.* (1993, pp. 50–97)].

[11]Inequalities in infant mortality rates were −0.284 in Brazil and −0.150 in Nicaragua. These values of the infant mortality concentration index are from Wagstaff (1999).

were more concentrated than the distribution of income in the cases of Brazil, Guatemala, Jamaica, Mexico, and Peru. In these countries, the share of private expenditure on health increased with level of income (income elasticity >1). In Ecuador the study found that the share of private expenditures on health was higher in the third and fourth quintiles than in the first, second, and fifth quintiles.

• Inequalities in the health status of the population were less pronounced than inequalities and inequities in access. Inequalities and inequities in access, in turn, were less pronounced than inequalities in private expenditure on health-related goods and services.

• The results suggest that financing of public health systems tends to be regressive (Ecuador, Guatemala, Jamaica, and Mexico) or, at best, neutral (Jamaica). Progressivity (or regressivity) in financing was undetermined in the case of Brazil and unknown in the case of Peru. Taxes (direct and indirect) were the main source of financing for government programs in Jamaica and Brazil. Contributions to social security were the main component of the public health system in Mexico. Taxes and contributions to social security were of equal importance in Ecuador, Guatemala, and Peru.

• The distribution of the benefits of government expenditures on health were pro-poor in the case of Jamaica, neutral in Peru, and pro-rich in Ecuador and Guatemala. No estimates were presented for the cases of Mexico and Brazil. In Jamaica, government expenditures represented 2.8% of GDP, 25% of which was received by the poorest 20% (first quintile) of the population. In Peru, MOH expenditures on health represented 1.5% of GDP, and each quintile received one-fifth of the benefits. In Ecuador and Guatemala, the MOH budget represented <1% of GDP, and around 30% of government expenditures benefited the richest 20% (the top quintile).

More detailed findings with regard to the various dimensions of health system inequalities are summarized below.

Inequalities in Health Status

Differences in self-reported health status by socioeconomic groups are relatively small compared with the large differences in health status measured by rates of disease incidence and prevalence and mortality (Zt). This is so even though low-income groups are more exposed to environmental risks, suffer illness more frequently than the rich, live shorter lives, and report more days of disability due to illness and accidents. This conclusion holds for almost all the countries, regardless of the variable used: SAH variables (subjective model) or self-reported SIA variables (medical model).

Figure 1 shows the slope of the relationship between these health status variables and income (by quintiles). The numerical values of these indices have been created for illustrative purposes only. The equality line indicates that all members of the population have similar health status, regardless of their income level. Points above the equality line indicate values of that particular indicator greater than the national average. Values below the equality line indicate values of the indicator below the national average. The slope or gradient of the illness distribution line is equivalent to the health status inequality coefficient. A negative slope indicates pro-rich inequalities in the distribution of ill health. Positive values—an upward sloping illness–income line—indicate pro-poor inequalities. Actual values of the concentration curves and inequality indices for different self-reported health status variables are shown in Table A3 in the Annex.

SAH. The Brazil and Mexico surveys included a qualitative question on SAH status that could be answered as excellent, very good, good, fair, or poor. The Brazil study found that the percentage of people reporting better-than-good health increased with income, from 76% in the lowest quintile to 87% in the top quintile (pro-rich inequalities). An opposite result was found in the case of Mexico: around 37% of the population in the lowest quintile reported good or very good health, whereas in the highest quintile the proportion was around 26%. In the case of Brazil, standardization enhanced the positive correlation between SAH and income. In the case of Mexico, standardization procedures yielded the opposite result: health

FIGURE 1. Inequalities in health status. Inequity index (gradient) by income quintiles or socioeconomic groups.

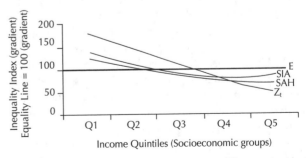

status improved with income, but there was little variation between percentage of population in the lower and upper quintiles. These findings are similar to those derived from an analysis of an early round of the Jamaican LSMS survey contained in one of the demonstration papers produced for the EquiLAC project (van Doorslaer and Wagstaff, 1998a).

The lack of significant pro-rich inequalities in SAH is reflected in the shape of the concentration curves, which are close to the equality line, and in the values of the concentration (C, $C^*/C+$) and inequality (I^*) indices, which are close to zero (see Table A3). The values of the coefficients are similar to those observed in Sweden and other developed countries with quite egalitarian health care systems (Wagstaff and van Doorslaer, 1998a).

SIA. In general, perception of SIA is inversely related to level of income and is much closer to the perfect equality line. Differences in the perception of illness or accident are relatively small compared with differences in the distribution of income or inequalities in the distribution of other socioeconomic variables.

In Brazil the relationship between SIA and income was negative: 27% of the population in the first (poorest) quintile versus 21% in the highest (richest) income quintile (the national average was 23.4%). In Ecuador the proportion of the population reporting SIA showed little variation across income groups or by urban and rural location. The population reporting SIA ranged from 40.3% in the second quintile to 42.8% in the third quintile. The proportions of population reporting SIA in the lowest and highest quintiles were similar—around 46%. For the population in urban and rural areas, the average was around 42%. Differences in the perception of SIA by different ethnic groups showed that indigenous populations, mainly rural and poor, reported less SIA than those self-classified as nonindigenous (36% versus 42%).[12]

The population in Jamaica reported fewer symptoms of illness or accidents than in other countries: 11.8%. No systematic variation seems to exist in the percentage of people reporting SIA by income group (quintiles) or by age group (adults and children). Reporting of SIA was more frequent in females than in males, and reporting of SIA was also higher in rural than in urban areas.

The Mexico case study found a negative relationship between percentage of population reporting SIA and income level, indicating some pro-rich inequalities. Standardization procedures resulted in a change in the slope of the relationship between these two variables (pro-poor inequalities) but, again, with little variation in the per-

centage of population by income group. In the case of Peru, the proportion of population reporting SIA in 1997 was 36%. Perception of SIA and income showed a positive correlation: the percentage of population reporting SIA in the poorest quintile was 33%, whereas the average for the highest-income quintile was 40%.

The relationship between SIA by type of symptom or illness and income, on the other hand, was not homogeneous. In the case of Brazil, the proportion of SIA related to respiratory illnesses (flu, cold, pneumonia) and digestive tract infections was higher in the lower-income group than in the higher-income quintile, signifying pro-rich inequalities. Reporting of SIA associated with infectious diseases, accidents, dental problems, and other nonspecified symptoms was positively correlated with income, again indicating pro-poor inequalities.

Although no clear relationship was found between overall reporting of chronic diseases by income level, some specific chronic diseases did show a correlation with level of income. In Brazil, chronic heart problems, hypertension, and diabetes were more prevalent in high-income groups, whereas chronic respiratory, digestive tract, and neuropsychiatric illnesses were reported more frequently in low-income groups. In the case of Mexico, both standardized and nonstandardized distributions showed pro-poor inequalities, with a positive relationship between overall reporting of chronic illness and income. Because standardized distribution corrects for differences in the demographic characteristics of different income groups, findings of pro-rich inequalities in the perception of chronic illness suggest that the poor may be less aware of chronic diseases. Lack of awareness of chronic conditions may be due to cultural or educational factors and to relatively low levels of access to or utilization of health care services.

Jamaica is the only country with continuous and systematic collection of data from 1989 to 1996 through LSMS-type surveys. Results from these surveys show a significant decline in the percentage of persons reporting SIA during the reference period: from around 17% of the population in 1989–1990 to around 10% in 1995–1996. The largest reduction in the perception of SIA occurred in the low-income groups. However, results with regard to protracted (extended period) illness or injury suggest a different pattern. The percentage of the population reporting protracted illness or injury has been increasing over time: from around 23% in 1989–1990 to 33% in 1995–1996. With the exception of the results for 1990, no systematic variation in the percentage of population reporting protracted illness by income group was found. However, over this period, the slope of the relationship between protracted illness by income group seems to have tilted upward, and the increase in the percentage of

---

[12]The percentage of population classified as indigenous is very low: only about 5% of the total population.

the population reporting protracted illness was greater in the high-income groups.

RAD. In Brazil, around 40% of the population reported an average of 3 RAD due to some symptom or health problem or accident. No significant variations existed in the percentage of the population reporting RAD by quintile. In Ecuador, the population reported an average of 6.7 days of inactivity due to illness or accident—more than twice the number of days reported in Brazil. Moreover, the number of RAD in Ecuador was inversely correlated with level of income. The lowest quintile reported an average of nine days of inactivity due to illness, whereas the average for the fourth and fifth quintiles was five days.

Inequalities and Inequities in Access: Pro-rich Inequalities in Preventive and Curative Care Services

Inequalities in access are relatively large and significant. Utilization of health care services is, in general, positively correlated with level of income. Inequities in access, measured by the gap between health needs and actual utilization of health care services, are inversely correlated with income level. The lower the level of income, the larger the gap between health needs and utilization of health care services. This finding holds regardless of the measure of health needs used (Figure 2). In addition, standardization procedures to derive the inequity-in-access index yielded similar results—namely, pro-rich inequities in access to health care services.

The Brazil study analyzed access/utilization of health care services by grouping questionnaire data on utilization into three types of health care services: curative, chronic, and preventive care. Pro-rich inequalities and inequities in access were more pronounced for preventive care than for chronic and curative care. For the three types of health care services, the study found a positive association between frequency of utilization of health care services and income levels (deciles or quintiles). Although there was little difference in reporting of SIA by different income groups, health care services were more frequently used by high-income groups than by low-income groups. The slope of the relationship between utilization and income declines as one moves from preventive to chronic to curative care.

The study also found significant differences by income group in the type of providers and facilities used. Health centers and public hospitals were more often used by poor and low-income groups, whereas use of private physicians, clinics, and hospitals was more frequent among higher-income groups. Nevertheless, the study found that the inverse relationship between income level and use of public hospitals did not hold in the case of specialized public hospitals. The higher-income group tended to make intensive use of specialized public hospitals, particularly those offering costly medical treatments and clinical procedures. The survey showed small differences by income group in the type of provider consulted.

In the Ecuador study, inequalities in access/utilization were assessed by comparing the use of outpatient and inpatient services by income group overall; by type of facility, hospital, clinic, or health center; and by geographic location of the facility (large metropolitan area, medium or small urban area, or rural area). Use of outpatient services by high-income groups (the top quintile) was more than twice that of the low-income group (the bottom quintile). Eighty percent of outpatient services were provided at hospitals and clinics and 20% in health centers; 70% of outpatient visits occurred in urban areas and 30% in rural areas. High-income groups made more intensive use of hospitals and clinics than low-income groups—between two and three times more. In both urban and rural areas, the poorest 20% of the population accounted for fewer than 12% of outpatient visits at hospitals and clinics. Variations in the use of health centers for outpatient consultations by income group were relatively small. The middle-income groups, those in the second to fourth quintiles, made more use of outpatient services at health centers than the population in the lowest and highest income groups. Inequalities in the utilization of inpatient services were more concentrated than utilization of outpatient services. Utilization of health care services by the high-income group was two to three times greater than that of the low-income group. The low-income group accounted for 8.4% of total inpatient services, and the high-income group accounted for 28.4%.

FIGURE 2. Inequity in the delivery/access to health care services: preventive, curative, and chronic care.

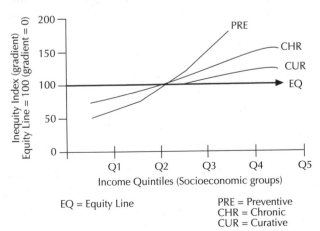

EQ = Equity Line

PRE = Preventive
CHR = Chronic
CUR = Curative

More than two-thirds (69%) of inpatient health care services were provided at clinics and fewer than a third (31%) were provided at hospitals. Approximately 77% of inpatient services were provided in urban facilities. The rural poor—the rural population in the lowest 20% of the income distribution—accounted for less than 5% of total use of inpatient services at hospitals and clinics.

The Peru study presents a breakdown of utilization by institutional and noninstitutional providers and utilization of institutional services by type of provider: Ministry of Health, social insurance, or private provider. No differences were found in the distribution of access to or use of institutional or noninstitutional providers, but there were large differences between income groups in the distribution of service use by type of providers. Although still favoring the rich, visits at Ministry of Health facilities were more equally distributed than visits to social insurance facilities and visits to private providers. Within the Ministry of Health services, visits to health posts and centers were more equally distributed than visits to hospitals (Gini coefficients of 0.0694 and 0.1793, respectively).

It was found that the poor in Peru made more intensive use of government services than did high-income groups: 61% of visits by low-income groups were to MOH facilities versus only 18% of visits by high-income groups. However, because of large differences in utilization rates between these two groups, there were only small differences in the distribution of public subsidies accruing to low- and high-income groups. Only 25% of the population with SIA in low-income groups sought medical attention, whereas this proportion was 62% in the high-income group. Inequalities in the use of prenatal care services by low- and high-income groups were even more marked: 1.4 prenatal visits per newborn in the lowest quintile versus 6 in the highest (Francke, 1998).

In the case of Mexico, the study found that, although health needs were evenly distributed across different socioeconomic groups, there were significant disparities and inequities in access to health care services. The Mexico case study reported utilization patterns for adults only (18 years of age and over) and for the total population. The study examined the utilization of hospitalization, curative care, and preventive care services. The reference period was one year for hospitalization and two weeks for preventive and curative services. Unstandardized data show a steep slope for utilization of all types of health care services by income group. The proportion of people reporting use of hospital and preventive services in the lower quintiles was half the proportion of those in the top quintile of the income distribution: 1.2% versus 2.1% in the case of preventive services, and 2% versus 4.2% in the case of hospital services. In terms of utilization of

curative health services, the proportion ranged from 40% in low-income groups to 61% in the high-income group. Standardized distribution of utilization of health care services—used as a proxy for health needs—showed little variation in the health needs of the population.

In all the countries studied, the poor used services provided at public-sector facilities (hospitals, clinics, and primary health care posts) more intensively. Use of private providers was positively correlated with income level. Higher-income groups used private-sector providers (visits and medical services at private physicians' offices, private clinics, or private hospitals) more intensively. Use of public clinics and health posts by high-income groups was minimal.

A separate study on health inequalities carried out recently in Chile with a similar methodology found that differences in the reporting of SIA across income groups were not significant. Although results from the EquiLAC project found pro-rich inequalities in access, the findings of this study suggest that utilization of health services is very similar across income groups (Sapelli and Vial, 1998).

Inequalities in the Financing and Distributive Impact of Government Expenditure on Health Care Services

Financing. Results from the country case studies suggest that financing of national health systems tends to be regressive or, at best, neutral. Full fiscal incidence analysis was limited by lack of current data or studies on fiscal incidence of different revenue collection instruments. Most of the empirical evidence on the fiscal incidence of different sources of revenue for countries of the region seems to show that, while direct taxes are progressive, indirect taxes are highly regressive (Inter-American Development Bank, 1999).[13] The country case studies bear out that finding. The argument is made that because government expenditure on health is financed with general tax revenues—mainly indirect taxes—the financing of the public component of national health systems is, in general, regressive.

However, the studies reveal that there are important differences in the way national health systems are financed. Taxes were an important source of financing for the national health systems of Jamaica and Brazil; they represented more than 2% of GDP. Contributions to social insurance systems were the main source of financing for the public health system in Mexico, accounting for

---

[13]The relationship between taxes and income (or any other ability-to-pay measure) is said to be regressive if the tax burden declines as income rises, proportional or neutral if the taxes constitute the same percentage of income at all levels, and progressive if tax increases as income increases.

FIGURE 3. Health financing mix in six countries of the Latin America and Caribbean region.

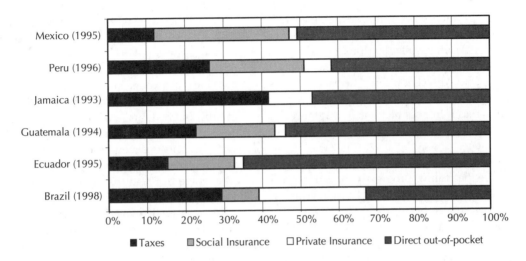

1.7% of GDP. Social insurance and taxes were of equal importance in the cases of Ecuador, Guatemala, and Peru (around 1% of GDP); they were of minor importance in the case of Brazil and nonexistent in the case of Jamaica (Figure 3).

In all the countries, direct out-of-pocket expenditures were a main source of financing for the national health care system, accounting for proportions that ranged from around 30% in Brazil to more than 60% in Ecuador. As a percentage of GDP, out-of-pocket expenditures fluctuated between 2.3% in the case of Guatemala to 3.3% in the case of Ecuador. Voluntary contributions to private insurance schemes as a source of financing were significant only in the case of Brazil: more than one-fourth of total financing or 2.3% of the GDP. Private insurance represented less than 0.5% of GDP in all the other countries.

For the countries of the Latin America and Caribbean region as a whole, the share of direct taxes as a percentage of total government revenues, or as a percentage of GDP, is relatively small compared with that in more developed countries (OECD countries). During 1986–1992 direct taxes on individuals represented less than 8% of government revenues, less than 2% of GDP in LAC countries. For OECD countries, this type of tax accounted for 28% of total government revenues, around 8% of GDP.

Contributions to social security are also more important in OECD countries than in Latin American and Caribbean countries. In 1986–1992, social security contributions in OECD countries accounted for 25.6% of government revenue, around 8.3% of GDP. For Latin American and Caribbean countries this source of revenue accounted for 17% of total revenue, less than 3% of the GDP. In most countries of Latin America and the Carib-

bean, indirect taxes, value-added taxes, excise taxes, and taxes on international transactions are the main sources of fiscal revenues.[14] In the same period, indirect taxes accounted for 58% of total revenues in Latin American and Caribbean countries. For OECD countries, indirect taxes were around 33% of total revenues during the same period.

The results of the case studies with regard to the incidence of different sources of revenue were mixed. In the case of Brazil, during 1995–1997, public sector health expenditures were financed from taxes on net profits of firms (direct) and from contributions to finance social programs (health, social security, and social welfare programs) that were raised from taxes on enterprises' gross revenues from sales of merchandise and services. In 1997, these two sources accounted for 70% of MOH financing. In 1996, a transitory tax on financial transactions was approved: a 0.20% surcharge on all financial transactions, the Contribuicão Provisória de Movimentação Financeira (CPMF), which was earmarked to finance the implementation of the Unified National Health System (SUS). By 1998 resources from the CPMF represented 46% of MOH revenues. Contributions from the Contribuição para o financiamento de Seguridad Social [tax for financing social security] (COFINS) represented 25% of overall revenues, and revenues from net profits from enterprises declined from 20% during 1995–1997 to 9% in 1998. Although there is general agreement that COFINS taxes are

---

[14]Also, for countries of the LAC Region, the share of government revenues as a percentage of GDP was around 19.7%, almost half that observed in OECD countries (34.3%, unweighted average) for the period 1986–1992 (International Monetary Fund, 1995, pp. 289–310).

regressive, the authors questioned the assumption that taxes on net profits would be regressive as well as preliminary empirical findings that indicated the CPMF was progressive. In fact, a detailed analysis of the incidence of these instruments is not available. Household surveys (LSMS or household income and expenditure surveys) do not capture data on direct or indirect taxes or on taxes levied on financial transactions to finance health programs, which makes it impossible to arrive at a precise estimation of the distribution of the burden of different revenue instruments.

The same is true of Jamaica: it was not possible to accurately measure the relative progressiveness or regressiveness of the two major components of government revenues used to finance health expenditure—income taxes (direct) and the general consumption tax (indirect). These two sources accounted for 67% of government revenues. Based on the characteristics of the income tax structure in Jamaica, the authors concluded that the income tax was nominally regressive. There is a flat rate of 33% for income above $Jamaica 10,400 and an effective 0% tax for the lowest income quintile. Estimates of the effective general consumption tax (GCT) rate by quintiles found it to be regressive; the effective GCT rate was 7.7% for the lowest quintile and 3.9% for the highest quintile. The authors' conclusion is that "...the public revenue source is dominated by two taxes which seem to be biased toward regressivity" (Theodore and Lafoucade, 1998).

In Ecuador, progressivity indices were estimated for the following three main components of government revenue: direct and indirect taxes and contributions to social security. The case study found that, while direct taxes were relatively neutral (progressive in rural areas and regressive in urban areas), indirect taxes were highly regressive. Contributions to social security were also found to be regressive. In Mexico, the case study reported that, although direct taxes appear to be neutral, indirect taxes are somewhat more regressive. Overall, the distribution of payments for health—including private out-of-pocket expenditure, which was found to be progressive—was assumed to be neutral.

Analysis of the source of financing for national health systems was not included in the reports from Guatemala and Peru. However, based on Guatemala's tax structure, the authors argue that the financing of government programs, including the public component of the national health system, tends to be regressive. Indirect taxes, which in general are regressive, accounted for nearly 80% of government revenues.

All the country case studies reported large differences in the level of private expenditures on health by income groups. Private expenditures on health were found to be progressive and more concentrated than the distribution of income in the cases of Brazil, Jamaica, Mexico, and Peru. In these countries the share of private expenditures on health increased with the level of income (income elasticity greater than one). The Mexican study reported that findings from the 1994 survey were different from those obtained in an earlier survey (1992), which found that the share of expenditures on health care services was higher in low-income groups than in the higher-income groups. In Guatemala, the most recent National Household Income Expenditure survey reported a similar result. The share of expenditure on health services increased with income, from 3.0% in the lowest-income group to an average of 6% in the higher-income groups.[15] In the case of Ecuador, the study found that the share of expenditures on health was higher in the third and fourth quintiles than in the first, second, and fifth quintiles. Cross-country comparisons of data on the composition of national health care expenditures suggest that the larger the share of government expenditure on health as a percentage of GDP (Jamaica and Mexico), the smaller the differences in overall consumption expenditures between low- and high-income groups (Brazil, Ecuador, Guatemala, and Peru).

Data on the share of private expenditures on health insurance and prepaid plans for these countries reveals that these are of some significance in the case of Brazil (around 3.5% of household income, in 1994–1995) for all income levels. For the other countries for which this information is available (Ecuador, Guatemala, Mexico, and Peru), private insurance expenditures represent less than 0.5% of total household income and are concentrated in the upper-income groups.[16]

Distribution of Benefits

In most cases, the studies revealed that public sector expenditures do very little to correct health care expenditure inequalities associated with private consumption and income inequalities. In four of the countries, the reports included an analysis or data that served to reveal the distribution of government expenditures on health-related goods and services (benefit-incidence): Ecuador, Guatemala, Jamaica, and Peru. The results are presented in Table 4 and Figure 4. The table shows the distribution of

---

[15]Income groups are classified by income range, not by quintiles or deciles. Results from this survey were not available when the Guatemala case study was completed (Instituto Nacional de Estadística, 1999).

[16]The estimates for Ecuador were 0.15% of household income in 1995; 0.03% in Guatemala in 1998; 0.14% in Mexico for 1995; and 0.15% in Peru in 1985–1986 (Suárez, 1995, 1998b). Data for Guatemala are from the Instituto Nacional de Estadística (1999).

TABLE 4. Distribution of the benefits of government expenditure on health: Ecuador, Guatemala, Jamaica, and Peru.

	Quintile 1	Quintile 2	Quintile 3	Quintile 4	Quintile 5	% of GDP[a]
Brazil	...	...	...	...	...	...
Ecuador	12.5	15.0	19.4	22.5	30.5	0.86
Guatemala	12.8	12.7	16.9	26.3	31.3	0.97
Jamaica	25.3	23.9	19.4	16.2	15.2	2.75
Peru	20.1	20.7	21.0	20.7	17.5	1.45
Mexico	...	...	...	...	...	...

... = not available.
[a]Ministry of Health budget only.
Sources: Benefit incidence estimates taken or derived from country case studies.

FIGURE 4. Distribution of benefits of government expenditures in health.

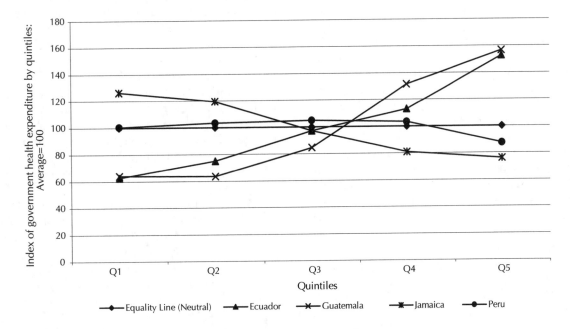

the benefits of government expenditures by income or socioeconomic quintiles. The last column indicates the amount of public expenditures being distributed as a percentage of GDP.

Jamaica (1996) is the only country in which a large part of government expenditure went to the lower-income groups; thus, it is the only country in which government expenditure inequalities were clearly pro-poor.[17] It was estimated that 25.3% of government expenditures went to the poorest 20% of the population. In the case of Peru, the distributive impact is neutral; all income groups benefited equally from government (Ministry of Health) expenditures on health care services. Results from Peru for 1997 are similar to the findings from earlier studies. A benefit incidence analysis of public expenditures on health in Peru, with data from a 1996 LSMS-type survey,

[17]The relationship between benefits and income (or any other ability-to-pay or wealth measure) is said to be pro-poor (pro-rich) if the distribution of government expenditures going to low-income groups as a proportion of overall government expenditures on health is more (less) concentrated in the low- (high-) income groups. The pro-rich and pro-poor definitions differ from the definition of

progressivity and regressivity of the distribution of the benefits of government expenditures. Progressivity (regressivity) requires, in the relative version, that the benefits as a share of household income increase (decline) as income rises. Distribution of the benefits is said to be proportional or neutral if the benefits constitute the same percentage for all income groups.

also found that these expenditures had little significant impact on overall health sector inequalities. Public expenditure was equally distributed among different income groups (Francke, 1998).

In the cases of Ecuador and Guatemala, a larger proportion of government expenditure on health went to high-income groups, leading to pro-rich inequalities. In these two countries, the richest 20% received more than 30% of the benefits of government expenditures on health. The lowest 20%, the poorest quintile, received around 13% of the benefits. The distributive impact of government expenditure on health care services was limited by the relatively low level of utilization of health care services by the poor. In addition, these two countries are among the countries in which Ministry of Health expenditure as a proportion of GDP was relatively low: less than 1% of GDP.

The results from the EquiLAC and IHEP studies are consistent with previous findings about the distribution of the benefits of government expenditures on health. Results for Argentina, Colombia, and Chile are presented in Table A5 in the Annex. These results show that a greater distributive impact of government health expenditures is found in Argentina and Chile, two countries whose systems can be classified as statutory national social insurance health systems (NHIS). In these two countries, 31% of government expenditures accrued to the population in the poorest quintile. The high-income group, the richest 20%, received less than 8% of the benefits of government expenditures on health. Historically, public sector expenditures on health have represented around 3% of GDP.

However, government expenditures in countries with MNHS also have the potential for achieving an important distributive effect. Results for Colombia for 1970, 1974, and 1993 show that the distributive impact of government expenditures can be changed in favor of the poorest group of the population (see Table A3). In the case of Colombia, the percentage of government expenditures that accrued to the lowest quintile increased from 21% in 1970 to around 28% in 1974 and 1993. However, these gains were made at the expense of the middle class, the population in the fourth quintile of the income distribution. The share of government expenditure going to that income group decreased from 26% in 1970 to 17.7% in 1974 and 15.9% in 1993. The percentage of government expenditure benefiting the top 20% of the income distribution almost doubled, rising from 6.8% in 1970 to around 12% in 1974 and 1993.

The qualitative results obtained by putting together the estimates and hypotheses on the incidence of the sources of financing and the distribution of the benefits of public expenditures on health are summarized in Table 5. In four

TABLE 5. Fiscal incidence of the financing and distribution of benefits of government expenditures on health.

	Financing	Benefits	Overall results
Brazil	?	U	U
Ecuador	R	PR	PR
Guatemala	R	PR	PR
Jamaica	R	PP	?
Mexico	R	U	U
Peru	U	N	U

R = regressive; P = progressive; ? = undetermined; U = unknown; PR = pro-rich; PP = pro-poor; N = neutral.

of the six countries included in the study, financing of the public component of national health systems was deemed regressive (ability-to-pay principle): Ecuador, Guatemala, Jamaica, and Mexico. It was undetermined in the case of Brazil and unknown in the case of Peru. Analysis of the distribution of the benefits of government expenditures on health found them to be pro-poor in the case of Jamaica. The share of government expenditures accruing to low-income groups was larger than that accruing to high-income groups. The benefits of government expenditures on health as a share of income declined as income rose (pro-poor). However, as the financing is regressive, the overall distribution of the benefits remains undetermined. The poor paid relatively more and received relatively more, but, it was not possible to determine whether they received more of what they paid for.

In the case of Peru, the benefits of government expenditures on health were equally distributed across income quintiles, with each quintile receiving around one-fifth. Therefore, government benefits as a percentage of income declined as income rose (progressive). Because no data on the fiscal incidence of the financing are presented, the overall impact of government expenditures on health is unknown.

In Ecuador and Guatemala, the overall distributive impact of the financing and benefits of government expenditures on health seemed to be pro-rich. In these countries the distribution of the benefits of government expenditures on health favored the rich. The first quintile, the poorest, received around 12% of government expenditures on health. The top quintile, the richest, received more than 30% of the benefits. As the financing of the system is regressive, the overall fiscal incidence seems to be regressive (pro-rich).

POLICY IMPLICATIONS OF THE FINDINGS

- Lack of significant differences in the perception of SIA among income groups suggests that service availability may not be a major constraint for the poor in accessing health care services.

In general, poor people do not feel sicker than rich ones. Although low quality of health care services available to the poor may be a deterrent to demand for health care services among the poor, results from the country case studies show that, in general, they do not suffer illness more frequently or more severely than the rich. This is in spite of strong evidence from morbidity and mortality data showing an inverse correlation between income and the incidence and prevalence of morbidity and higher rates of mortality among low-income groups.

- Increasing the availability of health care services may not result in an increase in utilization of these services, even if services are provided free of charge or at a low nominal fee.

For cultural reasons or because of a lack of education, the poor are not taking advantage of health care services provided by government institutions. Increasing awareness of the disproportionately high incidence and prevalence of disease among low-income groups is one mechanism for ensuring that the poor make full use of health care services where they exist.

- Low perception of SIA is also an indicator of the limited scope of "community participation" or demand-oriented policies that rely on people's perception of illness or health risks to decide on the type of services a community needs.

A more technocratic public health policy approach, based on an educated evaluation of the determinants of health status of different income groups, may provide a better understanding of the type of health policies and health care services that will be most conducive to breaking the cycle of disease and poverty.

- Community participation in financing, through cost recovery or fee-for-service schemes, may aggravate inequalities in access to quality health care services as measured by differences in the level of consumption expenditures by income group.

The relatively large magnitude of private expenditures as a proportion of overall national health care expenditures, coupled with an income-expenditure elasticity greater than one (share of expenditures as a percentage of total expenditures increases as income increases), suggests that inequalities in access are closely related to individuals' ability to pay. Inequalities in private consumption expenditures, which are more pronounced than inequalities in the utilization of health care services and overall socioeconomic inequalities, suggest that inequality and inequity indices are not capturing differences in the quality of services used by different income and socioeconomic groups as measured by the average expenditure for those services. Increasing the cost of access to public health care services through cost recovery or fee-for-service schemes will reduce the demand for those services and increase differences in the level of consumption by low- and high-income groups. The larger the share of out-of-pocket expenditures as a source of financing for health systems, the closer the relationship is between access and ability to pay and, therefore, the larger the inequalities in access/utilization of health care services.

- There is ample room to improve what governments can do to enhance the distributive impact of public expenditures on health: increasing the amount of resources, reducing regressivity in the financing of health systems, and—by redirecting public expenditures to intervention—inducing greater utilization of health care services by the poor.

The findings with regard to the distributive impact of government expenditures on health from the EquiLAC and IHEP projects, as well as other studies, suggest that the relative importance of government expenditures on health as a proportion of GDP matters. Government expenditures on health had some significant redistributive impacts (favoring the poor) in countries where they represented 2.5% or more of GDP (Argentina, Colombia, Chile, and Jamaica). Government expenditure on health was found to favor the rich in countries where it represented around 1% of GDP or less (Ecuador and Guatemala). Changing the financing of the system from an indirect tax-based system toward a direct tax-based system will reduce the regressivity of health system financing. In most countries, financing of the (public) system was regressive, as it was based on indirect taxes. Financing was considered progressive only in the case of Brazil, where in 1997–1998 an earmarked tax on financial transactions and direct taxes on net profits of businesses were the main sources of revenue for the Ministry of Health. Redirecting public expenditures toward policies aimed at improving individuals' perceptions of their own health status and health risks may be one effective way to reduce the gap between actual and self-assessed health status, make people aware of their health care service needs, and increase the demand for those services. Such policies also may help improve the distributive impact of government expenditures on health.

The results from the country case studies shed some light on the way applied research can be used to assess health system inequalities and inequities and to measure inequalities in health status and inequalities and inequities in the delivery/access to health care services. In addition, the studies show that general principles of fiscal incidence analysis can be applied to assess the likely distributive impact of government financing and expenditures on health care services. All these tools can be used for an empirically based assessment of the equity impact of health sector (reform) policies and programs.

However, the studies also raise many questions about conceptual and methodological issues, including conceptual issues relating to the definition of proxy variables for measuring health status, health needs, and access/utilization of health services; the concept of equity adopted; and the variables used in ranking socioeconomic groups. Some of the methodological issues are related to the models and standardization procedures used, the consistency between survey results and data from administrative sources, and whether the benefits of government expenditures on health should be assessed on a cost-of-services or a willingness-to-pay basis.

There is also the issue of international comparability of results. Wide variations in the coverage, contents, and quality of survey and primary data available in different countries impose some constraints on the accuracy and interpretation of summary statistics, as well as of inequality and inequity indexes across countries. Also, more research is needed to determine the impact that changes in the organization and financing of national health systems have on observed health care inequalities and how long it takes for such changes to translate into any measurable effect.

REFERENCES

Aronson JR, Johnson P, Lambert PJ. Redistributive effect and unequal tax treatment. *Economic Journal.* 1994; 104:262–270.

Bengoa R, Fernandez JM, Nuno R, Key P, Nichol D. *A Descriptive Review of the Health Systems of Latin American Countries.* International Health Partnership, a consortium of B & F Gestion y Salud, Dearden Management, and HMSU-University of Manchester. Prepared for the Equity in Health in LAC project; Human Development Network, The World Bank. Washington, DC: The World Bank Group; 1998.

Inter-American Development Bank. *Progreso económico y social en América Latina: América Latina frente a la desigualdad.* Informe 1998-99. Washington, DC: Inter-American Development Bank; 1999.

Fundación para la Investigación de Estudios Económicos Latinoamericanos. *El sistema de seguridad social: una propuesta de reforma.* Buenos Aires, Argentina: Fundación para la Investigación de Estudios Económicos Latinoamericanos; 1995.

Francke P. ¿Como hacer para que la salud publica lleguer a los pobres? Consultant report; Prepared for Abt Associates Inc. Washington, DC: Abt Associates, Inc; 1998.

Insituto Nacional de Estadística. *Encuesta Nacional de Ingresos y Gastos de los Hogares, 1998-99.* Guatemala: Insituto Nacional de Estadística; 1999.

International Monetary Fund. *Economic Policy and Equity: Issues Paper.* Paper presented at the Conference on Economic Policy and Equity, 8–9 June, 1998. Washington, DC: IMF Fiscal Affairs Department, Expenditure Policy Division; 1998.

Kakwani NC, Wagstaff A, van Doorslaer E. Socioeconomic inequalities in health: measurement, computation and statistical inference. *Journal of Econometrics.* 1997; 77:87–103.

May E. *La pobreza en Colombia: un estudio del Banco Mundial.* Bogota, Colombia: TM Editores, Banco Mundial; 1996.

Meldau EC. *Benefit Incidence: Public Health Expenditures and Income Distribution: A Case Study of Colombia.* North Quincy, MA: Christopher Publishing House; 1980.

Molina CG, Rueda MC, Alviar M, Gieidon U. *El gasto publico en salud y distribución de subsidios en Colombia.* Santa Fe de Bogota, Colombia: Fedesarrollo; 1993. Cited in World Bank. *Poverty in Colombia. A World Bank Country Study Report.* Washington, DC: World Bank; 1994.

Organization of Economic Cooperation and Development. Financing and delivering health care: A comparative analysis of OECD countries. OECD Policy Studies No. 4. Paris: OECD; 1987.

Pan American Health Organization. *Health in the Americas, 1998 Edition.* Washington, DC: PAHO; 1998.

Pan American Health Organization. *Health Situation in the Americas: Basic Indicators, 1998.* Program of Health Situation Analysis, Division of Health and Human Development, Pan American Health Organization. Washington, DC: PAHO; 1999.

Sapelli C, Vial B. Utilización y prestación de salud en Chile: Es diferente entre grupos de ingreso? *Cuadernos de Economía* 35 (106). Santiago: Universidad Pontificia Católica de Chile; 1998.

Selowsky M. *Who Benefits from Government Expenditures? A Case Study of Colombia.* Washington, DC: The World Bank. Oxford University Press; 1979.

Shome P (ed). *Tax Policy Handbook.* Washington, DC: Fiscal Affairs Department, International Monetary Fund; 1995.

Suárez R. *Cobertura y gasto en seguros de salud en America Latina: los seguros privados.* Washington, DC: Programa de Políticas Públicas y Salud, Organización Panamericana de la Salud; 1995.

Suárez R. *Health Systems in Latin America: A Taxonomy.* Prepared for the Human Development Network and Human Resources Management Unit of the Latin America and Caribbean Region. Washington, DC: The World Bank Group; October 1998a.

Suárez R. *National Health Expenditure Accounts, A SNA based approach: Concepts, Methods and Results.* Washington, DC: Paper prepared for the Human Development Network of The World Bank Group; March 1998b.

Theodore K, Lafoucade A. *Health Systems Inequality and Poverty in Jamaica.* Washington, DC: Prepared for the PAHO-UNDP Investment in Health, Equity and Poverty project and the World Bank Equity in Health in Latin America and the Caribbean Project; January 1998.

van Doorslaer E, Wagstaff A, Rutten F. *Equity in the Finance and Delivery of Health Care: An International Perspective.* Health Service Research Series No. 5, Commission of the European Communities. Oxford, UK: Oxford Medical Publications; 1993.

van Doorslaer E, Wagstaff. A. *Equity in the Finance and Delivery of Health Care: A Review of the ECuity Project Findings.* Washington, DC: Paper prepared for the Human Development Network and the Latin American and Caribbean Region Office of the World Bank; 1997.

van Doorslaer E, Wagstaff. A. *Inequity in Health: Methods and Results for Jamaica*. Washington, DC: Paper prepared for the Human Development Network and the Latin American and Caribbean Region Office of the World Bank; May 1998a.

van Doorslaer E, Wagstaff. A. *Inequity in the Delivery of Health Care: Methods and Results for Jamaica*. Washington, DC: Paper prepared for the Human Development Network and the Latin American and Caribbean Region Office of the World Bank; June 1998b.

Wagstaff A, van Doorslaer E, Paci P. Equity in the finance and delivery of health care: some tentative cross country comparisons. London: Oxford Review of Economic Policy; 1989, pp. 89–112.

Wagstaff A, van Doorslaer E, Paci P. On the measurement of horizontal inequity in the delivery of health care. *Journal of Health Economics*. 1991, 169–206.

Wagstaff A. *Inequalities in Child Mortality in the Developing World: How Large Are They? How Can They Be Reduced?* Washington, DC: Paper prepared for the Human Development Network of the World Bank; May 1999.

Whitehead M. (1998). *The Contribution of Health Policies and Improved Health to Poverty Alleviation and the Reduction of Inequalities in Access to Health Services: Experiences from Outside Latin America and the Caribbean*. Washington, DC: Paper prepared for the PAHO-UNDP Investments in Health Equity and Poverty Project; August 1999.

World Bank. *Chile: Poverty and Income Distribution in a High-Growth Economy, 1987–1995*. Washington, DC: World Bank; 1997a.

World Bank. *Social Indicators of Development* [CD-ROM]. Washington, DC: World Bank Group; 1999.

World Health Organization. Health Care Reform: Analysis of Current Strategies. Edited and written by Richard B. Saltman and Josep Figueres. Regional Office for Europe, World Health Organization. Copenhagen: WHO; 1997.

Zee H. *Taxation and Equity*. In: Shome P (ed). (1995). *Tax Policy Handbook*. Washington, DC: Fiscal Affairs Department, International Monetary Fund; 1995; pp. 30–34.

Annex

List of Country Case Studies, Members of Research Teams, and Their Institutional Affiliation.

Brazil

Equity in Health in LAC—Brazil; January 1999.
Investments in Health, Equity and Poverty in Latin America—Brazil; January 1999.
Prof. Antonio Carlos Coelho Campino*[†]
Prof. Maria Dolores M. Diaz[†]
Prof. Leda Maria Paulani[†]
Prof. Roberto G. de Oliveira[†]
Dr. Sergio Piola[‡]
Dr. Andres Nunes[‡]

* Project Coordinator
[†]Department of Economics, University of Sao Paulo, Sao Paulo, Brazil (USP)
[‡]Instituto do Pesquisas Económicas Aplicadas (IPEA)/Brazilian Research Insitute of Applied Economics

Ecuador

Equity in Health in LAC, Country Studies: Ecuador; November 1998.
Inversiones en Salud, Equidad y Pobreza; Estudio de Caso: Ecuador; November 30, 1998.
Ec. MSPH. Enrique Lasprilla*
Ec. Jorge Granda
Ingo. Carlos Obando
Lic. Eduardo Encalad
Sr. Christian Lasprilla

*Project Coordinator

Guatemala

Inversiones en Salud. Equidad y Pobreza: Guatemala, Informe Final; October 1998.
Ricardo Valladares
Edgard Barillas*
GSD Consultores Asociados; Ciudad de Guatemala, Guatemala

*Project Coordinator

Jamaica

Health and Equity in Jamaica; Investments in Health, Equity and Poverty in LAC (EquiLAC and IHEP); December 1998.
Prof. Karl Theodore*[†]
Prof. Dominic Stoddard[†]
Prof. Andrea Yearwood[†]
Prof. Wendell Thomas[†]

*Project Coordinator
[†]Health Economic Unit, University of West Indies, St. Augustine, Trinidad

Mexico

Equity in the Finance and Delivery of Health Care: Results from Mexico
June 1999.
Susan Wendy Parker*[†]
Eduardo Gonzales Pier[‡]

*Project Coordinator
[†]Progresa-Social Development
[‡]Mexican Institute of Social Security/Instituto Mexicano de Seguridad Social (IMSS)

Peru

Equidad en la Atención en Salud; Peru 1997. Informe Final; Enero 1999.
Margarita Petrera*[†]
Luis Cordero[‡]
Augusto Portocarrero[§]

*Project Coordinator
[†]Pan American Health Organization (PAHO)
[‡]Superintendencia de Entidades Prestadoras de Servicios de Salud (SEPS)
[§]Ministerio de Salud, Oficina General de Planificación (MINSA-Peru)

TABLE A1. Types of national health care systems according to institutional providers: LAC region.

Institutional configuration	Type I NHS		Type II NHIS			Type III MNHS
	I.1	I.2	II.1	II.2	II.3	III.
Public sector (statutory)						
Central government (MOH and other public institutions)*						
Local governments (state/provincial, municipal)†						
Social insurance systems (mandatory)						
Single (national)						
Multiple: provincial, departmental, occupational						
Mix-managed sickness funds (competitive, occupational)						
Private sector (voluntary)						
Institutional providers‡						
Individual providers‡						
Health insurance and repayment schemes						
Nonprofit institutions serving households (NPISH)						
Households						

*Other public health programs and institutions receiving transfers from the central government but operating with their own budgets.

†Countries with federal systems, in which local governments (provincial, state, departmental) play an active role in deciding on resource allocation and revenue collection.

‡Providers, in the public-finance sense, means individuals or institutions involved in the financing, production, or provision of health care services and health insurance plans.

(r) = restricted role.

Shaded cells indicate the degree of importance of the type of institution in the health system (darker shading indicates the institution plays a greater role); blank cells indicate the absence of that type of institution in the corresponding health system.

Source: Suárez (1998).

TABLE A2. EquiLAC-IHEP country case studies: data sources by country, year, type of survey, coverage, and institutions conducting the survey.

Country	Year	Type of surveys	Coverage	Institutions
Brazil	1996/97	LSMS (PPV)	Partial; urban and rural areas	IBGE/World Bank
Ecuador	1995	LSMS (ENCV)	National	INEC
Guatemala	1998/99	ENIG	National	INE
Jamaica	1993	LSMS	National	PIOJ INEGI
Mexico	1994	ENSA	National	
	1994	ENIGH		
Peru	1997	LSMS (ENIV)	National	Cuanto S.A. World Bank

ENCV = Encuesta Nacional de Condiciones de Vida (National Survey of Living Conditions).

ENIG = Encuesta Nacional de Ingresos y Gastos (National Income-Expenditure Survey).

ENIGH = Encuesta Nacional de Ingresos y Gastos de los Hogares (National Household Income-Expenditure Survey).

IBGE, INE, INEC, INEGI: National statistics offices of the corresponding countries. PIOJ = Planning Institute of Jamaica. Cuanto S.A. is a private consulting firm.

TABLE A3. Health status inequalities, summary of findings: SAH, SIA, and chronic illness.

Countries	C	C*	I*	(t statistic)
SAH				
Brazil			(< 0)	(n.a.)
Jamaica (1989)	−0.0919		−0.0345	(−6.3917)
Mexico	−0.2120		−0.0970	(−7.0410)
SIA/(curative care):				
Brazil* LSQ	−0.0402	0.0034	−0.0436	(−5.8491)
Logit	−0.0402	0.0034	−0.0436	(−5.8483)
Probit	−0.0402	0.0036	−0.0435	(−5.8306)
Ecuador*	0.0090	0.0075	−0.0015	(n.a.)
Jamaica (1993–1996)*	−0.0300		0.0018	(n.a.)
Jamaica[†]	−0.0458		−0.0042	(n.a.)
Mexico[‡]	0.0014		−0.0185	(−2.5110)
Peru[§]			(0.062)	
Chronic illness[§]		0.902		
Brazil	0.0424		−0.0420	(−5.6091)
Jamaica (1989)			−0.0603	(−2.4480)
Jamaica (1993–1996)	−0.0866		−0.0051	(n.a.)
Mexico	0.1660		0.0889	(−10.123)

*All individuals reporting SIA within the past four weeks.
[†]Number of days ill in the past four weeks.
[‡]All individuals reporting SIA within past two weeks.
[§]Reported as "long-term illness" or specific chronic conditions.
I* value refers to the value of the Gini coefficient. It indicates pro-poor inequalities in the distribution of SIA.
1989 data for Jamaica are from van Doorslaer and Wagstaff (1998a).
n.a. = not available.
Source: Prepared with information from the country case study reports and background papers.

TABLE A4. Inequalities and inequity in the delivery/utilization of health care services: curative, chronic, and preventive.*

Countries/variables	Cm	Cn	Hiwv
Curative care			
Brazil	0.0568	0.0401	+ 0.0969
Ecuador	0.07728	0.0090	+ 0.0682
Jamaica[†]	0.1670	−0.0032	+ 0.1700
Mexico	0.0820	−0.0040	+ 0.0860
Peru	0.1672	−0.0563	+ 0.1109
Chronic care			
Brazil	0.1192	0.0544	+ 0.0648
Hospitalization			
Mexico	0.1300	−0.0051	+ 0.099
Preventive care			
Brazil	0.1943	0.0122	+ 0.1821
Ecuador	0.1167	0.0099	+ 0.1077
Mexico	0.1220	0.0230	+ 0.1250

*Least squares estimates only. In general, the studies found little difference in estimates using alternative econometric techniques (Logit or Probit).
[†]Estimates derived from estimates of C* from Table A.3 and of C presented in the section on computation methods.
Source: Prepared with information from the country case study reports.

TABLE A5. Distribution of benefits of government expenditures on health in selected LAC countries.

	Quintile 1	Quintile 2	Quintile 3	Quintile 4	Quintile 5
Argentina	31.0	18.0	26.0	18.0	7.0
Brazil	...	...	...	...	...
Colombia, 1970	21.4	26.9	19.0	25.9	6.8
Colombia, 1974	28.0	22.0	20.1	17.7	12.2
Colombia, 1993	27.4	25.6	18.7	15.9	12.5
Chile	31.0	25.0	22.0	14.0	8.0
Ecuador	12.5	15.0	19.4	22.5	30.5
Guatemala	12.8	12.7	16.9	26.3	31.3
Jamaica	25.3	23.9	19.4	16.2	15.2
Peru	20.1	20.7	21.0	20.7	17.5
Mexico	...	...	...	...	...

... = not available.
Sources: Estimates for Ecuador, Guatemala, Jamaica, and Peru are taken or derived from EquiLAC-IHEP country case study reports. Estimates for Argentina are from Fundación para la Investigación de Estudios Económicos Latinoamericanos (1995). Estimates for Colombia for 1970 are from Meldau (1980)—distribution of health services benefits by income class estimated at cost-of-service basis; for 1974 from Selowsky (1979); and for 1993 from Molina *et al.* (1993) reported by May (1996). Estimates for Chile are from World Bank (1997a). Values for Argentina and Chile are rounded.

Health System Inequalities and Poverty in Brazil

Antonio Carlos Coelho Campino, Maria Dolores M. Diaz, Leda Maria Paulani,
Roberto G. de Oliveira, Sergio Piola, and Andres Nunes

Background

Brazil has one of the most unequal distributions of income in the world. According to the Inter-American Development Bank, the wealthiest 10% of Brazilians receive 47% of the national income, and the poorest 10% receive only 0.8% of the national income.

Although the Brazilian government is constitutionally charged with providing universal health care to its citizens, in practice the public health care system is inadequate and underfunded. A radical reorganization of the system from a centrally controlled system to a municipally controlled and operated system is ongoing—with mixed results.

Inequalities in income distribution are reflected in access to and utilization of health services as well as in the health conditions of individuals across income groups. Unfortunately, relatively little attention has been devoted to investigating these issues. One of the few studies analyzing the Brazilian health system is the 1995 World Bank study *"Organização, prestação e financiamento da saúde no Brasil: uma agenda para os anos 90"* (*"Organization, Delivery, and Financing of Health Care in Brazil: An Agenda for the 1990s"*). This study shows that the Brazilian health system differs sharply from others in developing countries. In Brazil, the public health care system provides 70% of ambulatory care, but 80% of hospital beds are in private institutions. The study also assesses health care expenditure in Brazil, which was estimated at 4.8% of gross domestic product in 1990, and describes the financing structure of public health care expenditures.

Although the World Bank study provides some important insights into the main challenges facing the public and private health care systems in Brazil, it does not investigate inequalities in health status and in access to health services. These issues will be examined in the following sections.

Health Care System

According to the 1988 Constitution, all Brazilian citizens have the right to obtain health care services. The Unified Health System (Sistema Único de Saúde; SUS) was created in 1989 to decentralize the provision of services and bring it closer to people. Within SUS, the municipal governments manage public health services, and the central government has more general responsibilities. However, this shift of responsibility to the municipal governments has been a slow process.[1] Economic, political, and administrative issues have further delayed decentralization.

Structure of SUS

Central Government

Within SUS, the central government defines the principal features of national health policy and regulates the provision of public and private health care services. In addition to the Ministry of Health, which directs SUS, two other institutions participate in decision-making and regulate the relationship between different levels of government. The first is the National Health Council (Conselho Nacional de Saúde), which is composed of representatives of consumers, public and private providers, government entities, and health sector workers. The Council serves as an advisory and auxiliary organ of the Ministry of Health, reviewing national health policy and supervising SUS management. The second institution is the Tripartite Management Committee (Comissão Intergestores Tripartite), a commission that coordinates the

[1]This is partly due to the fact that the country has so many extremely small cities. Brazil has more than 5,000 cities, 25% of which have fewer than 5,000 inhabitants.

three levels of SUS management in the implementation of national health policy.[2]

Role of State Governments within SUS

Under the original design of SUS, the role of state governments was not sufficiently defined. Subsequent revisions of the design made state governments responsible for coordinating the "municipalization process," which is defined as the gradual transfer of health care functions to municipal governments. During the first phase of this process, state governments are responsible for supporting municipal governments as they take on their new tasks. During the transition period, state governments are responsible for managing public health services in cities that have not yet adapted to the new requirements.

Once the municipal government is adequately managing public health services, the role of the state government is limited to coordinating health services and designing state health policy, following the general directives of national health policy. Coordination of municipal health services is a critical task, because many cities are very small and lack the ability to provide and manage a complete package of services.[3] To ensure the supply of services, especially complex ones, states must coordinate the use of facilities in larger cities by patients from rural areas and small towns. In addition to this coordinating role, state governments are responsible for controlling and inspecting the quality of health care services, both public and private. Each state has an organizational structure that parallels the national structure: the state health secretariat operates like the national Ministry of Health, whereas the state health council and the bipartite management commission (Comissão Intergestores Bipartite; CIB)[4] have structures and functions similar to those of the tripartite commission at the central government level.

Role of Municipal Governments within SUS

As previously noted, the principal change introduced by the creation of SUS is decentralization of public health services to the municipal level. Under this system, mu-
nicipalities manage and provide health care services directly. They are also responsible for ensuring the quality of these services, although they do not have primary responsibility for this function. The municipal organizational structure is similar to the central and state health care organizations, with the municipal health council overseeing local SUS management.

The private sector legally can participate in the SUS structure as a provider. The relationship between public managers and private providers is administered through contracts, and payments generally take the form of fee-for-service. In most cases, this type of relationship between private providers and SUS is restricted to second-level providers (hospitals).

Decentralization Process

The development of a regulatory scheme to guide the significant transfer of power and financial resources brought about by the decentralization process has been very slow. The Basic Operational Regulations of 1993 (Norma Operacional Básica de 1993; NOB93) were enacted five years after the new Constitution. This legislation established three distinct stages in the process of incorporating municipal governments into the SUS health care system: incipient, partial, and complete.[5] According to NOB93, the municipal governments should be fully managing health care services at the third stage. However, very few municipal governments have been able to meet the operational requirements at this stage. Between 1993 and 1997, fewer than 3% of Brazilian cities were in a position to assume management of health services at the most advanced stage.

The rules were changed in 1996 to accelerate the decentralization process. The Basic Operational Regulations of 1996 (Norma Operacional Básica de 1996; NOB96) established only two stages in the transfer of control: Complete Management of Basic Health Care (CMBHC) and Complete Management of the Health System (CMHS). To qualify for the first stage, the municipal government must have a health fund and an organized health database. It must also demonstrate the existence of a working municipal health council. NOB96 has yielded very positive results and has even exceeded some of its own goals. In the first half of 1998, more than 4,000 municipal governments qualified for the CMBHC stage and over 400 municipal governments qualified for the CMHS stage. This increase in the number of municipal governments that are fully responsible for health care service delivery, or that are tak-

---

[2]The central government still works as a provider and manages some facilities, such as national hospitals (particularly those linked to universities). Its role as a health care provider, however, is minor, which is in keeping with the changes introduced by SUS.

[3]For this reason, some state governments have retained their role as service providers despite the general tendency toward municipalization.

[4] CIB is charged with coordinating the municipal and state government levels in the execution of health policy.

---

[5]A literal translation of the third level is "semicomplete." The term "complete" is used here for the sake of clarity.

ing concrete steps toward full control, has important implications for the financing of health care in Brazil (see the section on health care expenditures and financing).

Relationship Between the Private and the Public Systems

As mentioned above, private health care providers may participate in the SUS structure by means of contracts.[6] However, these providers act more as competitors than as partners in delivery of services. Given the endemic problems with the public health services (waiting lists, shortage of doctors for basic care services, less comfort and fewer amenities than private services), the private system has had propitious conditions for growth. Recent studies show that about 37 million people (23% of the Brazilian population) use the private system.

Private health care is the preference of middle-class persons who buy their own health plans and of individuals in the formal labor market who are covered by employer-provided health plans. In most cases, the relationship between private insurers and providers is contractual, with very few cases of patient reimbursement in the system. The upper classes also buy health plans, but they also make substantial out-of-pocket payments to private providers, unlike the middle classes, which rarely incur out-of-pocket expenditures. Out-of-pocket payment is also quite common among poor people in the informal sector. The explanation for this paradoxical situation lies in the weakness of the public health system. Given that the public system pays service providers very little, patients often have to make additional out-of-pocket payments for health services in order to obtain them.

The middle and upper classes and people employed in the formal labor market tend to use private providers to obtain primary care and inpatient services. In the case of more complex services, even these classes use the public health services because they tend to be better than the private services, despite the lack of higher standards of comfort and privacy. This produces another paradoxical result: low-income people and workers in the informal labor market have less access to this type of public service. They often are unaware that they are entitled to the services or they lack the necessary information to obtain them.[7]

INEQUALITIES IN HEALTH CONDITIONS

The most recent and relevant source of data on Brazilian health conditions is found in the Living Standards Measurement Survey (LSMS) carried out by the Instituto Brasileiro de Geografia e Estatística from March 1996 to March 1997. The survey gathered information on various themes in the areas of education, health, housing, employment, fertility, contraception, migration, and time use, among others. Although the survey was quite extensive, the sampled population did not include all regions of the country. Therefore, the results are not completely representative of Brazil. Nevertheless, it is an important source of information on health and other social and economic issues.[8]

For the purposes of this study, the analysis focuses on distribution of responses to health issues across income quintiles. Table 1 presents a general overview of the perception of health status by the 19,049 individuals who participated in the survey. Perception of health improves slightly as income increases; the proportion of individuals who described their health as excellent, good, or very good increased from 76% for the first quintile to 87% for the fifth quintile. The inverse occurred with those who indicated their health status was average or bad.

A more unequal distribution is observed with respect to the practice of physical exercise. The proportion of individuals who exercise regularly or practice a sport more than doubles from the first to the fifth quintile (from 14.7% to 34.4%), a trend that can be attributed to increased leisure time, greater financial resources, and higher educational level of individuals in the high-income groups.[9] Reporting a chronic health problem increases slightly from the first to the fifth quintile; however, the proportion of those with a chronic health problem is greatest in quintile 3, which includes the main distribution. With respect to the type of chronic health problem, wealthier groups report a higher incidence of heart problems, hypertension, and diabetes. Respiratory, digestive tract, and neuropsychiatric illnesses are more frequent among low-income groups. The other types of chronic health problems do not show a very clear pattern in relation to income. The proportion of people who reported a health problem in the past 30 days decreases slightly with in-

---

[6]In fact, the private sector has little interest in participating in the SUS structure. In most cases, private providers consider the fees set by the central government for health services too low.

[7]The Brazilian system, therefore, is a blend of four models included in the taxonomy developed by the Organization for Economic Cooperation and Development. Its predominant features derive from the voluntary contract model and the public integrated model, but it also has features from the voluntary out-of-pocket model and the public contract model.

[8]The study concentrated on the northeastern and southeastern regions of the country. It included the following geographic areas: the Metropolitan Region of Fortaleza, the Metropolitan Region of Recife, the remaining urban area of the Northeast, the remaining rural area of the Northeast, the Metropolitan Region of Belo Horizonte, the Metropolitan Region of Rio de Janeiro, the Metropolitan Region of São Paulo, the remaining urban area of the Southeast, and the remaining rural area of the Southeast.

[9]A higher educational level is likely to be associated with a better understanding of the benefits of physical exercise.

TABLE 1. Perception of health status by income group, Brazil, 1997.

	Income quintile											
	1		2		3		4		5		Total	
Evaluation	No.	%	No.	%	No.	%	No.	%	No.	%	No.	%
Excellent	338	9.5	506	13.1	583	16.4	691	19.7	918	24.8	3,036	16.7
Very good	705	19.9	977	25.4	967	27.1	882	25.2	1,057	28.6	4,588	25.3
Good	1,659	46.8	1,578	40.9	1,289	36.2	1,284	36.6	1,263	34.1	7,073	38.9
Regular	678	19.1	632	16.4	580	16.3	566	16.2	419	11.3	2,875	15.8
Bad	154	4.3	152	3.9	141	4.0	76	2.2	40	1.1	563	3.1
Not evaluated	11	0.3	8	0.2	3	0.1	4	0.1	2	0.1	28	0.2
Does not know	2	0.1	1	0.0	...	...	1	0.0	...	...	4	0.0
Total	3,547	100.0	3,854	100.0	3,563	100.0	3,504	100.0	3,699	100.0	18,167	100.0

... = not available.
Source: LSMS, 1997.

come. Across all income groups, the most common health problem is in the category "flu-cold-pneumonia," followed by "pain" (14.4%) and "infection" (13.0%). Table 2 provides complete information. This variable is used in the definition of the variable curative need.

On average, 40% of the respondents reporting a health problem stopped their activities in the past 30 days. There was little difference across income groups in terms of the length of inactivity. A large majority of respondents (55%) were inactive for up to three days. The first and fifth quintiles present the same proportion of people who were away from their regular activities for up to 7 days (76%); the same occurred with quintiles 2, 3, and 4 (79%). Complete data are presented in Table 3.

HEALTH CARE EXPENDITURES AND FINANCING

In 1995[10] the combined expenditures on health care for the three levels of government totaled R$ 21.7 billion (about 3.3% of the gross domestic product). Annual per capita expenditure by the central government is close to US$ 100, and there are plans to raise this amount to US$ 170. The two largest categories of expenditure in the Ministry of Health budget are hospital services (35.9%) and medical and dental clinics (36.5%). A third category, public health services (which includes vaccinations, sanitation, nutrition, blood and related programs, information and screening, and communicable disease control), accounts for 12.8%.[11]

Private expenditures (including expenditures on health plans, out-of-pocket payments, medicines) reach about US$ 11 billion per year, which represents 50% of annual public health expenditure.

Sources of Financing for Public Health Care Expenditures

About 65% of public health expenditures in Brazil are financed by the central government. Other levels of government contribute 20% (states) and 15% (municipalities).[12] At the level of states and cities, resources come from general tax revenue. At the level of the central government, resources come basically from compulsory income-related contributions that are tied to individual wages, firm profits, and business turnover.

To cope with the permanent budgetary shortfall, a flat-rate tax of 0.2% on all bank account transactions by persons and firms was recently created (contribuição provisória sobre movimentações financeiras; CPMF).

The method whereby resources are transferred from the central government to states and municipalities depends on the services that are being financed and the stage the municipality has reached in the decentralization process (described in the section Health Care System).

When municipalities achieve the CMBHC stage they begin to receive monthly payments from the central government. These payments, referred to as the basic care floor (piso de atenção básica), have two components. The first is directed at financing basic ambulatory care (including sanitary actions) and payments are on a per capita basis.[13] This arrangement for transferring resources from the federal to the municipal levels constitutes a major

---

[10]This is the most recent year for which there is consolidated information on public health care expenditures.

[11]These figures are estimates based on a reclassification of the 1997 outlays reported by the Ministry of Health. The reclassification was based on the Manual on Government Finance Statistics, Part 2 (Classification of the Function of the Government) of the International Monetary Fund. Some aggregations and simplifying assumptions were necessary to complete this exercise.

[12] Article 198 of the Brazilian Federal Constitution (CF) prescribes that "the Single Health System (SUS) shall be financed, in the terms of Art. 195, with resources from the social security budget of the Union, the States, the Federal District, and the Municipalities, in addition to other sources." In other words, the CF does not connect specific sources of financing to health, thereby leaving open which taxes will finance SUS.

[13]The value of this per capita transfer is centrally defined.

TABLE 2. Type of health problem in the past 30 days by income group, Brazil, 1997.

| Type of health problem | Income quintile | | | | | | | | | | Total | |
| | 1 | | 2 | | 3 | | 4 | | 5 | | | |
	No.	%	No.	%	No.	%	No.	%	No.	%	No.	%
Cold-flu-pneumonia	470	49.3	417	46.7	417	50.0	350	44.8	372	47.1	2,026	47.7
Infection	103	10.8	118	13.2	109	13.1	112	14.3	112	14.2	554	13.0
Accident-injury	28	2.9	34	3.8	27	3.2	36	4.6	45	5.7	170	4.0
Digestive problems	47	4.9	45	5.0	32	3.8	33	4.2	27	3.4	184	4.3
Pain	160	16.8	142	15.9	117	14.0	100	12.8	92	11.7	611	14.4
Heart attack	...	...	1	0.1	0.20	...	...	...	...	...	3	0.1
Dental problem	15	1.6	19	2.1	11	1.3	20	2.6	20	2.5	85	2.0
Other	130	13.6	116	13.0	119	14.3	130	16.6	121	15.3	616	14.5
Total	953	100.0	892	100.0	834	100.0	781	100.0	789	100.0	4,249	100.0

Source: LSMS, 1997.

change with respect to the previous fee-for-service system, because it forces municipal managers of health care services to take costs into account. The second component of the basic care floor supports priority programs of the central government. In this case, the amount of resources transferred to the municipalities varies with the degree to which programs are implemented. The programs may be offered by municipalities themselves or by private providers by means of contracts. The specialized ambulatory care and hospital services are still paid by the Ministry of Health or by the State Health Secretary on a fee-for-service basis. Both public and private health care entities can provide these services.

When municipalities reach the next stage, the CMHS, they become responsible for all types of health services. Each month the central government transfers a fixed amount of resources. The amount is determined by average expenditures on health services in prior years.

The municipalities that have not qualified for either the CMBHC or the CMHS stage have no autonomy in the management of local health care; instead, they function as service providers, following a fee-for-service system. However, the fees do not go directly to the municipal government; instead they go to the state government, which then makes the payments. In these cases, the manager of SUS at the municipal level is the state government, and the municipal government receives no resources for sanitary actions and programs.

Financing of Central Government Expenditures

Resources for health care provided by the central government come primarily from the social security budget. In 1988, the Act of Transitory Arrangements established that "thirty percent, at least, of the social security bud-

TABLE 3. Days of inactivity due to illness by income group, Brazil, 1997.

| Days | Income quintile | | | | | | | | | | Total | |
| | 1 | | 2 | | 3 | | 4 | | 5 | | | |
	No.	%	No.	%	No.	%	No.	%	No.	%	No.	%
1	60	16.0	76	19.9	68	20.1	67	21.1	51	18.0	322	19.0
2	80	21.3	91	23.9	68	20.1	73	23.0	62	21.9	374	22.1
3	52	13.9	64	16.8	42	12.4	47	14.8	37	13.1	242	14.3
4	36	9.6	18	4.7	24	7.1	19	6.0	24	8.5	121	7.1
5	38	10.1	29	7.6	32	9.5	24	7.5	20	7.1	143	8.4
6–7	20	1.9	26	3.1	33	2.7	25	3.1	23	1.8	137	7.5
8–9	24	5.9	20	5.0	17	5.0	15	4.7	7	2.5	83	4.9
10–12	11	2.4	11	2.1	10	2.4	15	2.5	16	4.2	63	3.7
13–15	29	0.3	22	...	18	0.6	8	...	23	...	100	6.0
16–20	5	0.3	10	0.3	6	...	10	0.3	6	...	37	2.2
21–29	2	0.3	3	0.3	4	0.6	3	30	...	...	12	0.6
30 or more	18	4.8	11	2.9	16	4.7	12	3.8	14	4.9	71	4.2
Total	375	100.0	381	100.0	338	100.0	318	100.0	283	100.0	1,695	100.0

Source: LSMS, 1997.

get, excluding unemployment insurance, shall be destined to the health sector." However, the permanent Law of Budgetary Guidelines (LDO) did not mandate a percentage of revenue to be directed to health care. Subsequent LDOs have defined a nominal amount of resources for health care out of the social security budget, but there has been pressure to decrease this funding. In response, technical and political groups in the health sector have proposed earmarking revenue sources for health care financing or establishing a fixed percentage of the social security budget for health care expenditures.

In the past, an important source of financing for SUS was the employers' and laborers' contribution to social security, which historically represented the largest source of funds for medical assistance in the country. As of 1993, however, because of problems with social security, this participation was no longer available, which led to earmarking of other revenue sources to finance federal expenditures on health.

During the past five years, federal health care expenditures have been financed by five sources:

- The Social Contribution on Net Profit of Firms (Contribuição Social sobre Lucro Líquido; CSLL) financed 12.8% of the expenditures of the Ministry of Health in 1994 and approximately 20% during 1995–1997. The share dropped to 9.27% in 1998.
- The Social Contribution for Financing Social Security (Contribuição para o financiamento de Seguridad Social; COFINS) financed 49% of federal expenditures in 1995, but the figure dropped to 25% in 1998.
- The CPMF (the flat-rate tax of 0.2% on all bank account transactions, with revenues linked to health) has become increasingly important in the financing of the health sector since its creation in 1997. In 1998 it financed 46% of the Ministry of Health's budget.[14]
- The Fiscal Stabilization Fund (Fundo de Estabilição Fiscal [FEF]) contributed 12% of the Ministry of Health's resources in 1998.
- Other sources, with contributions that vary from year to year.

Inequalities in Public Health Care Financing

A broad analysis of the impact of social spending should also take into account the impact of taxation (direct and indirect taxes, fees, and contributions) on income distribution. Verifying the incidence of taxes and, further, the

degree of progressivity and regressivity of the sources of health financing, however, is a difficult task in Brazil because public health care is financed by several sources, as indicated in the preceding section.[15] Two of the financing mechanisms for public health expenditures are corporate taxes; a third mechanism is a tax on financial transactions. A detailed description of these three tax instruments follows, with an analysis of the regressive or progressive nature of each.

COFINS is a tax on the monthly revenue of firms. Because the tax is levied on all firms (producers, wholesalers, and retailers), it affects all stages of the productive process. This results in the so-called "cascade effect," which increases the tax load on the final product, cumulatively affecting its price. If it is assumed that the firm manages to pass on the full value of the tax through an increase in prices, the tax burden falls on consumers. Consequently, it can be classified as an indirect tax and very probably is regressive, considering that the tax incidence occurs regardless of the contributive capacity of the payer.[16] COFINS has also been criticized on several grounds, mainly because its tax base (turnover and gross operational revenue of firms) nearly coincides with another tax, the CSLL (see below). Other criticisms of COFINS are that it violates the principles of neutrality, equity, and competitiveness.

As a cascade tax, it distorts relative prices and encourages the vertical integration of firms in their production and commercialization phases. Vertical integration, in turn, inhibits specialization and negatively affects productivity. Also, two factors tend to aggravate the regressivity of COFINS. First, because the tax rate is fixed, it does not take into account the income levels of the population and therefore tax payments are proportionally greater for the poor. Second, as a cascade tax, it discriminates against products with an extensive production and commercialization cycle.[17]

CSLL, established in 1988, taxes the net profits of firms, but its incidence does not cascade along the chain of production. The tax base for a firm is gross profits (before

---

[14] This figure includes the resources that went to funds such as the Fiscal Stabilization Fund, which replaced the Social Emergency Fund, in 1997. These funds came from the retention of CPMF (the flat-rate tax of 0.2% on all bank account transactions).

[15] The great difficulty with this type of analysis is that household surveys, the most commonly used method in the country for measuring the incidence of social spending, do not capture expenditures on indirect taxes or on the contribution on financial transactions. This makes it impossible to analyze tax incidence by income class.

[16] Some authors (for example, Diana, 1995a) point out that the debate on equity and tributary progressivity can no longer simply be limited to direct versus indirect taxes. Nevertheless, for the purposes of this analysis, direct taxes are considered progressive because the burden increases with income. Indirect taxes, on the other hand, are considered regressive in the sense that they do not discriminate between consumers according to income, which causes the poor to bear a proportionally greater burden.

[17] Because of these problems, COFINS is quite likely to be replaced in the near future.

tax), with some adjustments. The tax rates in effect for the CSLL today are 10% for firms and 23% for financial institutions.

For this type of tax, it is difficult to precisely determine the degree of regressivity or progressiveness. The degree of regressivity depends on the firm's capacity to pass on the taxes to consumers. The share of CSLL in financing health has been reduced over the past few years, having reached its lowest level in 1998 (9%).

Temporary Tax on Financial Transactions (CPMF)

CPMF was instituted in 1996, exclusively destined to finance SUS. CPMF is a flat-rate tax of 0.2% on all financial transactions. In 1998, this tax provided about 46% of all Ministry of Health resources. CPMF has generated much controversy. Like COFINS, CPMF is an indirect tax and therefore should be regressive. However, some analysts point out that a tax on financial transactions may be progressive if there is a strong, positive relationship between income and utilization of financial transactions. A simulation carried out by Tavares (1995) supports the argument that CPMF is progressive.[18] This study found that the highest income strata, representing only 3.4% of the population, pays 63.5% of the CPMF tax. However, this and other findings rest on certain rather strict assumptions and many questions and issues remain to be investigated.[19]

Family Health Expenditures

Families also finance health care through out-of-pocket expenditures and private insurance schemes. Household survey data provide interesting insights into the type of financing used by different socioeconomic groups.

For example, a survey of living conditions in São Paulo (1994)[20] found that use of paid health services increased

significantly with income, from 3.9% among the indigent to 14.8% among the poor and to 25.8% for the highest income group. The use of prepaid services followed an increasing pattern also, from 14.8% in the case of the indigent to 62.3% among the highest income group. The indigent use free services at six times the rate of prepaid services (81% compared with 14.8%), whereas the second poorest quintile uses more prepaid services (44%) than free ones (41%).

Using the results of the LSMS once again, Table 4 summarizes the responses of individuals to the question of whether *they pay for the visit*. As expected, the proportion of those who pay grows with income, but what is surprising is the proportion. Only 19% of the people in the highest income quintile claimed that they pay for visits, yet the proportion of this group who do not seek public establishments was exactly the complement of this, 81%! From this contradictory information, it appears that many individuals who subscribe to health plans responded that they do not pay for visits, because their health plan reimburses the health care provider (they forgot they are the ones who pay for the health plan).

The LSMS also reveals that family health care expenditures (including insurance premiums, medications, consultations, hospital stays, and medical exams) grew dramatically with income. The highest income quintile spent on average 6.5 times the amount spent by the poorest quintile. The increase in expenditures is most significant between the fourth and fifth quintiles (it grew by 157%).

Coverage by a health insurance plan increases appreciably with income. Only 1.4% of the people in quintile 1 (the poorest) reported having a health plan. This percentage increased across quintiles, reaching 34% in quintile 4 and then almost doubling to 63.4% in quintile 5 (see Table 5).

The previously mentioned survey of living conditions in São Paulo (1994) found that 19% of the families classified as indigent reported that at least one of their members had health insurance. The average monthly expenditure on health insurance grows with income and, again, the increase is most significant between the top income groups, jumping 145% from the second highest to the highest income strata.

Returning once again to the LSMS, the number of people who had medical expenditures in the past 30 days grows with income as well as the amount of expenditure. As in the previous cases, the most substantial increase in expenditures (86%) is observed between the fourth and the fifth quintiles (see Table 6).

The number of people reporting expenditures on medical exams grows with income; the same occurs with average expenditures on exams and medication. Again,

[18]The simulations included only individual banking transactions, which represent only a portion of the total taxable base.

[19]For example, this study does not investigate the incidence of CPMF on firms, its indirect impact on individuals who do not use the banking system, its effect on interest rates, and how increases in the CPMF tax rate promote evasion through transactions outside the banking system.

[20]The 1994 Survey of Living Conditions was conducted by the State Service for Analysis of Statistical Data Foundation (SEADE), an organ of the Secretary of Planning of the State of São Paulo. The sample was limited to families living in metropolitan São Paulo. The population is classified into five socioeconomic strata by incorporating characteristics of housing, instruction, employment, and income by means of synthetic indicators that reveal privations or needs in each of these aspects. Thus, the groups can be differentiated among themselves by type and degrees of need they present and not merely by the variable income.

TABLE 4. Payment of medical consultations by income quintile, Brazil, 1997.

Medical consultation	Income quintile										Total	
	1		2		3		4		5			
	No.	%	No.	%	No.	%	No.	%	No.	%	No.	%
Patient paid	12	5.0	35	9.9	52	12.0	48	10.4	95	18.7	242	12.1
Patient did not pay	226	95.0	317	90.1	382	88.0	412	89.6	414	81.3	1,751	87.9
Total	238	100.0	352	100.0	434	100.0	460	100.0	509	100.0	1,993	100.0

Source: LSMS, 1997.

there is a jump from quintile 4 to quintile 5; expenditures on lab exams increase by 40% and expenditures on medication increase by 67%.

INEQUALITIES IN ACCESS TO AND UTILIZATION OF HEALTH SERVICES

The utilization of health services was divided into three categories: supervision of a chronic problem, curative care, and preventive care. This division is based on the assumption that individuals with different health care problems have distinct patterns of health service utilization. In the 1997 LSMS survey respondents answered a series of questions about the type of care, facilities and type of professional consulted, and time spent waiting to be seen. Following is a summary of the patterns of health care utilization for chronic, curative, and preventive care of the sampled population by income groups.

Utilization of Health Services in Treatment of Chronic Health Problems

Individuals who responded affirmatively to the question about whether they suffer from chronic health problems were asked to categorize their problem (heart related, hypertension, diabetes, respiratory, digestive, gynecological, prostate related, cancer, bone/muscular/joint, neuropsychiatric, hypercholesterolemia, and others). As discussed previously, there was a pattern associated with income level: individuals belonging to the upper quintiles

reported more heart problems, hypertension, and diabetes but fewer respiratory, digestive, and neuropsychiatric problems.

Among the survey participants, the percentage of people who use medical care and periodic exams to treat chronic health problems grows visibly with income; similarly, the percentage of individuals who have follow-ups with the same doctor for a chronic health problem increases with income (Table 7).

Among individuals with chronic problems, the response to the question *where do you get medical care* demonstrates unequivocal behavior, with the poorer quintiles seeking health care in public hospitals or clinics and higher income groups seeking care in private facilities (hospitals, clinics, and doctor's offices). The distribution does not have a smooth pattern; the percentage of individuals who go to public facilities in the first three quintiles is very similar (between 48% and 49%), but beginning with the fourth quintile there is a heavy decline. The use of public health centers or stations, however, decreases smoothly with income (Table 8).

When asked who cared for them, most people indicated that a doctor saw them (89%), a proportion that did vary significantly with income. Care by a nurse or pharmacist, however, decreased with income.

Utilization of Curative Services

The demand for curative health care services clearly grows with income. Only 47% of the people in the first quintile (the poorest) sought health care for curative rea-

TABLE 5. Population with health insurance by income group, Brazil, 1997.

Population	Income quintile										Total	
	1		2		3		4		5			
	No.	%	No.	%	No.	%	No.	%	No.	%	No.	%
Insured	50	1.4	191	5.0	598	16.8	1,210	34.5	2,347	63.4	4,396	24.2
Uninsured	3,497	98.6	3,663	95.0	2,965	83.2	2,294	65.5	1,352	36.6	13,771	75.8
Total	3,547	100.0	3,854	100.0	3,563	100.0	3,504	100.0	3,699	100.0	18,167	100.0

Source: LSMS, 1997.

TABLE 6. Expenditures (R$) on medical treatments and consultations in the past 30 days, by income group, Brazil, 1997.

Quintile	Average expenditure	Median expenditure	Maximum expenditure	Standard deviation	Number of observations
1	28.21	20.00	80.00	1.57	19
2	38.41	40.00	150.00	2.44	29
3	57.35	35.00	570.00	11.35	65
4	67.23	50.00	350.00	9.95	79
5	124.94	70.00	1,500.00	35.53	170

Source: LSMS, 1997.

sons, reaching 69% in the last quintile. Similarly, the results of the survey of living conditions in São Paulo (1994) show that the demand for health care in the preceding 30 days by the indigent is similar to that of the poor and middle strata (27%) but increases considerably in the highest income strata.

As in the case of chronic problems, poor individuals received curative care in public hospitals, health centers, and stations, and—in a much less significant proportion—pharmacies, whereas the wealthy went to doctor's offices, clinics, and private hospitals. Moreover, when individuals from the higher income groups seek care in public hospitals, it is often because the treatment involves high technology, is costly, and is not necessarily available in the private sector.

The time that people wait to be seen is a relevant variable in terms of equity because, from an ethical and medical viewpoint, waiting time should be a function of the severity of the case. Waiting time is also important from the viewpoint of accessibility; for some, waiting can be too costly and inhibit utilization. The results of the study are encouraging. Two-thirds of the interviewees reported

waiting less than an hour, but this proportion clearly grew with income, going from 50% in the first quintile to 81.5% in the fifth quintile. Extremely long waiting periods of 7–12 hours were not reported in the highest quintile.

QUANTIFICATION OF INEQUITY

The previous sections provide mixed evidence supporting the hypothesis that the poor in Brazil face disadvantages in terms of health conditions and access to health care compared with high-income groups. As income grows, the incidence of temporary illnesses diminishes, but the incidence of chronic illnesses increases slightly. However, the poorer income groups reported a worse perception of their health status than the higher income groups. Indicators of health care utilization showed a pattern favoring high-income groups.

According to Kakwani et al. (1997), an assessment of health care need and utilization cannot ignore the fact that biological and demographic factors decisively influence the patterns observed across income groups. The

TABLE 7. Indicators of medical attention for individuals reporting chronic health problems, Brazil, 1997.

LSMS question	Income quintile										Total	
	1		2		3		4		5			
	No.	%	No.	%	No.	%	No.	%	No.	%	No.	%
Have you seen a medical professional about this health problem?												
Yes	238	54.7	352	63.3	434	70.3	460	78.9	509	82.9	1,993	71.1
No	197	45.3	204	36.7	183	29.7	123	21.1	105	17.1	812	28.9
Total	435	100.0	556	100.0	617	100.0	583	100.0	614	100.0	2,805	100.0
Was there a follow-up visit with the same professional?												
Yes	123	51.7	207	58.8	285	65.7	336	73.0	411	80.7	1,362	68.3
No	115	48.3	145	41.2	149	34.3	124	27.0	98	19.3	631	31.7
Total	238	100.0	352	100.0	434	100.0	460	100.0	509	100.0	1,993	100.0
Do you have periodic exams for this health problem?												
Yes	145	60.9	230	65.3	305	70.3	357	77.6	420	82.5	1,457	73.1
No	93	39.1	122	34.7	129	29.7	103	22.4	89	17.5	536	26.9
Total	238	100.0	352	100.0	434	100.0	460	100.0	509	100.0	1,993	100.0

Source: LSMS, 1997.

TABLE 8. Place of treatment for chronic health problems, Brazil, 1997.

| Place of treatment | Income quintile | | | | | | | | | | Total | |
| | 1 | | 2 | | 3 | | 4 | | 5 | | | |
	No.	%	No.	%	No.	%	No.	%	No.	%	No.	%
Public hospital	114	47.9	173	49.1	213	49.1	158	34.3	76	14.9	734	36.8
Health center/post	102	42.9	112	31.8	97	22.4	71	15.4	21	4.1	403	20.2
Private hospital	2	0.8	7	2.0	13	3.0	27	5.9	34	6.7	83	4.2
Private hospital (with agreement with the government)	3	1.3	22	6.3	21	4.8	39	8.5	50	9.8	135	6.8
Private clinic (with agreement with the government)	9	3.8	16	4.5	37	8.5	88	19.1	162	31.8	312	15.7
Private doctor's office or clinic	7	2.9	16	4.5	47	10.8	70	15.2	157	30.8	297	14.9
Home	1	0.4	2	0.6			1	0.2	2	0.4	6	0.3
Other			4	1.1	6	1.4	6	1.3	7	1.4	23	1.2
Total	238	100.0	352	100.0	434	100.0	460	100.0	509	100.0	1,993	100.0

Source: LSMS, 1997.

analysis must take these factors into account through a standardization procedure (see the chapter titled "Inequity in the Delivery of Health Care: Methods and Results for Jamaica," which appears later in this section) that identifies the portion of the observed inequalities that result from demographic characteristics instead of income. Essentially, standardization creates variables to represent the health care needs and utilization of services of an individual based on his or her sex and age.

Using the model developed by van Doorslaer and Wagstaff, concentration indexes were constructed both for chronic need and for curative need (see the Annex at the end of this chapter for a more detailed discussion of estimation methods and results). The nonstandardized concentration indexes for curative need and chronic needs were calculated. Figure 1 presents the corresponding concentration curves.

In the case of chronic need, the concentration curve is situated below the line of equality. This shows that individuals in the higher quintiles of income distribution have a clear tendency to indicate the presence of chronic problems more frequently than those individuals in the first two quintiles. There are two possible explanations for this: either individuals with less purchasing power are less aware of their health status and thus report less chronic illness, or these individuals may, because of their demographic profile, have fewer chronic health problems. To better understand the underlying causes of this pattern, the age profile of the respondents was analyzed; the average age of individuals in the first quintile is 21 years and it grows systematically until it reaches 33.8 years for the highest income quintile. According to the demo-

graphic profile of the poorer population groups—essentially younger—the lower quintiles should report fewer chronic health problems than they do, whereas the higher income quintiles should report more chronic health problems than they do. This result may mean, for example, that, because of greater access to preventive health care services, chronic health problems are reduced among the higher income groups. This point is the target of analysis in the next section.

A second set of concentration indexes were estimated by the standardization procedure (see the Annex for detailed results).[21] The difference between the standardized and nonstandardized indexes for chronic need indicate that the most economically challenged group should report fewer problems than it does, whereas those who belong to the upper quintiles of income distribution should report more chronic problems than they do.

In the case of curative need (see Figure 1), the fact that the curve is slightly above the line of equality indicates that there is a tendency of individuals in low-income quintiles to report temporary health problems more frequently than individuals in high-income quintiles. The standardized index for curative need is slightly greater than the nonstandardized index but the difference is statistically significant. This means that individuals in the lower quintiles of income report greater temporary health problems than those in the upper quintiles and more than they should given their demographic profile. Once again, it can be hypothesized that reduced access to preventive

---

[21]Several models were used. For details see the Annex at the end of this chapter.

FIGURE 1. Concentration curves for health needs, Brazil, 1997.

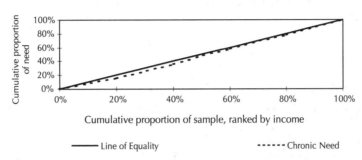

A. Concentration Curves for Chronic Need of Health Services

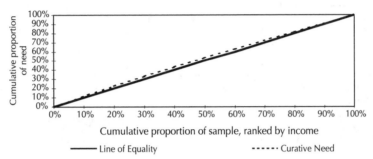

B. Concentration Curves for Curative Need of Health Services

health services may be generating greater curative need on the part of those in the less economically favored classes.

These inequalities in health status suggest the need to investigate whether unequal access to services, particularly preventive care, negatively affects the health of the economically disadvantaged in Brazil. When the concentration indexes are calculated for the three types of health care services (curative, chronic, and preventive), there is consistently greater utilization by the high-income groups than by the low-income groups, as illustrated by concentration curves below the line of equity (Figure 2).

The estimated differences between the standardized and nonstandardized indexes indicate the existence of pro-wealthy inequities in terms of utilization of health care services for all three categories.[22] These calculations show that actual use is lower than that determined by the need of the individuals in the lower quintiles of the income distribution. The greatest level of inequity is found in preventive health care utilization, which supports the hypothesis that the demand for this type of service by the poor is insufficient and may contribute to the

---

[22]The magnitude of the inequity varies depending on whether the model includes a variable representing chronic health need. See the Annex for more discussion of alternative models.

existence of pro-wealthy inequalities in the health status of individuals.

CONCLUSIONS AND CURRENT TRENDS IN PREVENTIVE HEALTH CARE

Conclusions

The analysis of household survey data demonstrates the presence of pro-wealthy inequalities both in terms of population health and in terms of utilization of health services. The analysis also revealed inequities in the utilization of health services, particularly for preventive services. One of the hypotheses raised is that inequity in the access to this type of service has serious implications for the health status of the lower income population.

Although universal health care is guaranteed by the constitution, health care expenditure per capita is quite low. Private health expenditures are 50% lower than public sector expenditures and individuals in low-income groups often resort to private services and pay out-of-pocket expenditures and health insurance premiums. Also, it is striking that preventive health care service has the most unequal pattern of utilization, yet it is one of the smallest categories of public health care expenditures.

FIGURE 2. Concentration curves for utilization of health services, Brazil, 1997.

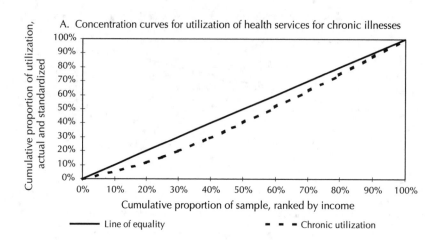

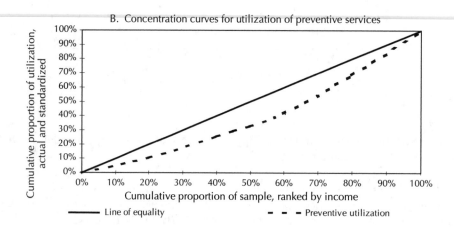

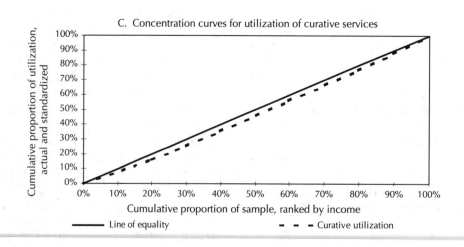

Preventive Health Care: Progress to Date

Given the inequalities in public financing and utilization, it is reassuring to note that the Ministry of Health has acknowledged the importance of projects that prioritize preventive health care services. Among the Ministry's program priorities are the Programs of Community Health Agents (Programa de Agentes Comunitários; PACs) and the Family Health Program (Programa de Saúde da Família; PSF).

Community Health Worker Programs

Inspired by previous experiences with disease prevention through information and with advisement on health care to high-risk groups, the Ministry of Health initiated the PACs in 1991. According to the information from the Ministry, by 1998 the PACs operated in all 27 states and the Federal District and were integrally tied to the ongoing process of municipalization and decentralization of health care.

Figures 3 and 4 illustrate the performance of PACs in the areas of preventive health care, prenatal care, and infant weight monitoring. As Figure 3 shows, the proportion of women with up-to-date prenatal care in areas served by PACs is higher than the national average of 56.4%, with the exception of Maranhão and Alagoas. Figure 4 shows the proportion of infants weighed at birth in areas served by PACs in northeastern Brazil. Again, only the states of Maranhão and Alagoas have percentages below the national average. These results suggest that implementation of the PACs program has improved some indicators of preventive care.

FIGURE 4. Proportion of children weighed at birth in areas covered by PACs in the Northeast, Brazil, 1994–1997.

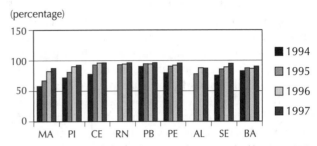

Source: Ministry of Health, Brazil, Program of community health agents (1998).

Family Health Unit (PSF)

PACs is part of an ongoing process in Brazil to reorient public health services toward a system based on the family health unit. The PSF has been officially described as "a public health unit, with a multi-professional team" that develops actions to promote health, prevent disease, and treat injuries. According to the Ministry of Health, by September 1998, 953 municipalities had formed a total of 2,616 family health teams. The descriptive document of the family health program emphasizes that the family health unit should focus on preventive care and provision of primary services. It should be connected to the network of services to guarantee integral attention to individuals and families and ensure reference and counterreference to the various levels of the system. PACs works within a defined territory and is responsible for the registration and care of the population enrolled in that area. The family health team is composed minimally by a general practitioner or a family doctor, a nurse, a nursing aide, and four to six community health agents.

Impact of the Municipalization of Health Care

It is hoped that the growing emphasis by the public sector on decentralization and primary care through the family health teams will have a positive effect on individuals' health and will reduce inequalities. An agency of the Secretary of the State of Health of São Paulo[23]

FIGURE 3. Proportion of pregnant women with up-to-date prenatal care in areas covered by PACs in the Northeast, Brazil, 1994–1997.

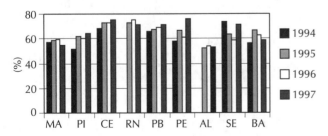

Source: Ministry of Health, Brazil, Program of community health agents (1998).

[23]The Nucleus of Investigation in Health Services and Systems of the Health Institute prepared the report and financing for the project was provided by the International Development Research Center, Canada.

evaluated the impact of decentralized management on various aspects of health services in 12 municipalities.[24] Interestingly, the researchers discovered that between 1994 and 1996 (during the period of implementation of the semicomplete management of the municipalities) there was an expansion of the supply of preventive services through several agents—family health teams, basic health units, dental clinics, health stations. In all the municipalities studied, the preventive and health-promoting actions were being developed in partnership with other sectors of municipal administration, such as education, sanitation, housing, culture, and sports. One project, Cidades Saudáveis (Healthy Cities), developed in Fortim, Diadema, and Santos, was identi-

fied as being the broadest in terms of intersector participation for preventive and health-promoting actions.

REFERENCES

Instituto Brasileiro de Geografia e Estatística. *Living Standards Measurement Survey*. Rio de Janeiro: Instituto Brasileiro de Geografia e Estatística; March 1997.

Kakwani N, Wagstaff A, van Doorslaer E. Socioeconomic inequalities in health: measurement, computation, and statistical inference. *Journal of Econometrics*. 1997; 77:87–103.

Tavares M. *Conceição, Tributação sobre Circulação Financeira*. São Paulo: Folha de São Paulo, edição de 24/09/95; 1995.

van Doorslaer E, Wagstaff A. *Inequity in the Delivery of Health Care: Methods and Results for Jamaica*. Paper prepared for the Human Development Department of the World Bank; June 1998.

---

[24]The specific objectives of the project were "to investigate the impact of decentralized management on the planning and scheduling process; on the structure and mechanisms of financing; on human resource administration; on the system of reference and counter-reference; on the supply of health services and care; and on people's participation and social control of the municipal health systems."

ANNEX: ESTIMATION OF INEQUITIES

ESTIMATION OF INEQUITIES IN HEALTH STATUS

The presence of a chronic health problem is represented by a dummy variable, NECCRON, whose unit value is associated to those individuals who responded affirmatively to the question about whether they suffer from a chronic health problem that requires constant medical care. The presence of a health problem within the past 30 days was represented by another dummy variable—NECCURAT; an affirmative response by an individual was taken to signal a curative need.

The nonstandardized concentration index for chronic need was 0.0424, with a t statistic of 4.71 (see Table 1A). The nonstandardized concentration index corresponding to curative need was –0.0402, with a t statistic of –5.3828 (see Table 2).

Both indices were obtained by means of the following model estimated by ordinary least squares (OLS) as demonstrated by van Doorslaer and Wagstaff (1998):

$$2\sigma_R^2[m_i / m] = \gamma_2 + \delta_2 R_i + u_i, \text{ with } 1 = i = N \quad (1)$$

where N is the sample size, R_i is the relative rank of the ith person, m_i is the value of NECCRON (or NECCURAT) of the ith person, m is the mean of NECCRON (or NECCURAT), and σ_R^2 is the variance of the variable R. The t statistic was obtained by means of the results obtained in Equation 1 for the standard error of δ_1.

Standardized concentration indices were calculated by incorporating the sex and age of the individual into the model to estimate the level of illness of individuals independent of their socioeconomic status. The standardized level of illness was obtained by means of three distinct models: OLS, Logit, and Probit.[25] The procedure consists of retaining the predicted values of the explanatory variable from the parameters estimated.

The standardized concentration index for chronic need varies from 0.083 to 0.09, depending on the method adopted (see Table 1A). It is important to note that the t statistics are very elevated, guaranteeing the represen-

---
[25]The results of the models (parameters, tests) are found in Tables 1–5 of this Annex.

TABLE 1A. Descriptive statistics for NECCRON, categorized by quintile values (included observations: 19,409).

Quintile	Actual Mean	Logit model Mean	Least squares Mean	Probit model Mean
1	0.122639	0.119721	0.115897	0.120177
2	0.144266	0.139910	0.139062	0.140312
3	0.173169	0.164339	0.163750	0.164200
4	0.166381	0.170624	0.172119	0.170740
5	0.165991	0.186963	0.189842	0.187060
All	0.155289	0.155289	0.155289	0.155532
C, C^*	0.0424	0.0840	0.0902	0.0831
t statistic	4.7129	26.3004	29.3974	27.0284
I^*	...	–0.0416	–0.0478	–0.0406
t statistic	...	–4.9337	–5.6091	–4.8134

tativeness of the results. In the case of curative need, the values of the standardized concentration index were situated around 0.0034, with the t statistic between 15.3 and 15.8 depending on the method of estimation (see Table 2A).

The variable I^*, which is simply $C - C^*$, measures the difference between the nonstandardized and standardized concentration indices. This variable provides an alterna-

TABLE 2A. Descriptive statistics for NECCURAT, categorized by quintile values (included observations: 19,409).

Quintile	Actual Mean	Logit model Mean	Least squares Mean	Probit model Mean
1	0.268678	0.233173	0.233165	0.233263
2	0.231448	0.234501	0.234499	0.234540
3	0.234072	0.235992	0.235994	0.235977
4	0.222888	0.236509	0.236512	0.236476
5	0.213301	0.237433	0.237438	0.237360
All	0.235458	0.235458	0.235458	0.235461
C, C^*	–0.0402	0.0034	0.0034	0.0033
t statistic	–5.3828	15.7872	15.8207	15.3841
I^*	...	–0.0436	–0.0436	–0.0435
t statistic	...	–5.8483	–5.8491	–5.8306

tive means of measuring the existent inequities.[26] The negative value of I^* for the case of chronic need indicates that the most economically challenged group should report fewer problems than it does, whereas those who belong to upper quintiles of income distribution should report more chronic problems than they do. Thus, there are indications to conclude that the existent inequities in the health of the population act in favor of the individuals who belong to those groups higher in the income distribution.

The results for curative need find a slightly positive value for C^*, the standardized concentration index; however, this value is not statistically different from 0. As verified from the analysis of the values in Table 2A, the standardized values for the variable NECCURAT, obtained by any of the three models, are quite similar for all the quintiles. This is represented by the near coincidence of the concentration curves for the standardized values with the line of equality (see text).

As in the case of chronic need, the curative need I^* is also negative and statistically different from 0.

Inequities in the Utilization of Health Services

The calculation of indices for the utilization of health services followed the same methodology described above. The dummy variable (UTILCRON) that represented utilization of services for treatment of chronic health problems was constructed from two questions in the questionnaire:

- Do you get medical care because of this problem?
- Do you do periodical exams as a result of this health problem?

An affirmative answer to either or both of the questions resulted in a unit value for UTILCRON. Using questions about the dates of most recent exams and consultations, it was verified that, in the vast majority of cases,[27] individuals who reported the use of services for chronic health problems had had at least one consultation or exam within the preceding year.

In the case of curative and preventive health care utilization, variables were constructed from the combination of answers provided for the following questions:

- Did you seek health care for treatment of a health problem you have had in the past 30 days?

- Did you seek health treatment for any other reason in the past 30 days?
- For what reason did you seek care?
  1. Accident or injury
  2. Dental problem
  3. Check-up
  4. Birth
  5. Obtainment of medical note
  6. Rehabilitation treatment
  7. Prenatal
  8. Vaccination
  9. Other

The dummy variable (UTILCURA) that characterizes curative care takes the unit value for every affirmative answer to the first of the three questions or when the affirmative answer to the second question is accompanied by the motives represented by items 1, 2, 4, 6, and 9 of the third question.[28]

The dummy variable (UTILPREV) that represents preventive care takes the unit value when there is an affirmative answer to question 2 combined with a selection of one of the remaining items in the third question.

It is important to highlight that the variables referring to utilization of health services are binary. Thus, the utilization will be represented by the fact of the individual having used some health service at least once.

In a manner analogous to that adopted in the measurement of inequities in the health of individuals, a standardization procedure for the utilization of health services was adopted. According to van Doorslaer and Wagstaff (1998) ". . . an equitable distribution of health care is one in which health care is allocated according to need."[29] Thus, it is necessary to construct a standardized variable of utilization that characterizes what would have been the utilization of health services simply as a result of elements that characterize need.

The following variables were used in construction of the variable that characterizes this standardized utilization of health services:

- Sex (1, female; 0, male)
- Age (completed years)
- Self-assessed health: set of five dummy variables to distinguish six categories—indeterminate (SAHINDET), bad (SAHRUIM), average (SAHREGUL), good (SAHBOA), very good (SAHMUIBO), excellent.
- Dummy (NECCURAT) representing the curative

---

[26]It should be remembered, however, that these were obtained, as demonstrated by van Doorslaer and Wagstaff (1998), by means of the following convenient regression:

$$2\sigma_R^2\left[\frac{m_i}{m} - \frac{m_i^*}{m^*}\right] = \gamma_2 + \delta_2 R_i + u_i, \text{ where } \delta_2 \text{ corresponds to } I^*.$$

[27]More than 90% in the case of consults and about 88% in the case of exams.

---

[28] This association of others to curative reasons was based on the discovery that the professional sought was usually a doctor (94%) or a pharmacist (2%).

[29]The authors agree that this is a controversial point and indicate other references dedicated to analyzing alternative viewpoints to address the definition of equity.

TABLE 3A. Need-predicted chronic visits, categorized by quintile income values (included observations: 19,409).

Quintile	Actual UTILCRON Mean	Logit model without NECCRON UTILCRONFLOG Mean	Least squares with NECCRON UTILCRONFLS Mean	Least squares 1 without NECCRON UTILCRONFLS1 Mean	Probit model without NECCRON UTILCRONFPRO Mean
1	0.067099	0.114043	0.084001	0.11479	0.114256
2	0.091334	0.112322	0.101019	0.109817	0.111816
3	0.121807	0.119805	0.123257	0.116677	0.119137
4	0.131279	0.111429	0.119005	0.110191	0.111045
5	0.137605	0.090503	0.119929	0.095135	0.091015
All	0.109949	0.109949	0.109949	0.109949	0.109833
Cm, Cn	0.1192	−0.0356	0.0544	−0.0323	−0.0356
HI_{wv}	...	0.1549	0.0648	0.1515	0.1548

need determined by the question: Have you had any health problem within the past 30 days?

- Dummy (NECCRON) representing the "need due to a chronic problem" determined by the question: Do you have a chronic health problem that requires constant care?

Three standardized indicators were estimated for each type of utilization—chronic, curative, and preventive. Each of the three indicators was estimated by using three methods: OLS, Logit, and Probit.[30] The idea is to obtain results that can be compared with those generated by analyses done in other countries.

The results of the three models used to estimate standardized utilization indices demonstrate coherence in relation to the importance of the variables sex, age, NECCURAT, and a subset of the variables representative of self-assessed health (Tables 3A to 5A). It should be remembered that these models play an intermediary role in estimation of the inequality coefficients, and the results should not be interpreted in terms of a structural relationship between the explanatory variables and the utilization of health services.

The calculation of the inequity index was obtained in a form analogous to that expressed in Equation 1 of the preceding section. The index HI_{wv}, which can be expressed by the equation,[31]

$$HI_{WV} = C_M - C_N$$

in fact was also obtained by a method equivalent to that presented in the preceding section for calculation of indicator I^*.

Tables 3A–5A present the results of the different models for the three classes of utilization: chronic problems, curative, and preventive. The values of the inequity index can be found in the last lines of each table.

The tables show that, in general, for the three types of utilization the different statistical models obtain similar results. The only exception is the model estimated by OLS for utilization for chronic problems, which differs significantly from the other models.

The result of index HI_{wv}, equivalent to index I^* from the preceding section, was positive in all the models estimated. The difference resides in the magnitude of the inequalities—that is, the index oscillated between 0.065 and 0.155. When considering the comparison of the actual situation given by the variable UTILCRON or by the chronic utilization curve, with the standardized, which is synthesized by index HI_{wv}, inequality favoring the group belonging to the upper quintiles of income distribution is verified. Indeed, the positive value of HI_{wv} indicates the existence of pro-wealthy inequities.

This can be easily visualized by comparing the mean of actual utilization with those obtained by means of standardization. Thus, it is clearly verified that actual utilization is lower than that determined by the need of the individuals belonging to the lower quintiles of the income distribution, with the reverse occurring in the situation of those belonging to the upper quintiles. Thus, regardless of the model utilized—that is, with or without the incorporation of NECCRON—the pro-wealthy inequity is unequivocally present. The distinction resides in the magnitude of said inequity.

---

[30]The estimation of the standardized index for chronic health care utilization was somewhat different. In this case, two models were estimated by OLS. The model that presents the best fit included the independent variable representing chronic need (NECCRON). Thus, estimation of a model by means of Logit and Probit was not possible. A choice was made to reestimate the model by the OLS method with a specification equivalent to that which generated the best results in the other two methods.

[31]It should be remembered, however, that these were obtained, as demonstrated by van Doorslaer and Wagstaff (1998), by means of the following convenient regression: $2\sigma_R^2 \left[\dfrac{m_i}{m} - \dfrac{m_i^*}{m^*} \right] = \gamma_2 + \delta_2 R_i + u_i,$

where δ_2 corresponds to HI_{wv}.

TABLE 4A. Need-predicted curative visits, categorized by quintile income values (included observations: 19,409).

Quintile	Actual UTILCURA Mean	Logit model UTILCURAFLOG Mean	Least squares UTILCURAFLS Mean	Probit model UTILCURAFPRO Mean
1	0.098393	0.133286	0.133699	0.133028
2	0.106902	0.118813	0.118596	0.11864
3	0.125175	0.119414	0.119596	0.119469
4	0.127568	0.114442	0.113718	0.114415
5	0.135712	0.106265	0.106653	0.106325
All	0.11912	0.11912	0.11912	0.119044
C_m, C_n	0.0568	−0.0399	−0.0401	−0.0394
HI_{wv}	...	0.0967	0.0969	0.0962

TABLE 5A. Need-predicted preventive visits, categorized by quintile income values (included observations: 19,409).

Quintile	Actual UTILPREV Mean	Logit model UTILPREVFLOG Mean	Least squares UTILPREVFLS Mean	Probit model UTILPREVFPRO Mean
1	0.014378	0.026347	0.026284	0.026348
2	0.01972	0.026536	0.026433	0.026531
3	0.021892	0.027375	0.027313	0.027375
4	0.037671	0.027951	0.027934	0.027949
5	0.041363	0.027648	0.027864	0.02766
All	0.027152	0.027152	0.027152	0.027155
C_m, C_n	0.1943	0.0108	0.0122	0.0107
HI_{wv}	...	0.1836	0.1821	0.1836

HEALTH SYSTEM INEQUALITY AND POVERTY IN ECUADOR

Enrique Lasprilla, Jorge Granda, Carlos Obando, Eduardo Encalad, and Christian Lasprilla

BACKGROUND

Ecuador's population (11.9 million in 1997)[1] is predominantly urban and relatively young. Approximately 62.4% of Ecuadorians live in urban areas and 37% are 14 years of age or younger; the annual population growth rate is 2.2%.[2]

Ecuador's economic performance has been disappointing since the onset of the debt crisis in 1982. Structural adjustment was pursued haltingly in the 1980s, but two natural disasters and a sharp decline in the terms of trade slowed economic growth. The implementation of adjustment policies was gradual, slow, and selective, and social conflict resulted in frequent setbacks (Berry, 1997).

The stabilization and reform programs carried out in the early 1990s reduced the public sector deficit, increased foreign exchange reserves, and lowered inflation. In 1995, however, the border conflict with Peru and a drought-induced electricity crisis had negative effects on economic activity and led to a deterioration of macroeconomic conditions. The sharp rise in nominal interest rates during the conflict placed considerable strain on borrowers and financial institutions. Although nominal interest rates returned to more normal levels in 1996, real interest rates remained high and many enterprises faced difficulties servicing their bank debts.

During 1996–1998 the country's economic problems were exacerbated by political instability (a president was ousted after six months in power and was succeeded by an 18-month interim administration) and low oil prices. Ecuador will end the decade with negative growth rates, widespread financial crisis, declining foreign exchange reserves, worsening fiscal and external imbalances, and the highest inflation rate in Latin America.

Income Inequality and Poverty

Ecuador has an extremely unequal distribution of income. In 1995, its Gini coefficient (0.57) was one of the highest in Latin America. The wealthiest 10% of the population received 44% of total household income. The poorest decile, on the other hand, received only 0.6% of total household income (Inter-American Development Bank, 1999).

According to various estimates, between 33% and 38% of Ecuadorians are poor (Table 1). The incidence of poverty is even higher in rural areas, where estimates range from 47% to 64%.

Health Care System: Public Sector

Within the public sector, health services are provided mainly by the Ministry of Public Health and the Ecuadorian Social Security Institute (Instituto Ecuatoriano de Seguridad Social; IESS). Several specialized public agencies, the municipal government of Quito, the Armed Forces, and the National Police also provide health services.

TABLE 1. Poor population by geographic area and by various measures of poverty (%), Ecuador, 1995.

Geographic area	Income-based poverty line	Consumption-based poverty line		
	Larrea*	Hentschel[†]	Roberts[‡]	Roberts[§]
National	33	35	38	38
Urban	17	25	24	20
Rural	56	47	58	64

Sources: Larrea et al. (1995); Jácome et al. (1997); Roberts (1998a).

*Based on LSMS (1995); income-based, purchasing power parity (PPP)-adjusted poverty line of US$2 (1985) per person per day.

[†]Based on LSMS (1995); consumption-based poverty line equivalent to the cost of 1.25 baskets of basic goods and services.

[‡]Based on LSMS (1995); consumption-based poverty line of 60,876 Ecuadorian sucres per person semimonthly.

[§]Based on projections using data from the national census of 1990 and consumption models developed using LSMS (1995).

---

[1]Inter-American Development Bank (1999: 229).

[2]Inter-American Development Bank estimates based on data from Latin America Demographic Center and United Nations Population Division.

Ministry of Public Health

The Ministry of Public Health designs and executes policies and health programs, regulates and coordinates the health sector, and administers units that deliver health services directly. As the regulatory entity of the health sector, the Ministry of Public Health presides over the National Health Council, the entity responsible for inter- and intrainstitutional coordination.

As part of the process of sectoral reform, the Ministry of Public Health is expected to expand its regulatory role and reduce its participation in the delivery of health services. Currently, however, the Ministry provides health services at three levels of complexity. Care at the first level is provided by various kinds of health centers, which are organized in "health areas;" care at the second and third levels is provided by general and specialized hospitals.

Other Public Sector Entities

Other entities in the public health sector include the National Malaria Eradication Service (Servicio Nacional de Erradicación de la Malaria; SNEM), the State Center for Drugs and Medical Supplies (Centro Estatal de Medicamentos e Insumos Médicos; CEMEIN), and the National Institute for the Child and the Family (Instituto Nacional del Niño y la Familia; INNFA). For the purposes of this study, INNFA was considered part of the central government because it is financed mainly by tax revenues.

Local Government

Traditionally, Ecuadorian municipal governments have not offered health services, except for the Quito metropolitan government. Several pilot projects were carried out recently in some municipalities (Cuenca, Tena, and Cotacachi), which could result in the establishment of permanent, government-managed health care units in the future. In addition, the Special Law on Decentralization of the State and Social Participation of October 1997 assigns responsibilities to the municipal governments in the area of primary care. Similarly, the law reforming the Free Maternity Care Law, enacted in August 1998, mandates the creation of local solidarity funds to provide care for pregnant women and for children.

The Quito municipal government provides health services mainly through the units of the Patronato San José (San José Foundation), which specializes in the care of senior citizens, maternal and childcare, pneumology, traumatology, and ophthalmology. In addition, the municipal government maintains various health programs, such as the School Health Program and the Health and Family Planning Program.

Ecuadorian Social Security Institute

IESS provides health services to urban workers employed in the formal labor market through a general insurance program and to rural families through a special rural social insurance program (Seguro Social Campesino; SSC). IESS covers about 18% of the Ecuadorian population.

The general insurance program covers about 10% of the population. It provides ambulatory and hospital services of various degrees of complexity. The services benefit workers in the formal sector who, along with their employers, make mandatory contributions to the social security system. The program does not cover other members of the workers' families except for children under 1 year of age.

SSC covers rural families, who make up about 8% of the Ecuadorian population. Unlike the general insurance program, it does cover all family members. SSC provides coverage for primary health services delivered through "medical dispensaries." Limited access to hospital services is available through referrals to the general insurance program. Families affiliated with SSC make minimal contributions to the system.

Armed Forces Social Security Institute

ISSFA offers services through health units of varying complexity and health centers and subcenters distributed throughout the country. The services are available to personnel of the different branches of the Armed Forces and their immediate families. ISSFA services are financed through obligatory contributions of Armed Forces personnel, budget allocations from the Ministry of Defense, and payment of user fees.

Police Social Security Institute

ISSPOL offers health services to police personnel, similar to those provided by ISSFA.

Health Care System: Private Sector

The private health sector includes for-profit establishments, NGOs, and informal providers. The for-profit sector provides services through private medical centers or hospitals, clinics, and doctors' offices. Deterioration in the quality of care provided by the Ministry of Health and the IESS has increased the demand for private services.

Various NGOs carry out health-related activities, but the most important are the Society to Combat Cancer (Sociedad de Lucha contra el Cáncer; SOLCA) and the Social Welfare Institute of Guayaquil (Junta de Beneficiencia Social de Guayaquil; JBSG). SOLCA provides ambulatory and hospital services in Quito, Guayaquil, and Cuenca, focusing on cancer prevention and treatment. It finances its operations through donations and user fees. JBSG provides hospital care, services for the elderly, and outpatient pediatric, maternal, and psychiatric services. It finances its operations through resources generated by the national lottery, investment income, and user fees.

Informal health care providers cover a significant portion of the country's rural and poor population. Most engage in traditional health care practices and are unregistered, unregulated, and subject to the drawbacks associated with working outside the formal health care structure.

Health Care System: Institutions That Serve the Poor

Of the entities listed above, those that serve predominantly poor populations are the Ministry of Public Health (particularly through the services provided by health centers and subcenters), SSC, INNFA, the municipal government of Quito, SOLCA, and JBSG. A study by Younger et al. (1997) on demand for health services provides information on the services available to the poor through the Ministry of Public Health. A study on INNFA provides evidence that this institution mainly serves the poor (Lasprilla et al., 1997a). SSC, SOLCA, JBSG, and the municipal government of Quito also target and subsidize health care for the poor.

INEQUALITIES IN HEALTH CONDITIONS

Epidemiological, Mortality, and Morbidity Profile

Preventable or easily treatable diseases are the main cause of premature death in Ecuador. Intestinal infections and various respiratory diseases are the primary causes of both infant and adult mortality (Instituto Nacional de Estadísticas y Censos, 1995). This profile suggests that early death is closely associated with poverty and lack of access to basic health care.

Ecuador's morbidity profile also reflects poverty and lack of access to basic health and sanitation services. The

main causes of infant morbidity are intestinal infections and pneumonia, with rates of 163 and 111 per thousand, respectively, whereas the main causes of general morbidity are obstetric infections, intestinal infections, and abortion (Instituto Nacional de Estadísticas y Censos, 1995). These outcomes reflect the lack of access to basic prenatal and maternity services in poor communities.

Self-Assessed Health

Data from the 1995 LSMS show that self-assessed health does not vary significantly across income groups. Approximately 41% of the poor and the nonpoor reported illness during the preceding month.[3] However, illness caused more days of inactivity among the poor than among the nonpoor: persons in the poorest income quintile reported an average of nine days of inactivity, whereas the number was eight for the second quintile and five for the remaining income groups. Preexisting debilitating conditions in poor communities and limited access to health services are the probable causes of this finding. Prolonged inactivity, in turn, perpetuates the vicious cycle of illness→poverty→illness, as the reduction in family income caused by loss of work days creates propitious conditions for the advent of new diseases and lessens the capacity to obtain the services that are necessary to treat them.

Other findings with regard to the health status of the population are the following:

- The indigenous population (defined as people who speak indigenous languages) reported fewer illnesses during the preceding month (36.6%) than the nonindigenous population (42.1%).
- The urban and rural populations reported illnesses in similar proportions (41.3% and 42.6%, respectively).

HEALTH CARE EXPENDITURES AND FINANCING

Health Care Expenditures

Ecuador's health care expenditures represent about 5.1% of gross domestic product (GDP), a figure below the Latin American average (7.3%). Per capita expenditure was US$ 71, one of the lowest levels in Latin America (PAHO, 1998).

Households account for the largest proportion of health care spending (37.0%), followed by the central govern-

---

[3]The poor were defined as those in the first income quintile. The nonpoor were defined as the population in quintiles 2–5.

ment (27.7%) and social security institutions (23.8%). Private insurance accounts for 4.6%, NGOs for 5.2%, and private companies for 0.8%. Figure 1 illustrates this distribution and Table 1 provides a more detailed breakdown.

The structure of health care expenditures (Tables 2 and 3) shows that the health system in Ecuador emphasizes curative care to the detriment of primary health care and public health services. Hospital services account for the largest share of health expenditures (34.4%), followed by clinics and medical services (23.6%), public health services (4.2%), drugs (36.6%), and research (0.9%).

At the household level, drugs account for most of the expenditure (73.8%), followed in importance by medical visits (20%) and hospitalization (6.3%). As Table 4 shows, there is an inverse correlation between level of expenditure on drugs and family income. This situation reflects the limited access of poor families to private and public insurance schemes and the limited coverage provided by the Ministry of Public Health for drugs. Out-of-pocket expenditures for medical visits, on the other hand, are positively related to family income. Hospitalization expenditures do not show any clear pattern among income groups.

Health Care Financing

As mentioned earlier, Ecuador's health care expenditures represent approximately 5.1% of GDP, a figure below the Latin American average (7.3%). Per capita expenditure was US$ 71, one of the lowest levels in Latin America (PAHO, 1998).

FIGURE 1. Health expenditures by institutional source, Ecuador, 1995.

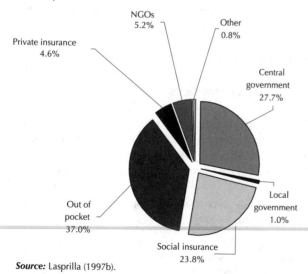

Source: Lasprilla (1997b).

As Figure 2 shows, the most important sources of financing for the national health system are fees paid directly by households (38.6%), contributions to the social security scheme by formal-sector employers and workers (24.1%),[4] tax revenues (15%), and oil revenues (13%). Less important sources include private insurance premiums (4.6%), payments of firms to private insurance, and the national lottery. A large proportion of the population are not covered by any insurance scheme, public or private.

Inequalities in Health Care Expenditures and Financing

The pattern of distribution of income and private expenditure in Ecuador's health sector is highly skewed. The two deciles with the highest income account for 59% of national income, 30% of private health expenditures, and 31% of government expenditure on health. On the other hand, the two deciles with the lowest income receive 3.0% of the national income and account for 13.7% of private health expenditures and 12.2% of public health expenditures.[5]

In all income groups except the wealthiest (the 9th and 10th deciles), the share of households in health expenditures is smaller than their share of national income. The 10th decile's share of national income is dramatically higher than its share of total public and private expenditures on health (see Figure 3).

Progressivity indices (Kakwani's indices) were calculated for the different sources of financing for the National Health Service Systems (NHS) (van Doorslaer and Wagstaff, 1998). The main results follow, and the computations appear in the Annex.

- Taxes. The Ecuadorian tax system is highly regressive because it relies primarily on indirect taxes, which were found to be regressive in both urban and rural areas. Direct taxes were found to be progressive in rural areas and regressive in urban areas (see Annex).
- Private insurance, out-of-pocket expenditures, and IESS contributions. The results show that out-of-pocket expenditures and private insurance are the most regressive sources of financing in both urban and rural areas. IESS contributions are less re-

[4]Includes contributions to the IESS, ISSPOL, and ISSFA.
[5]LSMS (1995); Instituto Nacional de Estadísticas y Censos (1995). The coefficients used for applying the concept of private expenditure per equivalent were as follows: zero children—1, one child—1.26, two children—1.52, three children—1.78, four children—2.04, five children—2.30, seven children—2.82.

TABLE 2. Types of health care expenditures by source, Ecuador, 1996 (percentages).

Expenditure	Central government MSP	ISSFA and ISSPOL	INNFA	Local government Quito municipal government	Social security funds General insurance	SSC	Private sector Households	Private insurance	Nonprofit institutions	Other	Total
Hospital services	44.8	0.9			24.6		6.7	7.6	15.0	0.4	100
Clinics and medical services	22.8	0.2	1.0	0.9	25.9	6.7	31.4	8.4		2.7	100
Public health services	83.8			16.2							100
Drugs, prostheses	4.2	0.6		0.2	20.4	0.4	74.1			0.0	100
Applied research	100.0										100
Total	26.9	0.6	0.2	1.0	22.1	1.7	37.0	4.6	5.2	0.8	100

Source: Lasprilla (1997b).

TABLE 3. Health expenditures of public and private institutions by type of service, Ecuador, 1996 (percentages).

Expenditure	Central government MSP	ISSPOL	INNFA	Local government Quito municipal government	Social security funds General insurance	SSC	Private sector Households	Private insurance	Nonprofit institutions	Other	Total
Hospital services	57.5	50.8			38.4		6.2	57.0	100.0	18.0	34.4
Clinics and medical services	20.0	9.1	100.0	22.3	27.6	91.3	20.0	43.0		81.5	23.6
Public health services	13.2			70.7							4.2
Drugs, prostheses	5.8	40.1		6.9	34.0	8.7	73.8			0.5	36.8
Applied research	3.5										0.9
Total	100.0	100.0	100.0	100.0	100.0	100.0	100.0	100.0	100.0	100.0	100.0

Source: Lasprilla (1997b).

gressive than private insurance at the national level and particularly in rural areas, because the rural social insurance program is subsidized and provides family coverage. Moreover, the IESS contribution scheme is directly proportional to the affiliates' income level in the five lower deciles of the income distribution.

TABLE 4. Household expenditures, by income deciles and type of expenditure, Ecuador, 1995 (percentages).

Deciles	Medical visits (%)	Drugs (%)	Hospitals (%)	Total (%)
Total	20.0	73.8	6.2	100
1	15.4	82.6	2.0	100
2	13.9	82.3	3.8	100
3	14.0	78.6	7.4	100
4	13.8	76.2	10.1	100
5	16.1	79.1	4.2	100
6	19.5	77.3	3.2	100
7	16.0	73.8	10.2	100
8	19.3	76.7	4.0	100
9	28.0	67.3	4.7	100
10	24.3	67.5	8.2	100

Source: LSMS, 1995; Income and Expenditure Survey, 1995.

FIGURE 2. Sources of financing of national health expenditures, Ecuador, 1995.

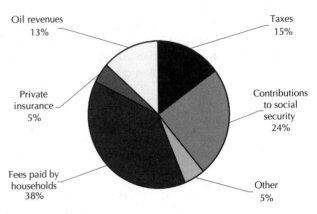

Source: National Health Expenditure Accounts.

Inequalities in Utilization of Health Services

Utilization of public and private hospitals and clinics increases with income (Table 5). Self-treatment in pharmacies and at home is common among all income groups but particularly among the poorest. The use of health

FIGURE 3. Income distribution compared with distribution of private and public expenditures on health, Ecuador, 1995.

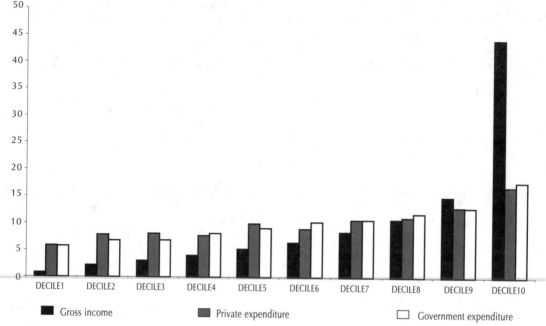

Source: LSMS, 1995; Instituto Nacional de Estadísticas y Censos, 1995.

subcenters administered by the Ministry of Public Health decreases with income.

High-income groups have greater access to physicians and dentists than low-income groups; self-treatment, on the other hand, is more frequent among the poor (Table 6).

The urban population has greater access to public hospitals, health centers, private clinics, and doctors' offices than the rural population. The latter received care at home more often. Similarly, the urban population has greater access to care by physicians and dentists than the rural

population, which relies on self-treatment more often (Tables 7 and 8).

The nonindigenous population used public hospitals, health centers, private clinics, and doctors' offices in larger proportion than the indigenous population (Table 9). The latter received care at home and at subcenters managed by the Ministry of Public Health more often.

In addition, the nonindigenous population has greater access to care by physicians than the indigenous popula-

TABLE 5. Place of medical visits during previous month by income quintiles, Ecuador, 1995.

Place of medical attention	Quintile 1 (%)	Quintile 2 (%)	Quintile 3 (%)	Quintile 4 (%)	Quintile 5 (%)	Total (%)
Public hospital*	6.19	7.68	8.75	9.46	9.53	8.35
Health center[†]	2.21	3.54	3.43	3.54	2.98	3.15
Health subcenter[‡]	5.64	6.18	4.50	4.82	2.94	4.79
Private hospitals, clinics, and doctors' offices	17.60	18.11	22.71	26.48	34.85	24.07
Pharmacies	10.99	13.51	13.62	12.82	8.05	11.80
Other	1.43	1.54	1.81	1.75	2.59	1.83
Home	55.94	49.45	45.19	41.13	39.07	46.01
Total	100	100	100	100	100	100

Source: LSMS, 1995; Instituto Nacional de Estadísticas y Censos, 1995.
*Ministry of Public Health, IESS, and Armed Forces.
[†]Ministry of Public Health and IESS.
[‡]NHS Ministry of Public Health.

TABLE 6. Health care providers during previous month by income quintiles, Ecuador, 1995.

Provider	Quintile 1 (%)	Quintile 2 (%)	Quintile 3 (%)	Quintile 4 (%)	Quintile 5 (%)	Total (%)
Traditional healer	2.47	1.67	1.28	1.61	1.48	1.69
Midwife	0.00	0.00	0.10	0.00	0.00	0.02
Pharmacist	10.56	13.78	12.91	12.45	7.60	11.45
Nurse/practitioner	1.11	0.91	0.69	0.46	0.59	0.75
Physician	26.98	31.11	36.52	41.20	47.31	36.80
Dentist	4.28	4.06	4.75	4.92	6.86	4.99
Self-treatment	54.60	48.47	43.76	39.36	36.16	44.31
Total	100.00	100.00	100.00	100.00	100.00	100.00

Source: LSMS, 1995; Instituto Nacional de Estadísticas y Censos, 1995.

tion (Table 10). The latter more often relies on self-treatment and traditional healers.

Utilization of outpatient services increases with income in urban areas (Table 11). However, the pattern reverses among the rural population, probably as a result of the low quality of these services in rural areas. It appears that high-income rural residents obtain outpatient services in urban areas.

The utilization of inpatient services also tends to increase with income in urban areas (Table 12). This is particularly true in the case of inpatient services provided by private hospitals and clinics (LSMS, 1995). The utilization pattern in the rural sector is unclear.

Quantification of Inequities

The ECuity method (see the chapter titled "Inequity in the Delivery of Health Care: Methods and Results for Jamaica," which appears later in this section) was applied

to test for inequities in health status and in the utilization of health services. When the variables were standardized, it was found that the system showed a clear pro-rich bias in the utilization of health services. Inequalities in the utilization of preventive services were greater than for curative services. However, no bias was found in health status. The standardization procedures are described in the Annex.

Conclusions and Policy Recommendations

- Households account for the largest proportion of health care expenditure (37.0%) followed by the central government (27.7%) and social security institutions (23.8%). Private insurance accounts for 4.6%, NGOs for 5.2%, and private companies for 0.8%.
- The health system in Ecuador emphasizes curative care, to the detriment of primary health care and public health services. Hospital services account for the largest share of health expenditures (34.4%) followed by clinics and medical services (23.6%), public health services (4.2%), drugs (36.6%), and research (0.9%).

TABLE 7. Place where medical attention was provided during previous month by area of residence, Ecuador, 1995 (percentages).

Place of medical attention	Urban areas	Rural areas	Total
Public hospital*	9.70	6.44	8.35
Health center†	3.75	2.30	3.15
Health subcenter‡	2.94	7.40	4.79
Private hospitals, clinics, and doctors' offices	27.31	19.48	24.07
Pharmacies	12.36	11.01	11.80
Other	2.21	1.29	1.83
Home	41.71	52.08	46.01
Total	100.00	100.00	100.00

Source: LSMS (1995), Instituto Nacional de Estadísticas y Censos (1995).
*Ministry of Public Health, IESS, and Armed Forces.
†Ministry of Public Health and IESS.
‡Ministry of Public Health.

TABLE 8. Health care providers during previous month, by area of residence, Ecuador, 1995 (percentages).

Provider	Urban areas	Rural areas	Total
Healer	0.99	2.67	1.69
Midwife	0.02	0.02	0.02
Pharmacist	11.78	10.99	11.45
Nurse/practitioner	0.36	1.30	0.75
Physician	41.51	30.14	36.80
Dentist	5.54	4.20	4.99
Self-treatment	39.80	50.67	44.31
Total	100.00	100.00	100.00

Source: LSMS, 1995; Instituto Nacional de Estadísticas y Censos, 1995.

TABLE 9. Place where medical attention was received during previous month by ethnicity, Ecuador, 1995 (percentages).

Place of medical attention	Indigenous population	Nonindigenous population	Total
Public hospital*	6.39	8.45	8.35
Health center†	2.39	3.19	3.15
Health subcenter‡	5.27	4.77	4.79
Private hospitals, clinics, and doctors' offices	14.64	24.53	24.07
Pharmacies	10.03	11.89	11.80
Other	2.04	1.82	1.83
Home	59.24	45.36	46.01
Total	100.00	100.00	100.00

Source: LSMS, 1995; Instituto Nacional de Estadísticas y Censos, 1995.
*Ministry of Public Health, IESS, and Armed Forces.
†Ministry of Public Health and IESS.
‡Ministry of Public Health.

- The most important sources of financing for the national health system are fees paid directly by households (38.6%), contributions to social security by formal-sector employers and workers (24.1%), tax revenues (15%), and oil revenues (13%). Less important sources include private insurance premiums (4.6%), contributions of firms to private insurance, and the national lottery. A large proportion of the population is not covered by any insurance scheme, public or private.
- The descriptive tables presented in this study show that the patterns of health expenditure and utilization of health services benefit the population in the higher-income groups. The computation of inequity indices related to use of health care facilities and financing of health services also shows that there is a bias favoring the wealthiest groups.

These conclusions lead to the following recommendations:

TABLE 10. Health care providers during the previous month, by ethnicity, Ecuador, 1995 (percentages).

Provider	Indigenous	Nonindigenous	Total
Traditional healer	2.36	1.66	1.69
Midwife	0.00	0.02	0.02
Pharmacist	9.12	11.56	11.45
Nurse/practitioner	1.87	0.69	0.75
Physician	22.99	37.47	36.80
Dentist	6.02	4.94	4.99
Self-treatment	57.63	43.66	44.31
Total	100.00	100.00	100.00

Source: LSMS (1995), Instituto Nacional de Estadísticas y Censos (1995).

TABLE 11. Use of outpatient services by income group and geographic location, Ecuador, 1995 (percentage).

Income group	Total	Big cities	Medium cities	Small cities	Rural sector
1	13.46	3.53	8.25	7.23	28.95
2	16.25	11.46	9.79	21.73	24.00
3	20.17	16.44	24.14	24.11	19.41
4	22.63	26.63	24.97	23.15	16.84
5	27.50	41.94	32.84	23.78	10.80
Total	100.00	100.00	100.00	100.00	100.00

- It is necessary to change the structure of national health expenditures by transferring resources from households to the social security system.
- The relative importance of direct taxation should be increased in order to reduce inequalities in health financing.
- It is important to provide more financial resources for the rural social insurance program in order to reduce the bias that exists against the rural population in the provision of health services.
- It is necessary to modify the structure of health care expenditure by reducing the importance of hospital services and improving and expanding public health services. In particular, more resources should be allocated for the provision of primary health care services by health centers and subcenters and for public health interventions.
- Public insurance schemes should be developed in order to address the needs of the population that is currently uninsured. These schemes should ensure coverage of children and mothers in order to reduce morbidity and mortality related to lack of access to health services by these segments of the population.
- Differential tariffs should be established for public health services on a sliding scale proportional to the users' income.

TABLE 12. Use of inpatient services by income group and geographic location, Ecuador, 1995 (percentage).

Income group	Total	Big cities	Medium cities	Small cities	Rural sector
1	8.40	5.91	7.82	3.34	15.69
2	24.06	19.58	12.95	0.15	30.84
3	18.78	27.08	13.87	1.04	18.86
4	20.34	21.27	28.75	2.46	13.49
5	28.43	26.16	36.61	93.01	21.12
Total	100.00	100.00	100.00	100.00	100.00

REFERENCES

Berry A. Contexto macroeconómico de las políticas para combatir la pobreza. In: Zevallos JV (ed). *Estrategias para reducir la pobreza en América Latina y el Caribe*. Quito: Programa de las Naciones Unidas para el Desarrollo; 1997, pp 29–104.

Instituto Nacional de Estadísticas y Censos. *Anuario de estadísticas vitales, 1995*. Quito: Instituto Nacional de Estadísticas y Censos; 1995.

Inter-American Development Bank. *Progreso económico y social en América Latina, Informe 1998–99* Washington, DC: Inter-American Development Bank; 1999.

Jácome L, Larrea C, Vos R. Políticas macroeconómicas, distribución y pobreza en el Ecuador. Quito: Programa de las Naciones Unidas para el Desarrollo [working paper]; 1997.

Larrea C. (ed.). *La geografía de la pobreza en el Ecuador*. Quito: Programa de las Naciones Unidas para el Desarrollo; 1995.

Lasprilla E. *Estudio sobre sistema tarifario de recuperación de costos y reinversión para los servicios del Programa de Acción Médica Solidaria*. Quito: Instituto Nacional del Niño y la Familia; 1997a. Mimeograph.

Lasprilla E, Granda J, Casas J, Cisneros O, Lasprilla C. *Gasto y financiamiento del sector salud en Ecuador, 1996,* Quito: Pan American Health Organization/World Health Organization; 1997b.

Pan American Health Organization. *La Salud en las Américas*. Washington, DC: Pan American Health Organization; 1998.

Roberts S. La distribución geográfica de la pobreza en el Ecuador. Metodología y resultados [unpublished]; 1998a.

Roberts S. Acceso y utilización de servicios públicos en el Ecuador: características geográficas, étnicas y económicas [unpublished]; 1998b.

van Doorslaer E, Wagstaff A. *Inequity in the Delivery of Health Care: Methods and Results for Jamaica*. Washington, DC: World Bank; 1998.

World Bank. *Ecuador Poverty Report, Vol. 1*. Washington, DC: World Bank; 1995.

World Bank, United Nations Development Program, Commission of the European Communities, International Monetary Fund, Organization for Economic Cooperation and Development. *System of National Accounts*. Washington, DC: CEC, IMF, OECD, UNDP, WB; 1993.

Younger S, Villafuerte M, Jara L. *Incidencia distributiva del gasto público y funciones de demanda en el Ecuador: educación, salud y crédito agrícola del BNF*. Quito: Facultad Latinoamericana de Ciencias Sociales; 1997.

ANNEX: QUANTIFICATION OF INEQUITIES IN HEALTH STATUS, HEALTH SERVICE UTILIZATION, AND HEALTH FINANCING IN ECUADOR

INEQUITIES IN HEALTH STATUS AND HEALTH SERVICE UTILIZATION

Standardized procedures based on regression methods were used to estimate "health needs" to derive the corresponding inequity in access indexes.

• Standardization procedure

Crude data on utilization of curative and preventive health care services were adjusted to obtain predicted needs for curative and preventive health care services at the national level. Estimation procedures were made in a segmented way for different age groups. Regression models (logit and probit) were used for each of the different age groups to compare the estimated needs with the observed utilization patterns (see Table 1A).

A summary of computations of distribution of need and utilization of curative and preventive health care by quintiles, standardized and not standardized, at a national level, as well as estimated Gini coefficients and health inequity indexes appear in Tables 2A and 3A.

• Findings

The results in Table 2A (national standardized) show inequity indexes (HI) favoring the rich. The inequity index is higher for preventive utilization than for curative utilization. When the unstandardized distribution indexes of inequity (HI) are used, results remain basically the same. The only difference is that the magnitude of the HI index for unstandardized regressions is a little bit lower than the standardized ones (Table 3A).

Apparently all income groups are in equal need, but higher income groups make more use of curative health care and even a higher use of preventive health care services. See the Gini coefficient in Tables 2A and 3A.

Comparisons of Gini coefficient and inequality indexes for the urban versus rural areas confirm that there are inequities favoring the richest in the population in both urban and rural areas. Inequalities are of greater magnitude for preventive than for curative health care. Inequalities in access to curative care seem to be more severe in rural areas. For preventive health care, inequity indexes for urban and rural areas are very similar (see Table 4A).

INEQUITIES IN HEALTH FINANCING

• Income distribution, private and government expenditures on health

In Ecuador, there is a highly skewed pattern of distribution of income and of private expenditure in health care–related goods and services. Segments of the population occupying the highest two deciles of income per capita concentrate 59% of the household income, whereas segments of the population occupying the lowest two deciles of income per capita represent only 3.0% of total household gross income. With regard to distribution of expenditure levels devoted to health, it can be said that the two segments of the population representing a higher level of income per capita concentrate approximately 30% of private expenditure per adult equivalent.[6] The first two deciles of income per capita participate in scarcely 13.7% of private health expenditures. In terms of the distribution of public expenditures on health, data show that larger percentages of government health expenditures go to the two higher income groups of the population than to the lower income groups.

For every decile of per capita income except the 9th and 10th, households devote a larger portion to health expenditure than their participation in the distribution of income. For the last decile, the level of income is much higher than the expenditures on health. These indicators

---

[6]The coefficients used for applying the concept of private expenditure per adult equivalent were as follows: no children, 1; one child, 1.26; two children, 1.52; three children, 1.78; four children, 2.04; five children, 2.30; seven children, 2.82.

TABLE 1A. Description of variables used to carry out the standardization of need for health services and utilization of curative and preventive health services.

Age group	Need		Curative utilization		Preventive utilization	
	Variables	Regression model*	Variables	Regression model	Variables	Regression model
Less than 1 year	Sex Vaccination	OLS	Illness Per capita income	OLS	Vaccination Sewerage	Logistic
1–4 years	Sex Vaccination Sewerage	OLS	Illness Per capita income Sewerage	OLS	Vaccination	OLS
5–14 years	Sex Sewerage Instruction level Per capita income	Logistic	Illness Per capita Income Insurance Sewerage	OLS	Per capita income Sewerage Instruction level	OLS
15–49 years	Sex Pregnancy Delivery	OLS	Illness Delivery Per capita income Insurance Sewerage	OLS	Sex Pregnancy Per capita income Insurance Sewerage	OLS
50 years and over	Sex Instruction level	OLS	Illness Per capita income Insurance Sewerage	OLS	Sex Per capita income Insurance Sewerage	OLS

Variables	Categories	Variables	Categories
Sex	1 = Man 2 = Woman	Per capita income	1 = First quintile 2 = Second quintile
Vaccination	1 = Received BCG, DTP, ATT, and measles† vaccinations 0 = Did not receive vaccination		3 = Third quintile 4 = Fourth quintile 5 = Fifth quintile
Sewerage	1 = Have sewerage in the dwelling 0 = Have no sewerage in the dwelling	Pregnancy	1 = Pregnancy, woman 0 = No pregnancy, woman
Instruction level	1 = None 2 = Primary school 3 = Secondary school 4 = High school	Delivery	1 = Women with delivery in 1995 0 = Women without delivery in 1995
Insurance	1 = With insurance 0 = Without insurance	Illness	1 = Insane or uncomfort 0 = Sane or comfort
		Curative use	1 = Used curative services 0 = Did not use curative service
		Preventive use	1 = Used preventive service 0 = Did not use preventive service *OLS = ordinary least squares.

†BCG = tuberculosis vaccine; DTP = diphtheria/tetanus/pertussis; ATT = tetanus antitoxoid.

represent a first approximation, which reveals the unequal distribution of private expenditure in the health sector.

- Analysis of the various sources of financing under the NHS, by means of progressivity indexes

Results of computations of progressivity indexes (Kakwani's) for different sources of financing the NHS, such as taxes, IESS contributions, private insurance, and out-of-pocket expenditures, are summarized below.

Findings show that direct taxes have practically a nil effect with respect to progressivity. Indirect taxes are highly regressive; this probably reflects the distortions found in the tributary system prevailing in the country, especially considering that indirect taxes are more important within the tax system of the country. Nevertheless, this should be compared with the progressivity of other sources of financing of the NHS. In urban and rural areas indirect taxes were also remarkably regressive; meanwhile direct taxes were found to be progressive in the rural area and regressive in the urban area.

TABLE 2A. Distribution of the need for health services, standardized national.

DISTRIBUTION OF THE NEED FOR HEALTH SERVICES

Quintile	Population in need	Distribution	Cumulative distribution	Optimal cumulative distribution	Estimated Gini coefficient
0	0	0	0	0	0
1	2948.87	0.195977011	0.195977011	0.2	0.019597701
2	2983.47	0.198276469	0.39425348	0.4	0.059023049
3	3011.72	0.200153918	0.594407398	0.6	0.098866088
4	3039.95	0.202030037	0.796437434	0.8	0.139084483
5	3063.01	0.203562566	1	1	0.179643743
Total	15047.02	1			**0.007569871**

DISTRIBUTION OF THE NEED FOR CURATIVE SERVICES

Quintile	Pop. actually using curative services	Distribution	Cumulative distribution	Optimal cumulative distribution	Estimated Gini coefficient
0	0	0	0	0	0
1	1033.84	0.161967473	0.161967473	0.2	0.016196747
2	1130.53	0.177115499	0.339082972	0.4	0.050105044
3	1306.69	0.204713764	0.543796735	0.6	0.088287971
4	1392.67	0.218183898	0.761980633	0.8	0.130577737
5	1519.28	0.238019367	1	1	0.176198063
Total	6383.01	1			**0.077268875**

DISTRIBUTION OF THE USE OF PREVENTIVE SERVICES

Quintile	Pop. actually using preventive services	Distribution	Cumulative distribution	Optimal cumulative distribution	Estimated Gini coefficient
0	0	0	0	0	0
1	969.73	0.146839794	0.146839794	0.2	0.014683979
2	1102.47	0.166939733	0.313779528	0.4	0.046061932
3	1293.38	0.195847971	0.509627498	0.6	0.082340703
4	1489.65	0.225567838	0.735195336	0.8	0.124482283
5	1748.77	0.264804664	1	1	0.173519534
Total	6604.00	1			**0.117823137**

DISTRIBUTION OF THE NEED FOR HEALTH SERVICES

Quintile	Cumulative distribution of the use of		Cumulative distribution of need	Optimal cumulative distrib.
	curative services	preventive services		
1	0.160582798	0.152180497	0.19645112	0.2
2	0.338398872	0.315112053	0.390177444	0.4
3	0.545824847	0.50938825	0.594204825	0.6
4	0.762024127	0.731526348	0.796637203	0.8
5	1	1	1	1
CM	0.077268875	0.117823137		
CN			0.007569871	
HI	0.069699004	0.110253267		

Source: ECV-95, INEC.
Note: Figure in bold = Gini coefficient.

TABLE 3A. Distribution of the need for health services, nonstandardized national.

DISTRIBUTION OF THE NEED FOR HEALTH SERVICES

Quintile	Population in need	Distribution	Cumulative distribution	Optimal cumulative distribution	Estimated Gini coefficient
0	0	0	0	0	0
1	2956.00	0.19645112	0.19645112	0.2	0.019645112
2	2915.00	0.193726324	0.390177444	0.4	0.058662856
3	3070.00	0.204027381	0.594204825	0.6	0.098438227
4	3046.00	0.202432379	0.796637203	0.8	0.139084203
5	3060.00	0.203362797	1	1	0.17966372
Total	15047.00	1			**0.009011763**

DISTRIBUTION OF THE USE OF CURATIVE HEALTH SERVICES

Quintile	Pop. actually using curative services	Distribution	Cumulative distribution	Optimal cumulative distribution	Estimated Gini coefficient
0	0	0	0	0	0
1	1025.00	0.160582798	0.160582798	0.2	0.01605828
2	1135.00	0.177816074	0.338398872	0.4	0.049898167
3	1324.00	0.207425975	0.545824847	0.6	0.088422372
4	1380.00	0.216199279	0.762024127	0.8	0.130784897
5	1519.00	0.237975873	1	1	0.176202413
Total	6383.00	1			**0.077267742**

DISTRIBUTION OF THE USE OF PREVENTIVE SERVICES

Quintile	Pop. actually using preventive services	Distribution	Cumulative distribution	Optimal cumulative distribution	Estimated Gini coefficient
0	0	0	0	0	0
1	1005.00	0.152180497	0.152180497	0.2	0.01521805
2	1076.00	0.162931557	0.315112053	0.4	0.046729255
3	1283.00	0.194276196	0.50938825	0.6	0.08245003
4	1467.00	0.222138098	0.731526348	0.8	0.12409146
5	1773.00	0.268473652	1	1	0.173152635
Total	6604.00	1			**0.116717141**

DISTRIBUTION OF THE NEED FOR HEALTH SERVICES

Quintile	Cumulative distribution of the use of		Cumulative distribution of need	Optimal cumulative distrib.
	curative services	preventive services		
1	0.160582798	0.152180497	0.19645112	0.2
2	0.338398872	0.315112053	0.390177444	0.4
3	0.545824847	0.50938825	0.594204825	0.6
4	0.762024127	0.731526348	0.796637203	0.8
5	1	1	1	1
CM	0.077267742	0.116717141		
CN			0.009011763	
HI	0.068255979	0.107705378		

Source: ECV-95, INEC.
Note: Figure in bold = Gini coefficient.

TABLE 4A. Distribution of the need for health services, standardized urban.

DISTRIBUTION OF THE NEED FOR HEALTH SERVICES

Quintile	Cumulative distribution of the use of		Cumulative distrib. of need	Optimal cumulative distribution
	curative services	preventive services		
1	0.167875339	0.149354782	0.196095125	0.2
2	0.352627035	0.328219126	0.393847898	0.4
3	0.562376041	0.5309191	0.596057007	0.6
4	0.776279312	0.752994789	0.796974606	0.8
5	1	1	1	1
CM	0.056336909	0.095404881		
CN			0.006810146	
HI	0.049526764	0.088594736		

DISTRIBUTION OF THE NEED FOR HEALTH SERVICES

Quintile	Cumulative distribution of the use of		Cumulative distrib. of need	Optimal cumulative distribution
	curative services	preventive services		
1	0.175714239	0.1660313	0.199000543	0.2
2	0.357933593	0.341095208	0.395539209	0.4
3	0.541545345	0.528714107	0.594101394	0.6
4	0.760616137	0.744411747	0.795497353	0.8
5	1	1	1	1
CM	0.065676274	0.087899055		
CN			0.006344601	
HI	0.059331674	0.081554454		

DISTRIBUTION OF THE NEED FOR HEALTH SERVICES

Quintile	Cumulative distribution of the use of		Cumulative distrib. of need	Optimal cumulative distribution
	curative services	preventive services		
1	0.178745268	0.1592089	0.196939537	0.2
2	0.364250946	0.336959209	0.392510575	0.4
3	0.576798269	0.541656366	0.601268972	0.6
4	0.783126014	0.754511743	0.801443145	0.8
5	1	1	1	1
CM	0.038831801	0.083065513		
CN			0.003135108	
HI	0.035696693	0.079930405		

DISTRIBUTION OF THE NEED FOR HEALTH SERVICES

Quintile	Cumulative distribution of the use of		Cumulative distrib. of need	Optimal cumulative distribution
	curative services	preventive services		
1	0.166480447	0.165298945	0.200171208	0.2
2	0.354562384	0.354044549	0.399629048	0.4
3	0.534450652	0.536928488	0.589242403	0.6
4	0.755679702	0.745603751	0.793693822	0.8
5	1	1	1	1
CM	0.075530726	0.079249707		
CN			0.006905407	
HI	0.068625319	0.0723443		

Source: ECV-95, INEC.

HEALTH SECTOR INEQUALITIES AND POVERTY IN GUATEMALA

Edgard Barillas, Ricardo Valladares, and GSD Consultores Asociados

BACKGROUND

Guatemala's population (8.3 million in 1994) is relatively young, predominantly rural, and ethnically complex (Instituto Nacional de Estadística, 1996b). Approximately 44% of Guatemalans are 14 years of age or younger, and 65% live in rural areas (Table 1). Nearly 80% of the rural inhabitants are indigenous peoples belonging to one of three major ethnic groups: Xincas, Garifunas, and Mayas; the last group speak 22 different languages. The regions of the country with a high proportion of rural and indigenous population tend to be the poorest.

TABLE 1. Distribution of population by area and ethnic origin, Guatemala, 1994.

| Area | Population (%) | | |
	Total	Indigenous	Nonindigenous
Urban	35.0	20.5	46.7
Rural	65.0	79.5	54.3
Total	100.0	100.0	100.0

Source: Instituto Nacional de Estadística (1996b).

public services and low coverage of social security in rural areas and marginal urban areas.

Income Inequality

Guatemala has an extremely unequal distribution of income. According to the World Bank, in 1989 the Gini coefficient for Guatemala (0.59) was the second highest in Latin America, surpassed only by that of Brazil (0.64). The most recent social and demographic survey revealed that the 10% of the population with the highest income accounted for 46.6% of national income, whereas the remaining 90% accounted for only 53.4%. The 20% of the population with the lowest income received only about 2.1% of total income (World Bank, 1997).

Income inequality is related to several factors: (a) the concentration of land ownership;[1] (b) the growing gap between the salaries of skilled and unskilled workers; (c) a regressive tax system;[2] (d) the concentration of public spending in metropolitan areas;[3] and (e) the paucity of

Poverty

According to government sources, 79% of Guatemalans are poor. The percentage is even higher in rural areas (85.7%) and in those regions of the country that are most deprived of basic infrastructure and social services (Northwest, 93.7%; North, 91.3%).[4]

Table 2 shows that the incidence of poverty and extreme poverty is greater for indigenous populations, the rural population, households with low educational levels, and workers in the agricultural sector.

Policies to Reduce Poverty

Since the mid-1990s, the three principal instruments for poverty reduction have been social investment funds, the various peace agreements signed in recent years, and the Government Plan, 1996–2000 (Programa de Gobierno 1996–2000).

---

[1]In 1979, 88.2% of the farms occupied 16.2% of the agricultural land; 2.6% occupied 65.1% of the total area.

[2]Nearly 80% of the tax revenues are generated by indirect taxes, the most important of which is the value-added tax (Ministerio de Finanzas Públicas, 1997).

[3]According to data for 1995, approximately half the budgets of the ministries of education and health were allocated to the Guatemala state, Metropolitan Region (Centro de Investigación y Estudios Nacionales, 1977; Ministerio de Finanzas Públicas, 1997).

[4]The distinction between poor and nonpoor was made on the basis of a poverty line equal to the cost of a basket of basic goods and services. The source of the figures presented is Secretaría General de Planificación (1996a).

TABLE 2. Variations in the incidence of poverty and extreme poverty, Guatemala, 1990.

Variable		Population (%)	
		Poor	Extremely poor
Ethnicity	Indigenous	92.6	81.3
	Nonindigenous	65.8	45.2
Place of residence	Rural	85.7	71.9
	Urban	57.2	33.7
Educational level of head of household	None	78.8	61.5
	Primary	48.1	24.3
	Secondary	16.1	7.0
	Higher	8.6	5.7
Sector of activity	Agriculture	85.5	71.8
	Manufacturing	61.6	36.3
	Commerce	50.0	28.0
	Service	38.8	19.9

Source: World Bank (1995).

The social investment funds promoted decentralization and community participation by channeling resources toward local governments, communities, and nongovernmental organizations (NGOs). The funds directed resources toward the poor, particularly in the form of infrastructure projects.

Poverty reduction is one of the four major goals of the third public policy instrument, the Government Plan 1996–2000. The plan's medium-term objective is to mitigate poverty by increasing the coverage and the quality of basic social services as well as the productive capacities of the poor. In operational terms, the antipoverty policy consists of three lines of action: (a) emergency programs directed toward priority groups and regions and implemented through the social investment funds; (b) institutional reforms aimed at increasing the effectiveness of the programs with the greatest impact on the poor; and (c) redirection of public spending toward the most vulnerable groups and regions, along with reduction of administrative costs and increased participation of communities and NGOs (Secretaría General de Planificación, 1996b). Within this general framework, the government's Action and Social Development Program (PLADES 1996–2000) establishes as priority goals the expansion of educational and health services for poor and vulnerable populations (Secretaría General de Planificación, 1996a).

The government's antipoverty strategies are reflected in the health sector in several ways. First, the social funds include health projects that provide for investment in infrastructure services, such as latrine building, drinking water supply, and community first-aid services (*botiquines comunitarios*), as well as personnel training. Second, the Ministry of Public Health and Social Welfare (Ministerio de Salud Pública y Asistencia Social; MSPAS) has undergone a process of financial decentralization and is adopting a new model of care known as the Comprehensive Health Care System (Sistema Integral de Atención de Salud; SIAS).[5] Third, both the Ministry of Public Health and Social Welfare and the Guatemalan Social Security Institute (Instituto Guatemalteco de Seguridad Social; IGSS) are making efforts to reduce the costs of service delivery. These efforts have led to the contracting of other providers and outsourcing of general services.[6]

HEALTH CARE SYSTEM

Coverage

Only 67% of Guatemalans have access to health services, and the figure drops to 49% for poor people living in rural areas (Instituto Nacional de Estadística, 1990). This low coverage reflects physical barriers (e.g., residence in a remote area, rugged topography in rural areas) as well as economic factors. Poor people often have difficulties covering even the nominal fees that are collected in public facilities. In addition, seeking services usually involves high transportation costs (relative to family income) and loss of working days. Forty-one percent of the rural poor must travel over 1 hour to reach a health care facility (Instituto Nacional de Estadística, 1990).

The low coverage also reflects the inefficient distribution of resources. The country has nearly one physician and one hospital bed per 1,000 people; however, 80% of the physicians and 50% of the nurses are based in the urban areas, which are home to only 35% of the population (Pan American Health Organization/World Health Organization, 1997).

Within the public sector, health services are provided by the Ministry of Public Health and Social Welfare, which is part of the central government, and the IGSS, which operates as a decentralized and autonomous entity. It has been estimated that the public health care system serves 48% of the population: the Ministry of Public Health and Social Welfare accounts for 32% of that figure, and the IGSS accounts for the other 16%. Approximately 20% of the population relies on private services,[7] leaving 33% of Guatemalans without health care coverage.

---

[5]Currently the first level of the system is being implemented in priority regions. See Unidad Sectorial de Planificación de la Salud, Ministerio de Salud Pública y Asistencia Social (1998b).

[6]See Unidad Sectorial de Planificación de la Salud, Ministerio de Salud Pública y Asistencia Social (1998b).

[7]Ministerio de Salud Pública y Asistencia Social (1996). Private for-profit health providers and NGOs cover 16% and 4% of the population, respectively (Pan American Health Organization/World Health Organization, 1997).

Public Health Care System

The Ministry of Public Health and Social Welfare is the main publicly funded health care provider. It operates through 28 area health authorities, which supervise the operation of 36 hospitals, 3 peripheral clinics, 256 health centers, and 857 health posts.

The IGSS, a semiautonomous entity, serves affiliated workers and their dependents as well as retirees. The IGSS administers 24 hospitals, 35 physicians' offices, 2 peripheral clinics, and 6 health posts.

There are other public sector entities that provide health services to specific populations, but their coverage is quite limited.[8]

Private Health Care Providers

The private health sector includes for-profit establishments, NGOs, and informal providers. The for-profit sector provides services through insurance companies, prepaid medical services, medical centers or hospitals, and clinics and doctors' offices in Guatemala City and other urban areas. Deterioration in the quality of care provided by the public sector (particularly during the crisis of the 1980s and the early 1990s) resulted in a boom in private establishments, mainly in the capital city. These establishments often recruited poorly paid public employees who were happy to supplement their income in the private sector, which led to widespread moonlighting by health care professionals. Around 1997, over 170 private hospitals and 1,786 private physicians' offices were in operation. One of the basic objectives of health reform at present is to increase the ability of the Ministry of Public Health and Social Welfare to regulate and control the activities of private health care establishments.

Of the 1,100 NGOs in Guatemala, 197 carry out health-related activities, primarily in the field of preventive medicine. Of these, 39 are devoted primarily or exclusively to providing treatment or preventive services, and together they cover all 22 departments of Guatemala (Consejo de Población, 1995; United Nations Development Program, 1997).

Informal health care providers cover a major segment of the country's rural and poor population. Most engage in traditional health care practices and are unregistered,

unregulated, and subject to all the drawbacks associated with practicing outside the formal health structure. Since the 1970s, some efforts have been made to integrate traditional health care providers into the formal health care system.[9] In recent years, naturopaths, chiropractors, allopaths, and others have joined traditional practitioners. Although it is difficult to quantify their importance, it is clear that there is a demand for their services and that they capture some of the out-of-pocket expenditures of the population.

INEQUALITIES IN HEALTH CONDITIONS

Inequalities in Reported Illness

The data on reported illness in Guatemala are contradictory. In a national survey carried out in 1989 (Instituto Nacional de Estadística, 1990), the poor reported less illness than the nonpoor, and individuals living in rural areas reported less illness than persons living in urban areas (Table 3). However, a more recent survey carried out in a region with high proportions of rural, indigenous, and poor population found that the perception of illness declined with income [Instituto Nacional de Estadística, 1997 (Figure 1)].

Data from the 1989 survey (Instituto Nacional de Estadística, 1990) indicate that in all areas of Guatemala the average number of days of inactivity due to sickness was higher among the poor (Table 4), probably because they often do not have access to health services or they receive low-quality services.

Inequalities in Health Indicators

Guatemala continues to have a morbidity and mortality profile in which infectious diseases and illnesses related to nutritional deficiencies have greater importance than chronic and degenerative diseases. The leading causes of illness and death are still upper respiratory infections, various perinatal disorders, and diarrheal diseases. This profile is a logical consequence of the poverty that affects many Guatemalan families and of other related determinants, such as illiteracy, inadequate sanitary infrastructure, and limited access to health services. Next to Bolivia, Guatemala has the lowest life expectancy at birth in Latin America (Table 5).

These figures—in themselves alarming—do not reveal the enormous disparities between the health conditions

---

[8]The Military Health Services (Sanidad Nacional) provide services to members of the army and their dependents. Municipal governments carry out infrastructure works in some communities to supply water and dispose of sewerage. Three social funds have made minor investments in health (the National Fund for Peace, the Solidarity Fund for Community Development, and the Social Investment Fund).

[9]For example, midwives were trained in the following areas: early identification of risks, safe and hygienic delivery, postpartum care, and referral of complications to formal health care establishments.

TABLE 3. Individuals reporting illness or accident during the past four weeks, by area of residence and economic situation, Guatemala, 1990.

Area	Extremely poor (%)	Poor (%)	Nonpoor (%)	Total (%)
Guatemala City	6.2	6.9	6.9	6.9
Other urban areas	4.5	4.9	7.0	5.6
Rural areas	4.5	4.5	6.5	4.8
All areas	4.6	4.9	6.8	5.3

Source: World Bank (1995, Annex 4; based on Instituto Nacional de Estadística, 1990).

of different groups. For example, neonatal, infant, and child mortality rates are notably higher in rural areas and among indigenous populations (Table 6).

The columns in Table 6 combine two variables: area of residence and ethnicity. This is done to call attention to a characteristic common to several indicators: there is a more or less fluid scale that goes from the most favorable conditions (in urban areas) to the worst conditions (among the indigenous population). Within this spectrum, indicators for the nonindigenous population are better than those for the rural population. Although these categories are not mutually exclusive, indigenous people are a majority in rural areas, whereas nonindigenous people are a majority in urban areas (see Figure 1).

Inequalities between urban, rural, indigenous, and nonindigenous populations follow the indicated pattern when other indicators related to health are examined (Table 7). Poverty rates, for example, display the same pattern: the urban population has the lowest rates and the indigenous population has the highest rates (Figure 2).

To examine the distribution of disease and death in the country, morbidity information by department[10] was analyzed in relation to a number of social variables. The main findings of this exercise were the following:

- The maternal mortality rate tended to be higher in departments with a high incidence of illiteracy, which is more common among the poor, indigenous populations, and rural populations.
- Child mortality rates were higher in departments with large proportions of indigenous population and in departments with high percentages of rural poverty.
- The percentage of death due to respiratory diseases tended to be higher in departments with predominantly poor and rural populations and in those with large proportions of indigenous population.[11]

---

[10]As reported by Ministerio de Salud Pública y Asistencia Social (1998b) and Instituto Nacional de Estadística (1990).

[11]Respiratory diseases are the principal cause of death in Guatemala. They accounted for 19% of all deaths reported during 1997 (United Nations, 1998).

FIGURE 1. Geographic distribution of indigenous and nonindigenous population, Guatemala, 1994.

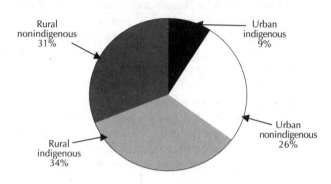

Source: Instituto de Estadística (1996b).

TABLE 4. Average days of inactivity due to illness, Guatemala, 1990.

Area	Extremely poor	Poor	Nonpoor	Total
Guatemala City	7.6	6.9	6.5	6.7
Other urban areas	6.8	6.3	4.9	5.7
Rural areas	7.5	7.4	5.4	7.0
Total	7.4	7.1	5.7	6.7

Source: World Bank (1995, Annex 4; based on Instituto Nacional de Estadística, 1990).

TABLE 5. Selected health indicators, Guatemala, 1995.

Indicator	Measurement
Crude birth rate*	37 per 1,000 population
General fertility rate*	176 per 1,000 women of childbearing age
Total death rate†	9.0 per 1,000 population
Population growth rate†	3.1%
Life expectancy at birth†	63 years
Infant mortality‡	51 per 1,000 live births
Neonatal mortality‡	26 per 1,000 live births
Child mortality‡	68 per 1,000 live births
Maternal mortality‡	19 per 10,000 live births
Low birth weight‡	9.7%

Source: Instituto Nacional de Estadística (1996a).
Reference period: *1993–1995; †1995; ‡1990–1995.

TABLE 6. Mortality by area of residence and ethnicity (per 1,000 live births), Guatemala, 1995.

Mortality	Urban area	Nonindigenous	Rural area	Indigenous
Neonatal	18	27	29	32
Infant (under 1 year)	41	53	56	64
Child (1–4 years)	55	69	74	94

Source: Instituto Nacional de Estadística (1996a).

TABLE 7. Selected health indicators by area of residence and ethnicity, Guatemala, 1995.

Indicator	Urban area	Nonindigenous	Rural area	Indigenous
Total fertility rate	3.8	4.3	6.2	6.8
Children with chronic malnutrition (%) (height-for-age)*	35.3	36.7	56.6	67.8
Children with acute malnutrition (%) (weight-for-age)*	18.2	20.9	30.6	34.6
Women of childbearing age without schooling (%)	14.2	16.0	39.2	53.4

Source: Instituto Nacional de Estadística (1996a).
*Malnutrition is defined as two standard deviations below the recommended international median.

• These findings confirm that the risk of illness and death is greater in poor, rural, and indigenous communities. This situation reflects the living conditions of poor families and their limited access to educational and health services.

HEALTH CARE EXPENDITURES AND FINANCING

The level of health expenditures in Guatemala is quite low compared with other countries, and in recent years it has declined as a percentage of GDP (Table 8). The low level of expenditures reflects the limited development of the health care infrastructure, the moderate growth of the health market, and the concentration of resources in the Guatemala City area. Data for 1990 show that private health expenditures in Guatemala were also well below the level in other countries of the region (Table 9).

FIGURE 2. Poverty rates (%) by area of residence and ethnicity, Guatemala, 1994.

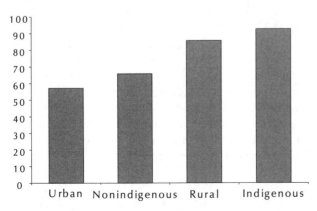

Source: World Bank (1995).

Flow of Financial Resources for Health Care

The financial resources for health care come from different sources and are channeled through intermediary agents to public and private providers of health services.

Sources

The government, international development organizations, private companies, and individual households provide the financial resources for health care. The government allocates between 8% and 10% of its budget to health expenditures; international development organizations provide loans and grants; private companies contribute to the social security regime and purchase private insurance for their employees; and households finance health care directly (through the purchase of goods and services) and indirectly (through contributions to the social security system). Table 10 shows how contributions from these four sources have varied in recent years.

Intermediary Agents

Within the public sector, the Ministry of Public Health and Social Welfare and the IGSS manage most financial resources for health care.[12] The Ministry of Public Health and Social Welfare receives funds from the government and international development organizations, whereas the IGSS is funded through mandatory contributions

---

[12]Social investment funds also operate with government funds, but the allocations they receive are relatively small. Other ministries (Interior and National Defense) have a minimum participation in national health expenditure through budget allocations for the operation of hospitals for their personnel and their families.

TABLE 8. Evolution of national health expenditures, Guatemala, 1990–1997.

Indicator	1990	1997
Per capita GDP (US$)	868.00	1,693.00
National health expenditure (thousands of US$)	265,491.00	409,627.00
National health expenditure (% of GDP)	3.33	2.30
Per capita health expenditure (US$)	28.87	38.93

Source: Suárez et al. (1994); Unidad Sectorial de Planificación de la Salud, Ministerio de Salud Pública y Asistencia Social (in press).

TABLE 9. Private health expenditures, Guatemala and selected countries, 1990.

Country	% of GDP
El Salvador	3.70
Nicaragua	3.42
Dominican Republic	3.28
Bolivia	3.10
Ecuador	2.80
Mexico	2.76
Peru	2.30
Guatemala	1.54

Source: Suárez et al. (1994).

TABLE 10. Sources of financing for health care, Guatemala, 1990, 1995–1997 (%).

Source	1990	1995	1996	1997
Government*	36.5	31.9	31.7	27.3
International cooperation[†]	NA	5.9	5.3	7.8
Households	48.3	43.0	44.2	42.9
Private companies[‡]	15.2	19.2	18.8	22.0
Total	100.0	100.0	100.0	100.0

Sources: Pan American Health Organization (1994) for the data for 1990; Ministerio de Salud Pública y Asistencia Social (1998) for the figures for 1995, 1996, and 1997.

NA = not applicable.

*Investments in water and sanitation are not included. The figure for 1990 [from the Pan American Health Organization (1994)] includes the contributions of international agencies.

[†]Includes loans and donations given to government entities.

[‡]Does not include the cost of purchasing group health insurance (accurate data are not available). The figure for 1990 [from the Pan American Health Organization (1994)] refers to health care expenditures of the social security system.

from employers and employees in the formal sector.[13] Both institutions then distribute resources among different health care providers.

Private resources for health care are managed by insurance companies and "second tier" NGOs. Insurance companies receive funds from households and firms in

---

[13]The Ministry of Public Health and Social Welfare also receives financial contributions from individual households in the form of payments for services. The IGSS should also receive government support, but this has not occurred for many years; as a result, the government has amassed a large debt to the IGSS.

TABLE 11. National health expenditure by agent, Guatemala, 1995–1997 (%).

Intermediary agents	1995	1996	1997
Ministry of Health	28.53	26.57	29.58
Other ministries	2.77	0.67	NA
Social investment funds	0.18	0.38	0.32
IGSS	27.82	30.22	30.54
Subtotal (public sector)	59.30	57.84	60.44
NGOs	3.99	4.29	4.17
Insurance companies	3.94	4.15	3.95
Households	32.78	33.73	31.44
Subtotal (private sector)	40.70	42.16	39.56
Total	100.00	100.00	100.00

Source: Ministerio de Salud Pública y Asistencia Social (1998).
Note: The definition of health expenditure does not include investments in water and sanitation.

the form of premiums and other charges, which are then transferred to health care providers in the form of payments for services rendered. Second tier NGOs are those that obtain resources from different sources and distribute them to other NGOs that provide services directly.

Table 11 shows the participation of public and private agents in national health expenditures. The Ministry of Public Health and Social Welfare and the IGSS manage similar amounts of resources; each accounts for approximately 30% of national health expenditure. The IGSS, however, covers a smaller population (formal-sector workers). NGOs and insurance companies together account for 8% of national health expenditures. The contribution of households is significant, accounting for more than 30% of total health expenditures.

Service Providers

Financial intermediaries distribute resources among public and private providers of services. The Ministry of Public Health and Social Welfare and the IGSS account for almost all public-sector health care expenditures (Table 12). NGOs contribute less than 3%, but this figure includes only activities that are exclusively related to health care. If multiprogrammatic NGOs were included, the figure would be higher.[14] Private, for-profit providers of health services do not report their income; the figures in Table 12 were calculated by distributing direct out-of-pocket expenditures among pharmacies and other service providers. Pharmacies capture 10% of expenditures and account for one-third of household spending for health services.

---

[14]The records of multiprogrammatic NGOs do not permit identification of health expenditures separate from other expenditures.

TABLE 12. National health expenditure (%) by service provider, Guatemala, 1995–1997.

Service provider	1995	1996	1997
Ministry of Health	31.24	27.40	28.59
IGSS	27.82	30.22	30.54
Hospital–National Police	0.25	0.00	0.23
Municipalities	0.29	0.01	NA
Subtotal (public sector)	59.61	57.63	59.36
NGO supplier	2.27	2.46	2.94
Private for-profit	23.93	25.14	23.49
Pharmacies	10.00	10.29	9.59
Subtotal (private sector)	36.20	37.89	36.02
Others	4.19	4.49	4.62
Total	100.00	100.00	100.00

Source: Unidad Sectorial de Planificación de la Salud, Ministerio de Salud Pública y Asistencia Social (1998a).

Note: The definition of health expenditure does not include investments in water and sanitation.

NA = not applicable.

Family Expenditures

Health expenditures by households vary according to income and place of residence (Figure 3). Among poor people in rural areas, more than 50% of health spending is for the purchase of remedies and drugs, whereas the figure for the nonpoor in urban areas is only 20%. On the other hand, spending on hospitalization and diagnosis is greater for groups that have better physical and economic access to health services: more than 50% of the expenditures of the nonpoor in urban areas fall into this

category, whereas the proportion for the rural poor is scarcely 10%.

Health expenditures represent between 2% and 5% of total household expenditures and between 3% and 11% of current expenditures (for basic goods and services). The proportion of both kinds of expenditure is greater for the population with better access to health services— that is, the nonpoor and urban population (Figure 4).

Poor families (predominantly members of indigenous communities living in rural areas) spend a smaller proportion of their income on health care than do the nonpoor (Instituto Nacional de Estadística, 1997). Individuals who are poor are less likely to seek professional help to deal with health problems; when they do decide to address them, most commonly they resort to self-medication. Financial constraints force poor people to ration the utilization of health services and to rely on less effective therapies. This in turn prolongs periods of inactivity due to illness, with the consequent loss of income.

Inequalities in Health Care Financing

The information needed to establish the exact contribution of different income groups to health care financing is not available (tax-related information is not broken down by socioeconomic categories and surveys of income and expenditures do not report these types of data). However, it is possible to derive a general picture of how contributions differ across groups based on existing information on the sources of health care financing.

Financing of Health Services Provided by the Social Security System

The social security system is financed by contributions of formal-sector employers and workers in amounts that

FIGURE 3. Distribution of household health expenditures (% of total health expenditure), Guatemala, 1997.

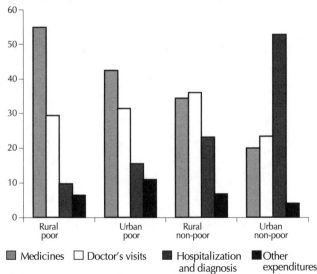

Source: Ministerio de Salud Pública y Asistencia Social (in press).

FIGURE 4. Health expenditure as a percentage of household expenditures, Guatemala, 1997.

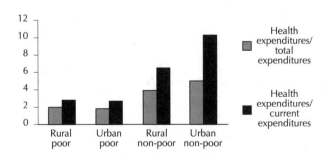

Source: Ministerio de Salud Pública y Asistencia Social (in press).

are proportional to wages. A recent study showed that the expenditures of the Guatemalan Social Security Institute on health care represent 0.7% of GDP and 30% of national health expenditures (Ministerio de Salud Pública y Asistencia Social, 1998a). However, the IGSS serves the families of only one-fourth of all Guatemalan workers (those employed in the formal sector). The services of the IGSS reach only a very small proportion of indigenous' and rural families.

The government is required by the Constitution to contribute to the social security system, but it has not done so for more than a decade. Payment of the cumulative debt would benefit formal sector workers but not the poorest and most unprotected workers in rural areas and in the urban informal sector.

Financing of Health Services Provided by the Central Government

Health expenditures of the central government are financed mainly through tax revenues. Guatemala's tax structure tends to be regressive. Indirect taxes on consumption (accounting for nearly 80% of all tax revenue) reduce the real income of the poor disproportionately relative to the nonpoor. The value-added tax (VAT) accounts for half of indirect tax revenue, and customs duties account for one-fourth of indirect tax revenue. Customs duties are normally transferred to consumers through the impact on the general price level.

Inequalities in Public Spending in Health

An examination of expenditure data across the country's 22 departments leads to the conclusion that public spending for health in Guatemala is very unequal and tends to be inversely related to poverty levels. Per capita expenditures range between 75.24 quetzals (Q75.25) in the Department of Guatemala (where the rural poor account for 75% of the population) and Q18.75 in the Department of Huehuetenango (where the proportion of rural poor is 97%). The inverse relationship between the level of spending and the degree of poverty is evident when departments are organized by quartiles, according to the proportion of the rural population living in poverty (Table 13).

As shown in column two of Table 13, the departments with the lowest percentages of rural population living in poverty receive the highest per capita allocations. This pattern reflects the distribution of expenditures on hospital care. As shown in the last column, per capita allocations of this type decline as the proportion of rural poor increases. Interestingly, per capita health care investments are higher in departments with a greater incidence of rural poverty.

This reflects the recent growth of investments in impoverished departments, a trend that ultimately could balance the distribution of public spending. Currently, however, nearly 70% of public funds are being used to fund hospitals. In departments with high percentages of urban and nonpoor population, the proportion rises to 83% (Table 14).

TABLE 13. Per capita expenditures (quetzals) of decentralized units of the Ministry of Health by departments grouped according to degree of rural poverty, Guatemala, 1996.

Departments (grouped according to degree of rural poverty)	Per capita expenditures on establishments that provide ambulatory services	Per capita expenditures on hospitals	Per capita health care investments	Per capita expenditures (all types)
Quartile 1*	9.94	54.59	1.00	65.52
Quartile 2†	12.86	30.43	1.14	44.43
Quartile 3‡	11.11	14.64	0.66	26.41
Quartile 4§	11.34	11.12	4.32	26.78
All departments	11.08	30.14	2.04	43.26

*Departments with the lowest proportion of rural population living in poverty (Izabal, Sacatepéquez, Guatemala, Escuintla, El Progreso, and Zacapa).

†Santa Rosa, Retalhuleu, El Petén, Jutiapa, and Quetzaltenango.

‡Jalapa, Sololá, Suchitepéquez, Chimaltenango, and Totonicapán.

§Departments with the highest proportions of rural population living in poverty (San Marcos, El Quiché, Chiquimula, Alta Verapaz, Huehuetenango, and Baja Verapaz).

TABLE 14. Distribution of the budget of the decentralized units of the Ministry of Health by department (grouped according to degree of rural poverty), Guatemala, 1996.

Departments (grouped according to degree of rural poverty)	Expenditures on ambulatory services (%)	Expenditures on hospital services (%)	Per capita health care investments (%)	Total (%)
Quartile 1*	15.16	83.31	1.52	100
Quartile 2†	28.94	68.48	2.57	100
Quartile 3‡	42.08	55.42	2.50	100
Quartile 4§	42.36	41.53	16.12	100
All departments	25.61	69.67	4.72	100

*Departments with the lowest proportions of rural population living in poverty (Izabal, Sacatepéquez, Guatemala, Escuintla, El Progreso, and Zacapa).

†Santa Rosa, Retalhuleu, El Petén, Jutiapa, and Quetzaltenango.

‡Jalapa, Sololá, Suchitepéquez, Chimaltenango, and Totonicapán.

§Departments with the highest proportions of rural population living in poverty (San Marcos, El Quiché, Chiquimula, Alta Verapaz, Huehuetenango, and Baja Verapaz).

Thus, an obvious way to reduce inequalities in the allocation of resources for health care is to increase the funding of the Ministry of Health, particularly for ambulatory services in poor rural communities. This Ministry is well suited to serve these communities through its broad network of services.

INEQUALITIES IN THE UTILIZATION OF HEALTH SERVICES

Access to health care is significantly lower among poor families in rural areas. According to 1990 INE data, fewer than 50% of the rural poor consulted health professionals when they were sick, compared with 75% in Guatemala City and 71% in other urban areas (Table 15). The most common places to obtain medical attention for all socioeconomic groups were private clinics, followed in importance by health centers in the case of the poor and hospitals in the case of the nonpoor (Table 16). Inequalities in access to and utilization of services vary according to the type of care, as shown below.

Reproductive Health and Maternal and Child Care

As Figure 5 shows, access to prenatal care is significantly lower among rural and indigenous communities. Fewer

TABLE 15. Patients who consulted health professionals during illness (%), Guatemala, 1990.

Area	Extreme poverty	Poor	Nonpoor	Total
Guatemala City	59.6	67.3	75.2	71.5
Other urban areas	66.2	65.4	70.8	67.7
Rural areas	47.7	48.9	66.0	52.2
Total	51.5	54.6	70.8	59.7

Source: World Bank (1995, Annex 4; based on Instituto Nacional de Estadística, 1990).

TABLE 16. Place where health services were received, by socioeconomic group (%), Guatemala, 1990.

Place	Extreme poverty	Poor	Nonpoor	Total
Hospital	22.5	21.0	18.1	19.9
Health center	30.6	26.0	9.4	10.8
Social Security Institute	4.2	7.0	9.4	7.9
Private clinic	32.5	35.9	51.1	41.6
Nurse's house	3.0	3.2	8.5	5.2
Others	7.3	6.9	3.4	5.6
All	100.0	100.0	100.0	100.0

Source: World Bank (1995, Annex 4; based on Instituto Nacional de Estadística, 1990).

pregnant women in indigenous communities are vaccinated against tetanus (to prevent complications caused by poor sanitary conditions during and after delivery). However, coverage is higher in rural than in urban areas, which reflects the impact of "vertical" vaccination programs targeted to rural communities without access to hospital services.

Information on the place where births occur shows that public and private entities tend to reinforce inequalities between social groups (Figure 6). Access to delivery care provided by the Ministry of Public Health and Social Welfare, the IGSS, and private clinics and hospitals is significantly lower among the rural and indigenous population. Nearly 90% of births in indigenous communities and 80% of births in rural areas take place at home. This pattern of service utilization subsidizes the nonpoor and helps to explain the higher maternal mortality rates in rural and indigenous communities.

Government efforts have expanded the coverage of immunization programs in rural areas, but the percentage of children without access to any form of immunization is still higher among indigenous and rural communities (Figure 7).

FIGURE 5. Gaps in prenatal care: access to prenatal examination by a physician and coverage of tetanus toxoid vaccine* (%), Guatemala, 1995.

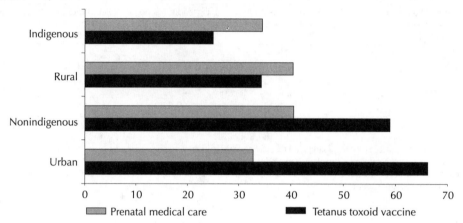

Source: Instituto Nacional de Estadística (1996a).
*Coverage with two or more doses.

The level of utilization of family planning methods is also significantly lower among the indigenous and rural populations (Instituto Nacional de Estadística, 1996a). Educational level influences most of the gaps between social groups. Utilization of prenatal services, medical care at delivery, and family planning increase with level of education (Table 17A). These services reach a very small percentage of rural and indigenous women, because their educational level tends to be very low (Table 17B).

The lack of access to education and health services increases the risks of illness and death in rural and indig-

enous communities. This is evident when data about AIDS are compared among women from different socioeconomic groups. Rural and indigenous women clearly know less about the disease and about ways to protect themselves (Figure 8).

Medical Treatment

A survey carried out in a region with a predominantly rural, indigenous, and poor population (Instituto Na-

FIGURE 6. Gaps in delivery care: place of birthing by ethnic group and area of residence, Guatemala, 1995.

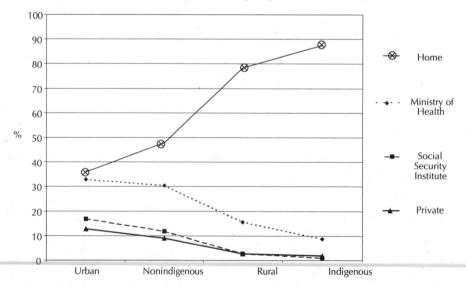

Source: Instituto Nacional de Estadística (1996a).

FIGURE 7. Gaps in immunization: percentage of children with complete immunization and with no immunization, by area of residence and ethnicity, Guatemala, 1995.

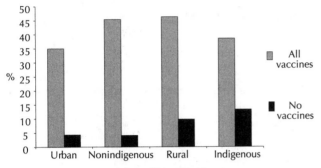

Source: Instituto Nacional de Estadística (1996a).

cional de Estadística, 1997)[15] found that 24% had perceived a health problem within the past 30 days,[16] and that the percentage of people who sought medical care increased with income (Figure 9). The same survey showed that self-medication is frequent, particularly among lower income groups (Figure 10), and that it is ineffective. The data indicate that 84% of individuals who took home remedies and 89% of those who took medicines purchased without prescription were unable to solve their health problem and had to take other action.

The incidence of diarrheal diseases does not show important differences between socioeconomic and ethnic groups. However, rural and indigenous children seek care less frequently and tend to reduce the intake of liquids and food during episodes of diarrhea (Figure 11). This fact suggests that their parents lack the necessary information to manage the disease at home.

CONCLUSIONS AND POLICY RECOMMENDATIONS

The risk of illness and death in Guatemala is greater among the indigenous and rural population. Awareness of this fact should facilitate the implementation of health policies aimed at correcting inequalities, because people with greater risks of disease and death can be located with relative precision throughout the country. However, the data presented in the study show that frequency of health interventions is inversely related to epidemiological and social risk. Guatemala's departments that have a greater proportion of indigenous and rural population

[15]Encuesta de Demanda y Gastos en Salud, carried out in the departments of San Marcos, Sololá, Totonicapán, and Quetzaltenango.

[16]An earlier survey at the national level (Instituto Nacional de Estadística, 1990) found that only 5.3% of the population reported illness during the previous 30 days (see Table 13).

(and, thus, of poor people) benefit from fewer interventions and receive smaller proportions of public resources than the nonindigenous population in urban areas.

The high risk of dying at an early age in rural and indigenous communities as a consequence of preventable or easily treatable diseases calls for reallocation of public resources. Investments in health should target the most neglected departments and municipalities through interventions with the greatest potential impact. However, the evidence presented in the study demonstrates that budgetary allocations for health care are inversely related to the health needs of the targeted population. The indigenous populations in rural areas receive a smaller proportion of public resources than the nonindigenous population in urban areas.

Data show that disease causes more days of inactivity among the poor than among the nonpoor. Preexisting debilitating conditions in poor communities and their limited access to health services are the probable causes of this finding. Prolonged inactivity, in turn, perpetuates the vicious cycle of illness–poverty–illness: the reduction of family income caused by loss of workdays creates conditions that are propitious for the advent of new diseases and lessens the family's capacity to obtain the services necessary to treat them.

This study suggests that lack of education limits the perception of disease and leads to a failure to seek timely care, with negative consequences (prolonged illness, financial losses, death). It follows that policies aimed at improving the educational level of poor families can help to improve the health and financial condition of their members. Concrete efforts in the field of health education can have a significant impact. For example, introduction of health education in the formal curriculum of schools can increase the ability to perceive disease adequately and to seek specialized care when the situation warrants it. Policies of this type can eliminate barriers to health care access and also contribute to poverty alleviation by reducing days of inactivity due to sickness.

The study demonstrates that rural and indigenous populations have less access to public services than other Guatemalans. In this regard, the performance of the public sector is very similar to that of the private sector—it favors those who have the least need—that is, the nonindigenous and urban populations. Health policies thus serve to exacerbate social inequities. Some measures that would contribute to the reduction of these inequities are:

- Strengthening the financial function of the Guatemalan Social Security Institute. This entity, because of the way it finances its activities, has the capacity to extend the coverage of health services expeditiously.

TABLE 17A. Utilization of reproductive health services and maternal and child care by educational level, Guatemala, 1995.

Service	Without education	With primary education	With secondary education	With higher education
Prenatal care by physician	26.0	47.3	89.6	99.8
Hospital birth	16.1	35.5	88.3	95.5
Know some method of family planning	65.4	87.1	99.8	100.0
Utilize some method of family planning	14.1	32.5	61.2	72.1

Source: Instituto Nacional de Estadística (1996a).

TABLE 17B. Distribution of rural and indigenous women of childbearing age by educational level, Guatemala, 1995.

Service	Without education	With primary education	With secondary education	With higher education
Rural women of childbearing age	39.2	50.5	9.1	1.2
Indigenous women of childbearing age	53.4	41.6	4.6	0.4

Source: Instituto Nacional de Estadística (1996a).

Experiences in other Latin American countries show that it is possible to use the resources available through social security institutes to establish innovative service delivery systems. To do so, the Guatemalan Social Security Institute has to concentrate its efforts on financing health services instead of providing them directly. To extend the coverage of health services to the most neglected communities, the institute needs a governmental subsidy to finance the purchase of health insurance for poor families. In addition, it must allow self-employed persons to participate.

- Targeting subsidies to the indigent. The contribution of the State to the social security system constitutes, in the final analysis, a subsidy to the formal labor force in urban areas. Although this population cannot be considered privileged from an economic standpoint, it undoubtedly faces less health risk than the indigenous population in rural areas. From an equity perspective, it is better to utilize the current State contribution to establish a sort of solidarity fund that would enable the IGSS to purchase a basic package of services for the indigent.
- Promoting the participation of NGOs in efforts aimed at extending the coverage of health services. This and other studies have demonstrated the ineffectiveness of traditional strategies in increasing the access of

FIGURE 8. Women of childbearing age who know about AIDS and percentage of those who are aware of protection methods, Guatemala, 1995.

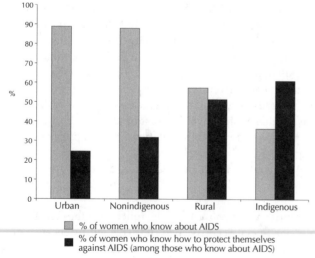

% of women who know about AIDS
% of women who know how to protect themselves against AIDS (among those who know about AIDS)

Source: Instituto Nacional de Estadística (1996a).

FIGURE 9. Population that perceived a health problem and percentage of those who sought medical help, by quintiles of income expenditure, Guatemala, 1996.

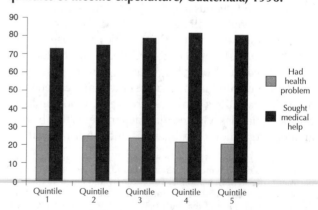

Had health problem

Sought medical help

Source: Instituto Nacional de Estadística (1996a).

FIGURE 10. Percentage of people who sought care by type of therapy and income group, Guatemala, 1996.

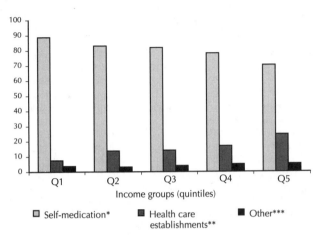

Source: Instituto Nacional de Estadística (1996a).

*Includes purchase of medicines in pharmacies without a prescription and consumption of home remedies and of medicines kept at home.

**Includes hospitals, clinics, health centers, and health posts.

***Includes attention at home, purchase of medicines with prescriptions, and traditional medicine.

rural and indigenous populations to health services. The new Comprehensive Health Care System has only recently designed a strategy to expand coverage based on contracts or agreements with NGOs. It is still too early to evaluate the impact of this initiative, but theoretically it seems appropriate to leave the delivery of services in the hands of entities that are physically and culturally close to the users.

The study indicates that the purchase of drugs (without consultation of specialized personnel) accounts for most of the private health expenditure of poor people. The rich, on the other hand, consult physicians more frequently and direct most of their private health expenditure to treatment services. The implication of this finding is that the health expenditures of poor families not only compete with other expenditures, many of which are fundamental for survival, but they are also highly inefficient in terms of solving health problems. Some public policies that could correct this situation are the following:

- Subsidizing essential drugs. The high cost of drugs affects the poor disproportionately. Subsidies to reduce the price of drugs with proven effectiveness in treating pathologies that are common among the poor would permit a more efficient use of resources by poor families. This, in turn, would improve both their health status and their living conditions.
- Informing the user. This study demonstrates that private health expenditure represents a high proportion of national health expenditure in Guatemala. The efficiency of private expenditure depends, to a large extent, on comparable access to information by both the user and the provider of services. It is reasonable to assume, therefore, that lack of information about health issues contributes to an inefficient pattern of expenditure by poor families. A key function of the State in this respect is to increase the access of poor families to health information, especially in the context of reforms that increase private-sector participation in the provision of services and give consumers more freedom of choice.
- Using native languages in health education. Some of the data presented reveal the negative impact of

FIGURE 11. Children who had diarrhea and percentage of those who received care and reduced the intake of liquids, by area of residence and ethnic group (%), Guatemala, 1996.

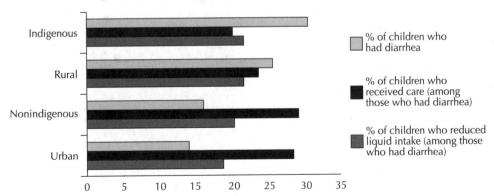

Source: Instituto Nacional de Estadística (1996a).

lack of health information (high rates of infant mortality caused by diarrhea, for example) and show that educational services make little or no contribution toward improving the health of the poor. It is critical to transmit this information and to do so in the native language of the target population.

The evidence presented suggests that "vertical programs" that depend more on supply than on demand are often more appropriate for attending to the health needs of the poor. The high coverage of the Expanded Program on Immunization supports this hypothesis. On the other hand, the limited progress achieved by projects aimed at increasing the utilization of contraceptives among rural and indigenous populations suggests that the sequence

education of the user →
identification of the need → spontaneous demand

is difficult to complete when the targeted population has low levels of schooling. Although it is clear that vertical interventions can be effective in terms of increasing the coverage of services and improving health indicators, they do not contribute to community self-determination or freedom of choice, which are fundamental ingredients of a long-term strategy to reduce poverty. Nevertheless, to address the health problems of poor Guatemalans in a pragmatic manner, a high degree of reliance on supply-dependent and vertical interventions seems inevitable, at least until it is possible to build a health system driven by the spontaneous demand of informed users.

REFERENCES

Centro de Investigación y Estudios Nacionales. *La educación en Guatemala.* Guatemala: Centro de Investigación y Estudios Nacionales; 1977.

Consejo de Población. *Inventario de ONGS que trabajan en el sector social de Guatemala, con énfasis en salud, mujer y desarrollo.* Guatemala: Consejo de Población, U.S. Agency for International Development; 1995.

Instituto Nacional de Estadística. *Encuesta nacional sociodemográfica: 1989.* Guatemala: Instituto Nacional de Estadística; 1990.

Instituto Nacional de Estadística. *Encuesta nacional de salud materno infantil 1995.* Guatemala: Instituto Nacional de Estadística; 1996a.

Instituto Nacional de Estadística. *República de Guatemala: características generales de población y habitación 1994,* X Censo de Población y V de Habitación. Guatemala: Instituto Nacional de Estadística; 1996b.

Instituto Nacional de Estadística. *Encuesta de demanda y gastos en salud 1997.* Guatemala: Instituto Nacional de Estadística; 1997.

Ministerio de Finanzas Públicas de Guatemala. *Presupuesto general de ingresos y egresos del Estado. Ejercicio fiscal 1997.* Guatemala: Ministerio de Finanzas Públicas; 1997.

Ministerio de Salud Pública y Asistencia Social. *PLADES 1996–2000: sector salud.* Guatemala: Ministerio de Salud Pública y Asistencia Social; 1996.

Ministerio de Salud Pública y Asistencia Social. *Cuentas nacionales de salud 1995–1997.* [Report on research project on national health accounts sponsored by U.S. Agency for International Development, Pan American Health Organization, and Harvard University]. Guatemala: Ministerio de Salud Pública y Asistencia Social; 1998a.

Ministerio de Salud Pública y Asistencia Social. *Situación de salud 1997 por departamentos.* Guatemala: Ministerio de Salud Pública y Asistencia Social; 1998b.

Pan American Health Organization. *National Expenditure and Financing of the Health Sector in Latin America and the Caribbean: Challenges for the 1990s.* Technical Report 30. Washington, DC: Pan American Health Organization; 1994.

Pan American Health Organization/World Health Organization. *Estudio sobre la red de servicios públicos de salud en Belice, El Salvador, Guatemala y Honduras.* Washington, DC: Pan American Health Organization/World Health Organization; 1997.

Secretaría General de Planificación. *Desarrollo social y construcción de la paz. Plan de Acción 1996–2000.* Guatemala: Gabinete Social; 1996a.

Secretaría General de Planificación. *Programa de Gobierno 1996–2000.* Guatemala: Secretaría General de Planificación; 1996b.

Suárez R, Henderson P, Barillas E, Vieira C. *Gasto nacional y financiamiento del sector de la salud en América Latina y el Caribe: desafíos para la década de los noventa.* Serie Informes Técnicos No. 30. Washington, DC: Pan American Health Organization/World Health Organization; 1994.

Unidad Sectorial de Planificación de la Salud, Ministerio de Salud Pública y Asistencia Social. *Bases de programación anual y el cumplimiento de los compromisos de gestión.* Guatemala: Unidad Sectorial de Planificación de la Salud; 1998a.

Unidad Sectorial de Planificación de la Salud, Ministerio de Salud Pública y Asistencia Social. *Informe anual de trabajo del Ministerio de Salud: 1997.* Guatemala: Unidad Sectorial de Planificación de la Salud; 1998b.

Unidad Sectorial de Planificación de la Salud, Ministerio de Salud Pública y Asistencia Social. *National health accounts: 1995–1997.* Research project sponsored by U.S. Agency for International Development, Pan American Health Organization/World Health Organization, and Harvard University; in press.

United Nations. *Guatemala: los contrastes del desarrollo humano.* New York: United Nations; 1998.

United Nations Development Program. *Directorio de ONGS y entidades de desarrollo y derechos humanos en Guatemala.* Guatemala: United Nations Development Program; 1997.

World Bank. *Guatemala, an Assessment of Poverty.* Report 12313-GU. Washington, DC: World Bank, Country Department II, Human Resources Operations Division, Latin America and the Caribbean Regional Office; 1995.

World Bank. *Informe sobre el desarrollo mundial 1997. El Estado en un mundo en transformación,* primera edición. Washington, DC: World Bank; 1997.

HEALTH SYSTEM INEQUALITIES AND POVERTY IN JAMAICA

Karl Theodore, Althea Lafoucade, Dominic Stoddard, Wendell Thomas, and Andrea Yearwood

BACKGROUND

Macroeconomic Context

Jamaica has a total area of 10,991 km² and a population of roughly 2.51 million. Per capita income is US$ 1,340 (1994), which puts it among the world's lower middle-income countries. After several years of adjustment entailing fiscal, monetary, wage, price, foreign exchange, trade, and institutional reforms, the Jamaican economy is still struggling to achieve the basis for macroeconomic growth and stability. The rate of unemployment, which declined considerably from about 25% in the 1970s and 1980s, stood at 16.2% in 1995, while the general price index continued its upward climb of about 29% per annum (Table 1).

One of the major macroeconomic challenges the government faces is the need to accelerate growth. The private sector has been identified as a key player in achieving this objective, and incentives for private-sector-led development continue to be provided. Another major issue is the need to stem the slide in the country's exchange rate parity, the value of which decreased by more than 19% from 1994 to 1995. The financial sector has undergone a near crisis in recent years with the collapse of several commercial banks and trust companies. Most probably this was due to insufficiently prudent regulation as well as to wider structural problems in the economy.

Another crucial challenge is the reform and modernization of the public sector. This, however, is being pursued within the constraints of a tight fiscal environment and an overall deficit, in 1995, of 5.35% of gross domestic product (GDP).[1] Divestment of state corporations and decentralization of key state functions therefore have

become important elements of the public sector reform program.

Poverty

Adverse economic conditions in Jamaica have resulted in high levels of poverty, which are aggravated by the country's unequal income distribution. Jamaica's national income traditionally has been unequally distributed. Declines in real GDP, high rates of inflation, and the contraction in public spending have led to declines in living standards and greater levels of poverty. During the 1970s and the 1980s, coinciding with the fall in bauxite production and the introduction of economic adjustment programs, there were higher levels of poverty than in the immediate postindependence era. Between 1989 and 1995, poverty levels oscillated within a relatively wide range. The percentage of the population unable to meet nutritional and other basic requirements during this period fluctuated from 29.3% in 1989, to 49.5% in 1991, to 32.3% in 1995 (Table 2).

Almost two-thirds of the poor live in rural areas; 23.4% live in the Kingston Metropolitan Area (KMA) and 16.6% live in other urban areas (Theodore et al., 1997). Among the poor, most (61%) are below the age of 25. For the country as a whole, poverty seems to be evenly distributed among females (51%) and males (49%). In the KMA, poverty is slightly more concentrated among females (53%). Interestingly, Jamaica has a relatively low unemployment rate among the poor (20% in 1993). This suggests the possibility of severe underemployment, exacerbated perhaps by low wage rates.

The level of poverty has been of great concern and the government has committed itself to a policy of poverty eradication. The government recognized that, in the wake of its efforts to balance the budget and meet high levels of debt service, inadequate investments in social infrastructure, such as water, sanitation, roads, and transpor-

---

[1]See pages 1.2 and 6.2 of *Economic and Social Survey, Jamaica* (Planning Institute of Jamaica, 1995).

TABLE 1. Macroeconomic indicators, Jamaica, 1988–1995.

Year	Consumer price index (×100)	Real GDP growth (%)	Unemployment rate (%)	Exchange rate (J$ = US$ 1)	Overall balance of fiscal account (J$ million)
1988	109.2	2.90	18.9	5.5	−262.9
1989	128.0	6.90	18.0	6.5	−1,206.4
1990	166.1	5.50	15.4	8.2	−398.7
1991	299.3	0.73	15.4	20.9	578.9
1992	419.6	1.50	15.7	22.2	1,542.2
1993	546.0	1.40	16.3	32.7	2,941.4
1994	692.3	0.74	15.4	33.4	4,329.9
1995	778.8	0.50	16.2	39.8	....

Source: Theodore (1997); World Bank (1996); Planning Institute of Jamaica (1995).

tation, may have occurred. This "public poverty" exists in addition to individual "private poverty"—i.e., the inability to meet nutritional and other basic needs. The National Poverty Eradication Program (NPEP), which commenced in 1995, targets poverty eradication through food security and development of human resource potential. This program uses the preexisting Food Stamp Program to target beneficiaries. Street and working children are also covered through the use of nongovernmental organizations (NGOs) and community-based organizations as outreach mechanisms.

The success of programs such as NPEP depends, among other things, on identifying the geographic location of the poor, as well as understanding their demographic and social characteristics. Toward that end, the Planning Institute of Jamaica measured national poverty in the various geographic regions, using five poverty indicators: water supply, toilet facilities, unemployment, education, and overcrowding (Planning Institute of Jamaica, 1996). The result of this work showed that the parishes with large urban centers, such as Kingston and St. Andrew, St. Catherine, and St. James, ranked better than the national average on all indicators (Table 3).

HEALTH CARE SYSTEM

Health services in Jamaica are provided by both the public and private sectors. The Ministry of Health is the main provider of secondary care, with approximately 95% of all hospital beds. At the secondary level, there are 27 hospitals that offer mainly curative care, with a total capacity of nearly 5,000 beds. Of these hospitals, 18 are acute-care facilities, 6 are specialty hospitals, and 3 are chronic-care hospitals. The acute-care institutions are classified according to types (A, B, and C), depending on the level and sophistication of the services offered. Primary health services are provided through a network of institutions spread across the island's four administrative units or regional health authorities. There are 371 health centers in total, which, like hospitals, are divided into five types.

The private sector is quite intensely involved in the delivery of ambulatory care. These services are provided mainly through private hospitals and doctors' offices. The private sector is also active in providing diagnostic services. There are six private hospitals on the island, with a total capacity of approximately 270 beds.

Health sector reform in Jamaica is not a new phenomenon. It began as early as 1984 with the introduction of revised service charges for public hospitals and the rationalization of the public sector's health delivery system. In 1991, the Health Reform Unit was created to coordinate and monitor sectorwide reform activities. Thus far, the reform process has concentrated on seven key areas: decentralization, quality assurance, private partnership, alternative financing, hospital restoration, human resource development, and legislative modernization to support the sectorwide changes.

TABLE 2. Poverty estimates, Jamaica, 1989–1995 (individuals).

Indicator	1989	1990	1991	1992	1993	1994	1995
Percentage poor	29.1	28.1	49.5	35.9	28.4	26.2	32.3
Poverty gap index	7.1	7.0	16.3	10.7	8.2	6.7	8.1
Poverty severity index	3.2	2.8	7.8	4.7	3.6	2.7	3.0

Source: Theodore et al. (1997).

TABLE 3. Ranking of parishes based on poverty indicators (average values), Jamaica, 1996.

Parish	% 15–29 with primary education only	% labor force 15–29 unemployed	% households without exclusive water closet	% households without piped water in dwelling
Kingston	17.19	25.80	57.03	47.64
St. Andrew	15.15	20.08	40.93	31.70
St. Thomas	27.91	26.20	78.88	81.76
Portland	42.96	30.61	76.23	80.49
St. Mary	34.75	30.45	80.00	81.11
St. Ann	38.86	22.46	67.71	71.87
Trelawny	41.64	26.22	79.43	84.38
St. James	27.24	21.78	61.09	58.15
Hanover	35.25	28.38	80.64	85.57
Westmoreland	35.80	26.44	81.83	86.88
St. Elizabeth	43.36	29.29	79.70	79.79
Manchester	39.93	27.70	73.97	76.44
Clarendon	36.06	30.59	80.56	83.04
St. Catherine	25.22	25.09	57.09	48.23
National average	30.79	25.70	72.97	65.62

Source: Planning Institute of Jamaica (1996).

Several institutions and programs are especially designed for disadvantaged groups. Some are *direct* programs within the health sector that target the poor, and others are *indirect* programs, which do not necessarily form part of the national health system but target the poor for health and health-related services.

Direct Programs of Primary Health Care

All primary health care services are provided to the entire population free of charge. Primary health care is a major component of the health care system. The objectives of the primary health care network are to promote healthy lifestyles and prevent disease by making care accessible to all. The physical infrastructure of the primary health care system consists of a total of 371 health facilities of the following types:

- Type I health centers (a total of 172 that serve a population of 2,000–4,000 people) provide basic maternal and child health services—prenatal, postnatal, child health, immunization, family planning, and nutrition counseling.
- Type II health centers (a total of 85 that serve a population of 4,000–12,000) provide curative, dental, and environmental health services in addition to the services given at the Type I facilities. However, these services are not provided on a full-time basis.
- Type III health centers (a total of 66 that serve a population of 12,000–30,000) provide the services given at the Type II facilities on a regular basis. In addition, some specialized services may be offered, such as treatment of sexually transmitted diseases and mental health services.
- Type IV health centers (a total of 5) provide services similar to those provided at the Type III centers. They are located in the capital townships of Spanish Town, Lucea, Port Antonio, and Falmouth.
- Type V health centers (a total of 4) provide comprehensive health care services for densely populated urban areas. Laboratory support and facilities for research and accommodation for zonal or parish administrative staff are also provided.
- Community hospitals/polyclinics (a total of 6) provide services similar to those provided in Type III centers but also have maternity wards for intrapartum (delivery) care.

Other Direct Programs

Although the primary health care system is available at no cost, user fees are charged at hospital facilities. The Ministry of Health has a schedule of exemptions, which seeks to respond to the needs of the indigent as well as other risk groups. This schedule identifies the indigent as persons on poor relief, persons whose income is less than the minimum wage, persons whose sole income is the national insurance pension, and individuals receiving food aid. Identified as vulnerable with special needs are persons who use the following services: family planning, immunization, prenatal visits, postnatal and nutrition clinics, and child health services.

The Ministry of Health introduced the Drugs for the Elderly Program as a means of subsidizing pharmaceuticals for major conditions that afflict the aged. Conditions include hypertension, diabetes, glaucoma, arthritis, and heart disease. This move was motivated by the high cost of drugs to the elderly, estimated in 1996–1997 to be approximately J$ 30 million (Jamaican dollars) (Ministry of Health of Jamaica, 1997).

The Ministry of Health also operates a number of outlets that provide lower-cost generic pharmaceuticals to the public. These outlets are available throughout the island.

Indirect Programs

The Diabetes Association, created in 1976, is responsible for developing and implementing a nationwide plan for treatment, education, and training of diabetic patients. The Diabetes Association is a private, voluntary, nonprofit organization. It monitors and evaluates the effectiveness of the country's public diabetes services and provides subsidized care to its members.

In 1984, the Jamaican Food Stamp Program was introduced after general food subsidies were eliminated. The Jamaican Food Stamp Program is a social program designed to transfer income in the form of food purchasing power to low-income households. The program aims at protecting target groups from the negative effects of the rising cost of domestic and imported food items and sustaining the nutritional status of these groups at a socially acceptable level. The program is financed by the central government and forms part of the wider social safety net. Those eligible are pregnant women, lactating mothers, children under 5 years old, the elderly, Poor Relief and Public Assistance beneficiaries, and indigent households. Over the period 1989–1996, the Jamaican Food Stamp Program served an average of 6% of the population (Planning Institute of Jamaica, 1996). In 1996, two categories of beneficiaries—children aged under 6 and the elderly/poor/disabled—accounted for 71% of the total value of stamps distributed (Planning Institute of Jamaica, 1996).

INEQUALITIES IN HEALTH CONDITIONS

Jamaica's health indicators are more favorable than those of most countries in the developing world. Life expectancy at birth was 73 years in 1994. The crude birth rate was 25 per 1,000; the crude death rate, 8 per 1,000; infant mortality, 15 per 1,000; and fertility rate, 3 per woman of childbearing age. The country's morbidity/mortality profile is indicative of a transition in epidemiology away from infectious diseases. Chronic noncommunicable diseases are the main threat to the health of the adult population.

Cardiovascular disease, cerebrovascular disease, malignant neoplasms, and diabetes mellitus rank as the top causes of death. Accidents and trauma also contribute significantly to the overall disease burden.

Gender and Age Variations

The disease pattern in Jamaica, as is the case in other countries, is gender and age specific. Over one-third of all morbidity and mortality among males is caused by injury, whereas among women, noncommunicable diseases accounted for 70%. Among children under 5, communicable diseases are the leading causes of death and disability, and among persons 45 and over the leading cause is noncommunicable chronic illness (World Bank, 1996).

Differences across Socioeconomic Groups

Differences in health status across socioeconomic groups are found in many countries. Several factors may account for this, including differences in access to and utilization of health services, nutritional imbalances across groups, and unevenness in the quality of care or use of preventive services. Action or nonaction by the central government—such as poor maintenance of the medical infrastructure—also may affect the health status of low-income groups, who are greatly dependent on publicly provided services. Private as well as public poverty, therefore, can influence health outcomes.

The percentage of the population reporting an illness or injury decreased by six percentage points over the period 1989–1996 (Table 4). What this suggests, in a most general sense, is that either the health status of the population improved or the perception of illness changed over the survey period. There is very little geographic difference in the level of self-reported illnesses, except that the numbers in KMA were just below those in rural areas and other urban areas. The percentage of the population reporting illness during the four-week reference period averaged 14% in other urban areas and in rural areas and 11% in KMA.

The issue of the perception of illness also arises when we note that cases of reported illness/injury are greater among the nonpoor sections of the population. In fact, when one compares the results for the poorest and the wealthiest consumption quintiles for each year the survey was conducted, there is an unexpected positive correlation between the level of illness/injury reported and consumption levels. This seems to conflict with other empirical findings of this report that suggest that pro-rich inequalities exist. The latter results of this report are

TABLE 4. Percentage reporting illness in a four-week reference period, Jamaica, 1989–1996.

Classification	1989	1990	1991	1992	1993	1994	1995	1996
Area								
KMA	12.0	17.4	11.8	9.3	10.7	11.2	8.9	10.0
Other urban	18.2	22.3	17.7	11.1	13.3	11.9	8.4	8.9
Rural areas	18.2	17.5	13.3	11.1	12.4	14.4	11.0	12.0
Quintile								
Poorest	14.9	17.3	12.1	10.1	12.1	13.5	10.4	9.6
2	17.1	16.0	14.4	9.8	12.8	13.6	10.5	11.0
3	17.1	16.3	14.1	11.0	12.5	13.9	7.5	10.2
4	17.9	22.1	11.7	10.8	10.4	11.3	10.1	10.6
5	17.1	19.8	16.0	11.4	11.3	12.2	10.7	12.2
Sex								
Male	15.0	16.3	12.1	9.9	10.4	11.6	8.3	9.7
Female	18.5	20.3	15.0	11.3	13.5	14.3	11.3	11.8
Age								
0–4	....	....	....	....	....	....	....	....
5–9	....	....	....	12.8	9.7	11.8	8.3	11.1
10–19	....	....	....	5.9	6.7	6.5	4.9	5.6
20–29	....	....	....	4.7	6.3	8.2	5.5	5.6
30–39	....	....	....	7.0	8.1	8.0	6.4	7.4
40–49	....	....	....	10.5	11.0	12.9	8.2	9.6
50–59	....	....	....	13.5	13.2	16.0	15.1	14.7
60–64	....	....	....	18.2	26.0	21.8	15.8	14.6
65+	....	....	....	28.6	33.0	30.0	26.8	22.2
All Jamaica	16.8	18.3	13.7	10.6	12.0	12.9	9.8	10.7

Source: Planning Institute of Jamaica (1996).

.... = not available

largely in line with those obtained by Wagstaff and van Doorslaer (see chapter titled "Inequity in the Delivery of Health Care: Methods and Results for Jamaica," which appears later on in this section). As Table 4 indicates, the reduction in reported illness/injury was greater for respondents from the poorest consumption quintile (5.3 percentage points) than for those from the wealthiest quintile (4.9 percentage points). There is an obvious need for further research on these findings.

Data for reported illnesses by age cohort were available only from 1992 to 1996. These show the more familiar positive link between age and ill health, with as much as 28% (average for 1992–1996) of the 65-and-over age cohort reporting illness or injury. With respect to gender, the numbers reporting illness/injury were higher for women than for men.

For the 1989–1996 period, the mean number of illness days remained very stable (Table 5), declining only from 11.4 days in 1989 to 10.0 days in 1996. The 1996 figure was the lowest mean number of illness days reported since the survey began.

The Jamaican Survey of Living Conditions (SLC) allows two interesting indicators of health status to be analyzed. The first relates to the degree of incapacitation suffered because of the illness/injury and the second relates to the chronic nature of the condition. In the first

case, the number of days of restricted activity within the four-week reference period that resulted from the illness/ injury is identified. This allows data on the mean number of days of impairment by all variables—age, sex, and geographic region—to be examined. In the second case, the survey asks whether the illness/injury began before the four-week reference period, thereby allowing a distinction between acute and protracted (long-term) conditions. However, this does not provide an indication of severity or seriousness in the clinical sense. It should also be noted that persons who suffer from recurring spells of minor ailments are included among the positive responses to this question.

TABLE 5. Mean number of days of illness/injury and impairment, Jamaica, 1989–1996.

Year	Mean number of days of illness	Mean number of days of impairment
1989	11.4	5.5
1990	10.1	4.7
1991	10.2	4.9
1992	10.8	6.0
1993	10.4	6.3
1994	10.4	6.2
1995	10.7	5.6
1996	10.0	6.0

Source: Planning Institute of Jamaica (1996).

The number of days of restricted activity in 1996 was 9% above the mean number of days reported in 1989 (Table 5). The number reporting protracted illness increased significantly between 1990 and 1996. In 1990, about 20% of those reporting illness/injury also reported that it began before the four-week period; in 1996, this figure climbed to 33%. Females reported a higher incidence of protracted illness/injury than did men, and the elderly (65+) reported higher levels than all other age groups (Table 6). These results meet our *a priori* expectations because they are in keeping with the country's epidemiologic profile, reflecting increases in chronic noncommunicable diseases. It is important to take into account such differences inherent among the demographic groups before making judgments about health inequalities.

Protracted illnesses/injuries are concentrated in the lower-income groups. On average, the poorest consumption quintile reports a higher incidence of protracted illness/injury than the richest quintile. However, the increase in protracted illness/injury over the six years was much greater for those in the wealthiest quintile—a 16.3 percentage point increase for quintile 5 as opposed to 8.3 percentage points for quintile 1 (Table 6).

If we were able to manipulate the data set to restrict attention to protracted illnesses instead of illnesses/injury, we could gain a better understanding of what may appear to be inequalities. This is because there are associations between employment, conflict management, and injury. Unskilled, semiskilled, and skilled manual and nonmanual workers are prone to occupational injury, and violence is rampant among the poor in the inner-city areas of Kingston, the capital city. The unknown effects of these associations complicate this analysis. We will address this situation later in the study with data for 1993.

It must be noted that the usefulness of the data in measuring health inequalities is somewhat limited because of the absence of information about disease types. In other words, a better index of health status would be provided if the results could be interpreted within the context of specific medical conditions. Questions about chronic medical conditions were asked in the health module for 1991. Of those surveyed, 8.5% reported that they had hypertension, and 2.4% had diabetes. Of course, chronic noncommunicable diseases are age specific. As many as one-third of those over the age of 50 reported that they had hypertension, and 10% percent reported that they had diabetes. The prevalence of hypertension was higher among women and among the highest-income quintile. However, this may reflect better detection rates, as the higher-income groups often tend to use more preventive services. The prevalence of diabetes was also higher

TABLE 6. Percentage reporting protracted illness/injury, Jamaica, 1990–1996.

Classification	1990	1991	1992	1993	1994	1995	1996
Area							
KMA	18.2	23.1	31.3	28.5	36.8	36.0	29.8
Other urban	15.5	25.9	27.4	33.6	27.6	31.6	27.7
Rural areas	22.1	26.4	37.5	40.2	28.9	30.0	36.8
Quintile							
Poorest	24.9	26.8	40.8	37.1	32.8	25.0	33.6
2	24.8	27.8	31.6	34.6	29.8	30.4	27.3
3	17.6	34.5	35.2	26.1	26.4	35.4	34.6
4	16.9	23.9	35.4	43.9	36.4	34.0	39.3
5	15.5	15.9	28.6	36.7	26.2	36.3	31.8
Sex							
Male	18.4	25.4	31.6	35.0	26.3	28.4	30.4
Female	20.6	25.5	36.2	35.8	34.4	34.6	35.6
Age							
0–4	....	....	....	15.2	15.6	12.9	14.8
5–9	....	....	16.5*	20.4	20.0	18.1	25.1
10–19	....	....	15.2	19.4	17.0	17.5	18.0
20–29	....	....	18.5	22.5	21.6	12.0	22.6
30–39	....	....	22.4	29.4	27.7	29.4	28.3
40–49	....	....	39.4	32.8	26.2	26.4	46.8
50–59	....	....	46.1	41.3	38.7	44.9	47.8
60–64	....	....	57.3	61.4	43.2	53.5	46.5
65+	....	....	63.4	62.4	61.3	66.8	66.2
All Jamaica	19.6	25.5	34.8	35.5	30.9	32.0	33.3

Source: Planning Institute of Jamaica (1996).
*Percentage protracted illness for children 0–9 years.
.... = not available

TABLE 7. Hypertension and diabetes prevalence, by quintile, residence, sex, and age, Jamaica, 1991.

Category	Hypertension	Diabetes
Quintile		
Poorest	8.2	1.8
2	8.0	2.2
3	7.8	2.7
4	7.8	2.3
5	10.0	3.0
Sex		
Male	5.6	2.0
Female	11.9	2.8
Age group		
0–9	0.0	0.1
10–19	0.5	0.1
20–24	1.6	0.2
25–29	3.5	0.9
30–34	5.4	1.0
35–39	7.5	0.9
40–44	11.2	2.7
45–49	11.9	3.5
65+	34.1	10.7
All Jamaica	8.5	2.4

Source: Armstrong (1994).

among females and among the higher consumption quintiles (Table 7). It is safe to assume that these population characteristics had not changed significantly by 1993.

HEALTH CARE EXPENDITURES AND FINANCING

Public Health Care Expenditures

Expenditures of the Ministry of Health Based on Official Estimates

According to estimates of expenditures of the Ministry of Health,[2] 62.1% of public health funds are allocated to secondary care—i.e., hospital services. In contrast, only 19.6% of the funds are utilized for primary health care. Other items in the national health budget include pharmaceutical services[3] (6.8%), administrative costs of the Ministry of Health (4%), health services support[4] (3.6%), training (2.3%), family planning[5] (1.2%), and regional and international cooperation (0.4%).

[2]Estimates of the Ministry of Finance and Planning for the financial year 1992/1993. We assume that a similar breakdown holds for more recent years.
[3]"Pharmaceutical services" includes the procurement, storage, and supply of pharmaceuticals and medical sundries by the agencies delivering health care and by the public.
[4]"Health services support" covers surveillance (prevention and control activities aimed at reducing the occurrence of endemic diseases), paramedical services, and hospital maintenance.
[5]Operated by the National Family Planning Board.

We reclassified expenditures based on the COICOP[6] system, which identifies four categories of individual consumption as follows:

- medical and pharmaceutical products and therapeutic appliances and equipment,
- nonhospital medical and paramedical services,
- hospital services, and
- sickness and accident insurance services.

Only the first three categories are relevant because in Jamaica there is no health insurance system, which fuels public spending. We also included the category "other" for expenditures that are not directly related to the provision of services. The results of the reclassification exercise are shown in Table 8. The central government spends the largest share of the health budget on hospital services (49.43%). Medical and pharmaceutical products, therapeutic appliances, and equipment account for about 24%, and nonhospital and paramedical services account for 16.6%. Other miscellaneous spending takes up 10.29% of the national health budget.

Health Care Financing

Structure of Health Financing

Table 9 summarizes the structure of health financing in Jamaica. The data indicate that the financing burden is shared almost equally between the public sector and private individuals and that these two contributors account for the lion's share—85%. Social security, as already indicated, makes no direct contribution to health financing in Jamaica. This is one of the major changes being considered by the health sector reform program.

Evaluating Progressivity of Sources of Financing

In the case of taxation, although it was not possible to measure the extent of progressivity of the different components, a few general comments are in order. To begin with, the personal income tax structure seems to contain both progressive and regressive elements. In 1993, income was taxed at a flat rate of 33% for all income above

[6]Classification of Individual Consumption by Purpose (COICOP) was developed by the Organization for Economic Cooperation and Development and is used to classify individual consumption expenditures of households, nonprofit institutions serving households, and general government. "Individual consumption expenditures" are defined as expenditures made for the benefit of individual persons or households.

TABLE 8. Expenditures of the Ministry of Health based on the Classification of Individual Consumption by Purpose (COICOP), Jamaica, 1992–1993.

Category	Expenditure fiscal year: 1992–1993 (thousands of J$)	%
Medical and pharmaceutical products, therapeutic appliances, and equipment*	299,733	23.95
Nonhospital medical and paramedical services†	204,213	16.32
Hospital services‡	618,538	49.43
Other	128,836	10.30
Total	1,251,320	100.00

*Medical and pharmaceutical products and therapeutic appliances and equipment include purchase of goods and services and purchase of equipment and capital goods from the following programs: primary health care, secondary health care, health services support, and pharmaceutical services.

†Nonhospital medical and paramedical services include expenditure of the primary health care system, excluding purchases (goods and services and capital items)—that is, compensation to employees, travel and subsidies, rent, public utilities, awards, and grants.

‡Hospital services cover expenditure of the primary health care system, excluding purchases (goods and services and capital items)—that is, compensation to employees, travel and subsidies, rent, public utilities, awards, and grants.

J$ 10,400. This means that for the lowest quintile the effective income tax rate was zero. However, it also means, if we assume diminishing marginal utility of income, that for the other quintiles the utility cost of the tax system declines with income. The personal income tax system is therefore nominally regressive.

Turning to the indirect tax, the general consumption tax (GCT), although the overall rate was 12.5% for 1993, the effective rate for the different quintiles varies depending on the way the different exemptions or zero ratings affect their budgets. Table 10 presents estimates of the effective quintile-related rates of GCT based on a review of purchases recorded in the survey of living conditions.

TABLE 9. Structure of health financing, Jamaica, 1993.

Source	Amount (million J$)	%
Taxation*	2,890	0.43
Out-of-pocket†	2,800	0.42
Private insurance	760	0.11
NGOs	75	0.01
Social security	0	0.00
Other	221	0.03
Total	6,746	1.00

Source: Theodore (1997).

*Includes income, indirect, and other taxes, and there is no earmarking for health.

†Based on a doubling of the figure derived from the 1993 Jamaican Survey of Living Conditions. This is still more than 40% smaller than Boston University estimates of J$ 4,920 million, derived on the basis of a few interviews with health providers.

TABLE 10. Effective consumption tax rates, Jamaica, 1993.

Quintile	Effective GCT rate (%)
1	7.7
2	6.1
3	4.7
4	4.1
5	3.9
Average	4.6

The fact that the rates decline as incomes rise is a feature of most indirect tax systems. This is the manifestation of nominal regressivity in this type of system.

In 1993, income taxation and the GCT accounted for 67% of all government revenues (J$ 19,500 million of J$ 29,100 million). The other major contributors were customs duty (J$ 3,640 million), stamp duty (J$ 1,610 million), education tax (J$ 1,050 million), and special consumption tax (J$ 1,990 million). Other taxes accounted for J$ 1,840 million.

Without knowing the income and payment profiles of all taxpayers, it is difficult to comment on the progressivity of the financing mechanisms for the health system. We do know that the sources of public revenues are mainly two taxes that seem biased toward regressivity. Therefore, the issue is whether public expenditure on health care counteracts regressivity in the tax system. In this sense, the focus of inequality analysis should be on the uses of public funds. In other words, the real issue in the context of Jamaica is whether the utilization of public health facilities has the potential to modify the overall level of inequality. This issue is examined in the next section.

INEQUALITIES IN ACCESS TO AND UTILIZATION OF HEALTH SERVICES

The Question of Equality of Access in Policy Documents

Policy documents reveal that the public sector provides a spread of services, which are geographically situated to serve defined populations. The physical facility network was generally found to be equitably distributed. However, when both supply and demand factors are taken into account, some concerns emerge from a review of the literature. This is because, despite the evenness of services supplied by the public health system, variations in quality between the private and public sector compromised equity principles (Armstrong, 1994; Lalta, 1995; Bicknell, 1994). It was generally noted that private care was demanded by those able to afford such services, and public services that failed to meet acceptable standards were reserved for the poor. Project HOPE (1985) and Bicknell (1994) noted, furthermore, that unevenness also existed within private service utilization across broad economic groups, because wealthier persons could afford either domestic or foreign private services, whereas other groups were limited to private domestic care.

Bicknell (1994) and Armstrong (1994) addressed equality of access as it relates to rationing. They noted that in Jamaica, because doctors are allowed to care for private patients at public facilities, inpatient care in fact was being rationed through the market mechanism. Persons able to pay often were allowed to jump queues, which resulted in a "crowding out" effect. These studies also observed that the distribution of physicians' time between private (paying) patients and public (nonpaying) patients appeared to be unjust.

The opportunity cost of time was found to be instrumental in reducing the likelihood of particular economic groups utilizing services (Armstrong, 1994). It was pointed out that some persons did not possess the ability to pay, either directly for private care or indirectly (in the form of waiting time) for public sector care. For such persons, self-treatment or nontreatment may be substituted for medical attention. This type of inequity is perhaps higher for informal-sector workers who were unable to abandon their jobs to wait extended periods for attention.

Utilization Patterns

Based on the findings of the various surveys of living conditions, the percentage of persons reporting illness/ injury and seeking care has been increasing since 1989 (Table 11). As many as 54.9% of those persons sought care in 1996. There continues to be roughly a 60:40 distribution in the utilization of private and public health services. Although this ratio has remained relatively stable since 1989 (Table 12), it should not be taken as an indicator of ability to pay for health care services, because many low-income households deplete assets or forgo other basic needs to purchase health services (World Bank, 1994). More of the ill or injured from rural areas (66%) were found to utilize private health care providers than was the case for their counterparts from other geographic regions (Planning Institute of Jamaica, 1996). This may be because the well-equipped public facilities are located in metropolitan areas, leaving rural communities with little choice but to seek care from private providers.

For persons utilizing the services of private providers, the mean individual expenditure on visits was J$ 598.30 (Table 13). However, mean expenditures were highest in the rural areas (Planning Institute of Jamaica, 1996). Mean annual expenditure for private care was also found to increase with consumption quintile. However, the highest mean private patient expenditure was observed for individuals 65 years and over (Planning Institute of Jamaica, 1996), which obviously reflects the greater need for care among the aged.

Equity in the Distribution of Health Benefits

Financing of the health system should not create access barriers to those in need of health care. Horizontal equity demands that health services be distributed according to need. To provide a sense of the extent of the need, the utilization findings of the 1993 Survey of Living Con-

TABLE 11. Percentage of ill/injured seeking medical care by area, consumption quintile, and sex, Jamaica, 1989–1996.

Classification	1989	1990	1991	1992	1993	1994	1995	1996
Area								
KMA	56.7	40.5	48.0	58.8	60.1	55.9	52.6	53.8
Other urban	45.5	40.9	45.6	52.4	51.6	59.0	57.5	55.5
Rural areas	47.2	36.8	48.6	47.1	47.2	47.0	62.8	55.4
Quintile								
1 (poorest)	43.7	35.7	38.7	34.7	39.0	44.3	55.4	53.4
2	49.8	38.0	52.0	45.8	48.7	44.6	60.1	45.6
3	47.5	38.8	48.7	53.5	45.4	50.8	58.4	51.1
4	52.7	40.2	50.6	55.9	63.4	56.8	63.4	59.0
5	51.6	39.7	47.8	60.3	60.3	63.4	58.4	63.0
Sex								
Male	44.7	37.9	48.5	49.0	48.0	49.0	59.0	50.5
Female	52.8	39.2	47.4	52.5	54.7	53.4	58.9	58.5
Jamaica	49.0	39.0	47.7	50.9	51.8	51.5	58.9	54.9

Source: Planning Institute of Jamaica (1996).

TABLE 12. Use of public/private sector by ill/injured for medical care, purchase of medication, and hospitalization during the four-week reference period, Jamaica, 1989–1996.

Year	Percentage of those seeking medical care		Percentage purchasing medication			Percentage hospitalization of those seeking medical care		
	Public	Private	Both	Public	Private	Both	Public	Private
1989	39.0	61.0	NA	NA	NA	NA	NA	NA
1990	39.4	60.6	NA	NA	NA	NA	NA	NA
1991	35.6	57.7	6.7	NA	NA	NA	NA	NA
1992	28.5	63.4	8.1	8.9	58.5	2.4	1.0	NA
1993	30.9	63.8	5.3	15.9	79.9	4.2	6.9	0.5
1994	28.8	66.7	4.5	21.4	75.6	3.0	4.6	0.8
1995	27.2	66.4	6.3	16.4	81.9	1.7	6.0	0.2
1996	31.8	63.6	4.6	19.1	78.0	2.9	5.1	0.5

Source: Planning Institute of Jamaica (1996).
NA = not applicable.

ditions are summarized in the tables and in Figure 1. It is apparent that almost one-half of those reporting illness did not seek care, which raises the question: Is this a perception-of-illness result or is it a problem of access barriers and therefore a problem of equity?

Health benefits delivered through the public health system include the services available at both primary and secondary care institutions. Figure 1 presents the general utilization patterns observed for 1993. Table 14 summarizes these patterns across income groups and allocates expenditures accordingly; the table indicates the number of days of reported illness and the corresponding treatment "hits" at public facilities.

Table 14 shows that the distribution of benefits clearly favors the lower-income groups. The lowest quintile enjoys more than twice the benefits (29%) enjoyed by the wealthiest quintile (12%). This means that, although more persons in the top quintile sought medical attention, they clearly showed a preference for private facilities. Almost by default, the public facilities became the haven for the lower-income groups.

To assess the impact of the public health expenditure we have sought to compare, under two scenarios, the distribution of consumption expenditure of those who sought attention at public facilities. In the first scenario, we consider the distribution including the tax component only. In the second scenario, we allow for the presence of both the tax and the health benefit. Presumably, the latter scenario comes closer to capturing the net benefit incidence of the public health benefit. Table 15 shows the structure of consumption under the two scenarios.

Of course there are two factors at work here. On the one hand, distribution of the health benefit itself clearly favored the lower-income groups. On the other hand, the share of the health benefit in the combined consumption/health welfare package was extremely large. The ratio of

TABLE 13. Mean patient expenditure on health care in public and private facilities in the four-week reference period, Jamaica, 1989–1996.

Year	Visits				Drugs		
	Private nominal (J$)	Private real 1990 (J$)	Public nominal (J$)	Private real J$ 1990	Private nominal (J$)	Private real 1990 (J$)	Public nominal (J$)
1989	57	74.0	11	14	48	62	5
1990	72	72.0	11	11	43	43	4
1991	82	44.0	11	6	95	51	8
1992	167	63.0	14	5	234	88	17
1993	298	85.0	115	33	331	94	131
1994	461	109.0	91	21	417	98	163
1995	496	98.8	130	26	509	101	234
1996	598	103.6	148	26	685	119	176

Source: Planning Institute of Jamaica (1996).

FIGURE 1. Perceptions of persons suffering from illness over the past four weeks and level of utilization of health services, Jamaica, 1993.

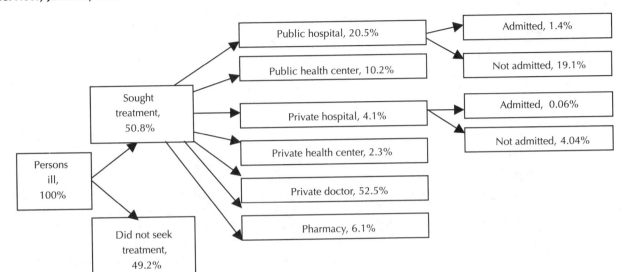

the health benefit to the consumption of those accessing public facilities is almost 4:1. In other words, the health benefit is large enough to make a difference.[7]

Table 15 shows an example of perfect rank reversal—literally, the first becomes last, and the last, first. On the face of it, the health benefit could not be asked to do more. The final share of the lowest quintile more than doubled and that of the next lowest quintile increased by more than 25%. The shares of the other three quintiles fell at an increasing rate, as progressivity requires.

This result raises a number of questions. Although it suggests that the health system in Jamaica has the potential to make a difference to the overall equity situation in the country, persons with a working knowledge of the system point to a high degree of dissatisfaction among those seeking care in the public system. The reason is most probably one highlighted by Wagstaff and van Doorslaer (see the chapter titled "Inequity in the Delivery of Health Care: Methods and Results for Jamaica," which appears later in this section)—*the equity measures being used do not capture the quality of the services delivered.* Linked to this is the second question raised by the results. Why is the number of persons seeking care in the public sector less than half those who seek care in the private sector, even though

care in the public sector is free at the point of service? Again, the issue seems to be one of the perceived quality of care in the public sector. It would be useful if future living standard surveys were to seek to capture this quality perception, as this information could be a useful guide to policy making.

In closing, it also must be noted that, in spite of the apparent perception of lower service quality in the public health system, the nonpoor continue to seek services there. The explanation for this phenomenon appears to lie in the fact that public providers not only have the option to engage in private practice but in some cases this practice takes place in the public facilities. Thus, it is quite possible that services of different quality are being provided in the same facility. This is one of the main challenges the health reform process faces, because that process is grounded on the principle of universal provision of a basic package of health services of equal quality for all citizens, regardless of income status.

QUANTIFICATION OF INEQUALITIES

The ECuity method (see the chapter titled "Inequity in the Delivery of Health Care: Methods and Results for Jamaica," which appears later in this section) was applied to test for biases in health status and in utilization of health services. When the variables were standardized, it was found that the system showed a clear pro-rich bias in three of four health status indicators and an unambiguous pro-

---

[7]Of the 7,316 persons in the 1993 sample, 865 (11.8%) reported being ill, 438 (6%) sought care, and 135 (1.8%) chose to go to a public facility. This fraction (1.8%) corresponds to the consumption level used in Table 15—that is, J$ 776.6 million or 1.4% of total consumption of J$ 56,800 million.

TABLE 14. Use of public health facilities by income quintiles, Jamaica, 1993.

Quintile	Days of illness	Treatment at public facilities	Primary no.	Value (million J$)	Secondary no.	Value (million J$)	Combined (million J$)	Distribution
1	790	393	261	186.5	132	561.1	836.2	0.289
2	1,096	419	352	166.5	67	459.0	729.0	0.252
3	960	306	188	93.2	118	612.1	557.5	0.193
4	1,026	178	72	66.6	106	510.0	428.8	0.148
5	1,028	209	165	86.6	44	153.0	343.1	0.119
Total	4,900	1,505	1,038	599.5	467	2,295.2	2,894.7	1.000

rich bias in the utilization of health services. The standardization procedures are described in the Annex.

CONCLUSIONS AND POLICY RECOMMENDATIONS

Jamaica's economic context is one of a country struggling to regain balance in its key accounts. Since 1990, the country has barely managed to achieve 1% annual growth and the level of unemployment seems to have settled at around 15%–16%. The average rate of poverty between 1989 and 1996 has been 35%, and the mean consumption ratio between the highest and the lowest quintile was more than 7:1. In other words, the situation has been one in which the growing demand for social services and a strong safety net have been met with a weakening capacity to respond.

Nevertheless, it is important to point out that the Jamaican government has sought to respond in two ways that are relevant to the health equity concerns of this project. First, the government has put in place a fairly extensive poverty alleviation program, including a food stamp program that covers a wide cross section of the indigent population. This measure was taken in response to growing evidence that the ongoing structural adjustment program was having a deleterious effect on child nutrition. Second, the government has embarked on a health sector reform program that has three main elements: decentralization of services in an effort to reach

the rural population better; refurbishment and restructuring of the public sector primary care system; and introduction of a national health insurance program that will make a basic package of health services available to all citizens regardless of income.

Because the national health system operates within an environment of poverty and inequity, it is not surprising to find that the system itself is infected with these social characteristics. This project attempted to determine the inequality bias of the health system with respect to three specific concerns:

- The health status of the population: Is the system pro-poor or pro-rich with respect to its health outcomes?
- Access to or utilization of health services: Is the system responding to the health needs of the population with a pro-rich or a pro-poor bias?
- Financing of the system: Is the system progressive or regressive in terms of sources and allocation of its finances?

With regard to health status, there were three salient survey results:

- According to the surveys of living conditions from 1989 to 1996, with the exception of 1995, the poor consistently reported less illness than the nonpoor. This may be an illness perception phenomenon that merits further investigation.

TABLE 15. Distribution of consumption with and without tax and health benefits, Jamaica, 1993.

Quintile	Consumption with tax but no health benefit (million J$)	Share	Consumption with tax and health benefit (million J$)	Share
1	93.9	0.121	930.2	0.253
2	147.4	0.190	876.5	0.239
3	154.4	0.199	711.9	0.194
4	165.6	0.213	595.4	0.162
5	215.2	0.277	558.3	0.152
Total	776.6	1.000	3,672.3	1.000

- With regard to protracted illness, however, the pattern was clearly one in which the poor were more severely affected.
- With regard to chronic illness, the 1993 survey showed no clear picture; the poor were neither more nor less afflicted than the nonpoor.

In applying the EquiLAC methodology to test for biases in health status, it was found that, when the variables were standardized, in three of four health status indicators the system showed a clear pro-rich bias.

With regard to utilization of health services there were also three salient survey results:

- Using the variable "illness days," it was found that, although the very poor reported less illness, they used the public facilities much more than the nonpoor.
- However, it was observed that even the very poorest Jamaicans were heavy users of private sector health services—almost half their services were sought in the private sector.
- For all quintiles except the first, the use of private sector facilities was almost twice the use of public sector facilities.

In applying the EquiLAC methodology to test for bias in the utilization of health services, again, standardization of the variable showed an unambiguous pro-rich bias.

These results are somewhat puzzling when we recall that the Jamaican public health system is an open-access system. Primary care services are free on demand, one section of the public sector drug service is free, and, although there are fees at hospitals, the range of persons exempted is so large that the secondary care system is also substantially free.

Seemingly, these results are consistent with a two-tiered health system in which even the very poor feel more confident about getting the quality of service they need in the private sector. The fact that some of the nonpoor use the public system points to the possibility of queue jumping and differential treatment at public sector facilities. This is consistent with the known practice in Jamaica of allowing public sector doctors to engage in private practice within the confines of public facilities.

As for financing, there were three noteworthy findings:

- On the sources side, taxation and out-of-pocket expenditures accounted for 85% of all health financing in Jamaica, with an almost even split between the two.

- Because out-of-pocket payment is known to be regressive, and because both the proportional income system and the main consumption tax (GCT) in the country are also deemed to be regressive, the *prima facie* conclusion is that there is regressivity on the sources side. In the absence of data on the distribution of the income tax burden, this study accepted this inference.
- On the usage side, the 1993 survey shows that the use of the public health facilities was strongly skewed in favor of the lower quintiles, with the lowest quintile accounting for almost one-third of the public resources applied to health.

This last result appears to suggest that the public health system has the potential to correct any prior regressivity that may result from the way the health system is financed. Assuming that the mode of financing is reflected in the overall distribution of income or consumption, we conducted an analysis that showed that, in fact, the public health system could change a regressive distribution of benefits into a progressive one.

Having found this, however, a number of questions remain unanswered. Why are so few persons using the "free" health service? Why are so many of the poor making the sacrifice to gain access to private sector facilities? Why do the nonpoor use the public health system at all?

It would seem that the answer to these questions lies in the quality of services available within the public health system. In fact, the answer probably lies in the differential quality of public sector services. With a multitiered system of hospitals and health centers it would seem that those who seek attention in the public sector are not guaranteed an acceptable basic quality of health services. In other words, although the public health system clearly needs to be made more attractive to the poor, it also must seek to avoid service differentiation between the poor and the nonpoor. This is one important means by which the apparent "correction" by public financing will be translated into better health status for the poor.

In a system in which only a small number of persons seek care in the public sector and in which poverty levels are very high, there is a distinct possibility that more and more poor people are seeking care in the private sector—a private sector that not only employs many of the same providers as the public sector, but one in which the price of services over the full range of health services needed is known to present access barriers to large segments of the population. Patients may barely manage to find the funds to visit a doctor, but then they are unable to pay for lab tests and prescriptions.

It is important to note that the welfare impact of the health system depends on three factors: the availability of epidemiologically appropriate services, the accessibility of these services to all citizens, and the quality of these services. Moreover, in a society in which the informal sector is becoming more and more important and more and more competitive, people simply are not willing to wait long hours at public facilities. It is important for overall equity improvements and for health status improvements among the poor that steps be taken to make the public sector facilities more attractive to those in need of health services. A public health system that attracts more patients will be in a position, given its size, to set price and quality standards for the entire health care system.

Finally, and most importantly, the government should invest in upgrading public health facilities and existing systems in order to expeditiously meet the health needs of the population.

REFERENCES

Armstrong J. *Jamaica Health Sector Review: Present Status and Future Options*. Report 13407 JM. Washington, DC: World Bank; 1994.

Bicknell WJ. *Jamaica Health Sector Assessment: Policy Implications and Recommendations*. Report prepared for the Ministry of Health under contract by Touche Ross Management Consultants. London: Touche Ross Management Consultants; 1994.

Blaxter M. A companion of measures of inequality in morbidity. In Fox J. (ed.) *Health Inequalities in European Countries*. London: Gower, Aldershot and London; 1989.

Lalta S. *Review of Health Financing in Jamaica and a Survey of the Feasibility of National Health Insurance*. Study funded by the U.S. Agency for International Development through the Latin America and Caribbean Health Nutrition Sustainability Project. Washington, DC: U.S. Agency for International Development; 1995.

Ministry of Health. *Jamaica Green Paper on the National Health Insurance Plan*. Kingston: Ministry of Health; 1997.

Planning Institute of Jamaica. *Economic and Social Survey Jamaica, 1995*. Kingston: Planning Institute of Jamaica; 1995.

Planning Institute of Jamaica. *Survey of Living Conditions, 1996*. Kingston: Planning Institute of Jamaica; 1996.

Project HOPE. *Health Insurance Options*. Millwood, VA: Project HOPE; 1985.

Theodore K. *Macroeconomic Implications of a National Health Insurance Programme for Jamaica*. Report for the Ministry of Health. Kingston: Ministry of Health; 1997.

Theodore K et al. *Health and Poverty in the Caribbean*. Report for the Caribbean Development Bank. 1997. Bridgetown: Caribbean Development Bank. Mimeograph.

World Bank. *Jamaica: Achieving Macro-stability and Removing Constraints on Growth*. Country Economic Memorandum. Washington, DC: World Bank; 1996.

ANNEX: STANDARDIZATION OF VARIABLES

EQUITY AND MORBIDITY

In the analysis of health care outcomes, data from the Jamaican 1993 SLC were used.[1] As with other living conditions inquiries, the main socioeconomic variable was per capita expenditures, adjusted for adult equivalents by a factor of 0.75, which yielded 1.00, 1.40, and 1.68 for a couple, a couple with one child, and a couple with two children, respectively. No specific distinction was made for morbidity patterns between adults and children and the effective sample size was 7,316 cases.

In 1993, reported morbidity was 11.8%, with approximately 7.7% reporting acute illnesses and 4.1% reporting chronic illness. There were no questions about the degree of self-assessed ill health in the 1993 survey. Of those reporting illness, 42.8% were male and 57.8% were female. This corresponds to 10.3% of the male respondents and 13.3% of the female respondents. Averages for adults and children showed a similar pattern in that 10.5% of those reporting ill health were adults and 12.8% were children.

Observed morbidity did not vary significantly by consumption decile. However, at higher levels of aggregation, differences were evident (see Figure A1). Grouped by per capita consumption quintile adjusted for adult equivalent units, observed morbidity showed significant variation.[2] Noteworthy in this respect, morbidity did not decline gradually as one moved upward in the consumption scale. Instead, the two highest quintiles showed higher-than-expected morbidity rates relative to the other consumption groups.

Morbidity patterns are likely not to vary simply in terms of socioeconomic differences but also by demographic factors. This gives rise to the notion of morbidity that can be eliminated—i.e., variation in morbidity across income groups adjusted for differences in age and gender. This adjustment is on the whole necessary because age and ill health are necessarily correlated, but more importantly income and age often manifest a statistically significant relationship. This can be further compounded when differences in attitude on the basis of gender determine whether one perceives oneself ill. Indices of health inequality therefore adjust for these differences. In this study, we have used the standardization procedure for ungrouped data articulated by Wagstaff and van Doorslaer (see chapter titled "Inequity in the Delivery of Health Care: Methods and Results for Jamaica," which appears later in this section) to derive a measure of C and C^*. The derivation is as follows:

Assuming that the illness concentration curve is piecewise linear, we can represent the concentration index C by

$$C = \frac{2}{\mu} \sum_{t=1}^{T} f_t \mu_t R_t - 1$$

FIGURE A1. Chronic illness rates by income quintile, Jamaica, 1993.

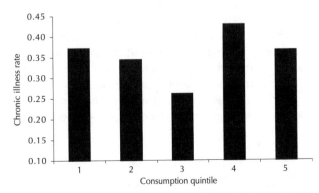

Source: Planning Institute of Jamaica, Survey of Living Conditions, 1993.

---

[1] In addition to providing a rich data set, the survey can be considered an improvement on its predecessors in that it benefited from several refinements, which led to a higher response rate and enhanced survey execution.

[2] Not adjusted for demographic differences.

where the mean morbidity rate is

$$\mu = \sum_{t=1}^{T} f_t \mu_t$$

and R_t is the relative rank of the tth socioeconomic group and f_t is the fraction of segment t in the entire population.

FRAMEWORK FOR ANALYSIS

Inequality in health care outcomes may be assessed in a number of ways. Notable among them is the framework proposed by Blaxter (1989). Three models are proposed in this schema: (1) a medical model, which considers illness/injury affecting the respondents' physical well-being; (2) a functional model, which ranks physical incapacitation by degree or extent, measured by the inability to perform what are considered normal functions; and (3) a subjective model, in which ill-health is assessed subjectively compared with persons of similar age. The 1993 SLC poses several limitations on the strict application of these models in that the subjective model could not be evaluated as the question about the degree of self-reported illness was omitted. In addition, no useful distinction could be made between illness per se and injury.[3]

Table A1 details the available indicators. The main results for the medical model are presented in Table A2 and Figure A2. For all the indicators except illness/injury, in the past 4 weeks the inequality index (I^*) reflects a bias against the poor. The standardized health status concentration curve is shown in Figure A3. All prevalence rates and means of illness days, except for long-term illness, show a decline with rising expenditure levels—again, a bias against lower-income groups.

Table A3 shows pro-poor inequality—a positive concentration index (C^*) with respect to the health status indicator (i.e., reported illness); however, the estimator is not statistically significant. This is in contrast to the indicator of utilization; it clearly shows a pro-rich pattern, which, although not by any means severe, is statistically significant. I^* also shows a similar pattern for utilization.

The cumulative distribution of utilization by consumption quintiles is shown in Figure A4. We have not tabulated the unstandardized measures, because the unstandardized indicator of utilization as measured by the concentration (Gini) index (reported below) was similar

in order of magnitude to the standardized concentration index, measuring 0.167, and was similarly insignificant.

What can be observed in general is that demographic standardization does indeed influence the measure of existing health inequality to the extent that the index changes from pro-rich to pro-poor. This result creates some discomfort, because an experimental raw data cross-tabulation to determine whether the gender of the respondent affected the seeking of medical attention generally showed no significant variation across the sexes. However, when age was superimposed, it was evident that it accounts for a substantial degree of the variation. For example, for children under 5 years of age, a poor child was more than 3.5 times as likely to seek medical attention as his/her counterpart from the highest quintile. For persons between the ages of 16 and 59 years, however, only 9.7% of the poorest 20% sought medical attention, compared with 31.2% of the wealthiest 20%.

COMPUTATION METHODS

In all cases, the indirect method of standardization was used and indices were computed on individual level data. Standard errors were not computed along the lines of the refinements suggested by Wagstaff and van Doorslaer (1998) but were derived directly from the regression estimates. In addition to those included in Table A3, unstandardized estimates for the health services utilization concentration index were derived as follows:

Health care utilization
$$C = 0.167 \qquad t(C) = 0.047 \qquad Se(C) = 3.542$$

Standardizations were confined to age and gender, as it was often the case that other demographic variables—specifically, education—did not account for significant variation in either observed morbidity or the choice to seek medical attention (the utilization variable used in the analysis).

INTERPRETATION

For health inequity indices (I^* and C), negative values indicate distributions favoring the nonpoor, and positive values indicate distributions favoring the poor. However, the size of the standard errors and the t statistics are to be considered in determining the reliability of the results.

---

[3]A filter variable identifying ill-health due to injury would be used.

TABLE A1. Health indicators in Jamaica.

Indicator	Definition	Mean
Medical model		
Illness/injury in past four weeks	Have you had an illness or injury in the past 4 weeks? For example, have you had a cold, diarrhea, injury due to an accident, or any other illness?	0.118
No. of illness days during past four weeks	For how many days during the past four weeks have you suffered from this illness or injury?	6.349
Acute illness	Have you had an illness/injury during the past 4 weeks?	0.649
Long-term illness	Have you had an illness/injury during the past four weeks that started more than four weeks ago?	0.351
Functional model		
No. of restricted-activity days	For how many days during the past 4 weeks were you incapacitated because of illness or injury?	6.35
Activity limitation	Does your health limit you from running, walking, eating, bathing, climbing stairs, etc.?	NA
Major limitation	Does your illness/injury limit you severely from any of the above activities?	NA
Minor limitation	Does your illness/injury limit you slightly from any of the above activities?	NA

Source: Planning Institute of Jamaica, Survey of Living Conditions, 1993.
NA = not applicable.

TABLE A2. Inequality index values and *t* values for medical model.

Health indicator	C	t(C)	Se(C)	I*
Illness/injury in past four weeks	–0.0300	–1.131	0.026530	0.0018
No. of days ill in past four weeks	–0.0458	–5.347	0.008570	–0.0042
Acute illness	–0.0341	–1.835	0.018579	–0.0010
Long-term illness	–0.0866	–5.184	0.016702	–0.0051

FIGURE A2. Medical model: unstandardized means for expenditure quintiles.

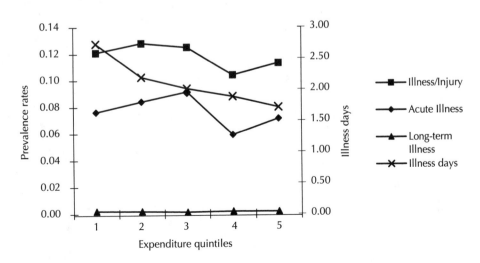

FIGURE A3. Health status concentration curve (standardized).

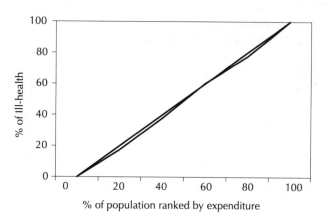

FIGURE A4. Utilization by consumption quintiles.

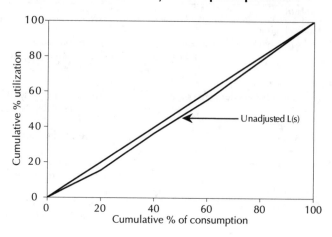

TABLE A3. Standardized health inequality indicators for service utilization and health care status.

Standardized indicators	Health status	Health care utilization	Inequality index	Health care utilization
C^*	0.100	−0.00032	I^*	−0.0319
$t(C^*)$	−0.874	−0.50900	$t(I^*)$	−4.9270
$Se(C^*)$	0.115	0.00063	$Se(I^*)$	0.006473

HEALTH SYSTEM INEQUALITIES AND POVERTY IN MEXICO

Susan Wendy Parker and Eduardo Gonzales Pier

BACKGROUND

Macroeconomic Context

Mexico has an area of approximately 1.96 million km^2 and a population of 94 million. A per capita annual income of US$ 8,370 places it among the world's upper middle-income countries. Since 1994, the country's economy has grown steadily, with the gross domestic product (GDP) increasing by 7.3%. Unemployment stood at 6.2% in 1995, but it fell to 3.3% by the end of 1997. There has been an upturn in domestic demand as well as in exports. Inflation has declined continuously over the past four years, but so have real wages, largely because of the sharp declines registered in the manufacturing sector every year since 1995. Still, economic growth has boosted job creation.

The financial crisis in Southeast Asia has had some repercussions on Mexico's financial markets. The slowing of capital flows, for example, has resulted in adjustments in exchange rates and increases in interest rates. Although these developments have not affected overall macroeconomic outcomes, they have no doubt accounted for the uneven performance of the country's productive base. Large firms, exporters, and companies that have access to external financing have performed quite well, but small firms geared toward the domestic market have had difficulty obtaining financing and therefore achieving their former levels of activity. This situation has had a greater impact on people in the poorest groups of society, who tend to be employed in smaller business enterprises and in the informal sector.

Poverty and Inequality

Despite some favorable economic trends, poverty levels in Mexico have hovered around 24% of the population since 1990. Rural poverty, at 36% in 1997, was much higher than the urban rate (19%). This situation also has implications for inequalities in health status between the poor and nonpoor in rural and urban areas.

HEALTH CARE SYSTEM

The Mexican Constitution makes health care a fundamental right of all persons. Although there have been considerable improvements in the health status of the population, inequalities in access, utilization, and financing of health care persist. Mexico is undergoing a protracted demographic transition. Life expectancy is increasing and the elderly population is growing in relative and absolute terms. The proportion of persons under 15 years of age is expected to decrease from 39% to 30% between 1990 and 2030, and the number of people over 65 is expected to increase threefold during the same period. The economic progress of the past few decades has had uneven effects across the different regions. The wealthier northern states have experienced significant increases in living standards, while the southern and more rural states have lagged behind. Large regional differences in the pace of economic development and demographic transition have resulted in the coexistence of two epidemiologic profiles: malnutrition, maternal and perinatal deaths, and the reemergence of communicable diseases commonly associated with poverty and underdevelopment prevail in the rural and southern states, whereas chronic conditions, cardiovascular disease, and mental health disorders are the most common health problems in the urban northern and central states.

The observed inequalities in health status are compounded by an equally uneven distribution of resources and supply of quality care. In general, higher-income groups in urban centers and northern states receive higher quality medical care and also enjoy broader consumer choice. At the same time, lower-income Mexicans in southern rural states are left with limited choice among mostly public providers with long waiting lists and chronic shortages of medical supplies and qualified personnel. The uneven distribution of hospital beds, physicians, and nurses is only partially explained by the greater purchasing power of the wealthier northern and urban dwellers. Inefficient, centralized "top-down" management, coupled with insufficient planning and collaboration across independent public system delivery networks, has led to duplication of resources and excess capacity in urban areas. Budget allocations based on historical spending rather than on health needs, including inflexible line-item budgeting practices, have meant that poorer states—which have the highest burden of disease—receive less spending per beneficiary. As a result, the differences in supply of health care between the poor and the nonpoor have persisted.

Organizational problems in the Mexican health care system generate inequities in health, health care delivery, and health financing. Although, in principle, all Mexicans have access to basic public health care services free of charge (or for a nominal user fee) at the point of service delivery, in practice, some 10 million people in need of health care have limited or no access. Others are required by law to contribute to and receive coverage from one of several social security institutes. Additionally, many workers employed in the formal sector and their families, who are covered by the social security system, find the available services inferior in quality and scope. Those dissatisfied with the public alternatives and groups that lack access to public health care services choose, or are forced, to pay out of pocket to private providers for health care.[1] As a result, although more than 90% of the population is covered by some form of public health care service, almost half of the national health expenditure each year occurs through the private sector.

National Health System

The reasons for the fragmented nature of the Mexican health care system can be traced to its historical development over the past 50 years. Currently, the network of health services includes the Ministry of Health (Secretaría de Salud; SSA) and the Mexican Social Security Institute (Instituto Mexicano de Seguridad Social; IMSS). The Ministry is the coordinating authority for the whole sector. It is concerned with public health, epidemic control, and health care delivery to the urban poor—a rapidly expanding segment of the population. The IMSS was created to respond to the needs of a newly industrialized labor force. New legal and organizational arrangements have enhanced its responses to demands from special population groups. In 1956, a separate social security institute (Instituto de Seguridad Social de los Trabajadores del Estado; ISSSTE) was created for public sector workers, while the national oil industry (Petróleos Mexicanos; PEMEX) and the armed forces (Instituto de Seguridad Social de las Fuerzas Armadas Mexicanas; ISSFAM) continued to operate their own independent health care facilities. More recently, the IMSS-Solidaridad program was established to address the needs of the rural poor. Alongside this public network, the private sector offers care on a mostly out-of-pocket, fee-for-service basis to those without public coverage or who are dissatisfied with the quality of public services.

Hence, the national health system in Mexico comprises three major components, each with a distinctive health care financing arrangement:

- Social security institutions are vertically integrated providers financed by compulsory employment-based insurance paid for by employers and workers through a payroll tax and complemented by general public funds.
- Governmental providers, who cover the uninsured population and are financed mostly from general tax revenues and partially by user fees.
- The private sector, which relies mostly on out-of-pocket payments and insurance premiums.

Each of these sectors runs its own services and is separately financed and regulated. Therefore, each determines independently the amount of care it will provide to its beneficiaries.

Social Security Institutions

The IMSS is the largest social security provider, covering formal private-sector workers, retirees, and their families—a population of about 40 million.[2] Health care is delivered directly by the Institute's own vertically integrated network of medical units, which are staffed by full-time salaried physicians. Theoretically, the entire continuum of care, from preventive to tertiary services, is covered. The IMSS provides not only health care but

---

[1] The 1994 National Health Survey reports that about one-third of those who are eligible for social security benefits regularly pay out of pocket to receive private health care.

[2] Although the IMSS insures mostly formal-sector workers and their families through compulsory employment-related contributions, recent legal changes have allowed for voluntary "opt-in" enrollment of informal workers and other workers who do not hold regular salaried jobs (mostly small businesses, the self-employed, and agricultural workers).

also a variety of social security benefits, including injury compensation for workers; old age, severance, and retirement pensions; and child care benefits.

The ISSSTE is the second-largest social security institute, covering federal, state, and municipal public sector employees, retirees, and their families—approximately nine million beneficiaries. ISSSTE is similar to IMSS in terms of the services it offers and the organization of its health care delivery.

Two other public sector institutions form part of the social security system. The national oil corporation (PEMEX) and the armed forces (ISSFAM) operate as integrated financiers and providers of health care and other social security benefits. PEMEX covers a total population of 0.6 million oil industry workers, retirees, and their families, and ISSFAM covers 0.8 million beneficiaries.

Public Sector Providers for the Uninsured

The Ministry of Health (SSA) combines the role of regulator of the health care system—including strategic planning, monitoring of food and drug safety, public health campaigns, and control of communicable diseases—with health care delivery as the largest provider of health care services for the uninsured population. Public services are supplied in exchange for a small user charge, which seeks to take into account the economic situation of the patient. Although in principle all Mexicans are eligible to receive SSA services, in practice those without access to SSA facilities—in particular, the rural poor and those with private insurance or social security coverage—do not normally use these services. Estimates of the Ministry's coverage are therefore difficult to obtain. The official figure is approximately 30 million persons.

IMSS-Solidaridad is a recently established program run by the IMSS but funded with federal tax revenues. The program, which operates in only 17 of the 32 states, is free of charge at the point of delivery and targeted to the rural poor who do not have access to alternative public providers. Again, difficulties in tracking beneficiaries make it difficult to estimate the program's actual coverage. According to official statistics, it is delivering basic health care to 10–12 million people living in the 140,000 very small poor rural communities scattered throughout the country.

Other smaller governmental health care institutions include the decentralized services in the Department of the Federal District (Mexico City); the National Indigenous Institute (Instituto Nacional Indigenista; INI), which provides health care services in areas with large indigenous populations, as part of its mission to support socioeconomic development of indigenous groups; and

the National Comprehensive Family Development System (Sistema Nacional para el Desarrollo Integral de la Familia; DIF), which provides health and social services to socially disadvantaged groups, including women, children, the disabled, and the elderly. These institutions also operate their own facilities and deliver services free of charge. Their total combined coverage is estimated at fewer than 1.2 million.

Private Sector

A significant portion of the population relies on the private sector as its primary source of health care or as an alternative to social security health care coverage. The private sector is made up of a collection of small urban hospitals and ambulatory clinics, physicians, newly formed managed care organizations, and practitioners of traditional medicine. This sector accounts for approximately 45% of total health expenditures. Although a total of just over two million indemnity health insurance plans exist, fee for service is by far the most prevalent payment arrangement.

Private insurers offer coverage that is generally purchased by the wealthiest 10% of the population. Indemnity insurance covers only about 3%–4% of the population and is relatively concentrated in large urban areas and among fewer than four insurance companies and some large hospitals. A few sectors (e.g., the banking sector) have been allowed by law to opt out of the IMSS and maintain their own arrangements for provision and financing of health care. A few private charitable institutions, including the Mexican Red Cross and church groups, provide services throughout the country. In addition, a significant number of Mexicans living in rural areas regularly seek care from traditional healers (curanderos) to treat their health needs. Unfortunately, estimates of coverage and costs are difficult to obtain from available data.

INEQUITIES IN HEALTH CONDITIONS

There are three main variables of health status identified in Table 1 for all individuals and for adults over 20 years of age:

- The indicator "self-assessed health," ranging from very good to very poor, shows a slight to moderate pro-rich bias and is further elaborated in Tables 2 and 3.
- The indicator "illness/injury in the past two weeks"—i.e., health problems affecting each mem-

TABLE 1. Health indicators in the Mexican National Health Survey, 1994.*

Indicator	Definition	Mean, all individuals	Mean, individuals over the age of 20
Self-assessed health	In general, would you say your health is very good, good, fair, poor, or very poor? (1–5)	Slightly pro-rich[†]	Moderately pro-rich[†]
Illness/accident in past two weeks	In the past two weeks, have you had any health problem due to disease or injury?	0.0912	0.111
Chronic condition	Do you have any of the following conditions: diabetes, hypertension, arthritis, asthma, heart disease, ulcer, rheumatic fever, Parkinson disease, mental health problem, disabilities including blindness, deafness, paralysis	0.0599	0.100

*Estimations are for the entire population and for adults over the age of 20 only, as children tend to suffer from different health problems.
†Shown more explicitly in Tables 2 and 3.

TABLE 2. Self-assessed health by income categories, adults over 20 years of age and all individuals, Mexico, 1994.

	Adults 20 and over only		All individuals	
Decile	Unstandardized	Standardized	Unstandardized	Standardized
1	0.441	0.389	0.357	0.321
2	0.498	0.393	0.392	0.327
3	0.443	0.391	0.399	0.331
4	0.432	0.389	0.364	0.333
5	0.396	0.388	0.359	0.337
6	0.396	0.388	0.340	0.338
7	0.391	0.394	0.349	0.344
8	0.364	0.395	0.320	0.349
9	0.317	0.395	0.284	0.349
10	0.239	0.398	0.216	0.356

TABLE 3. Self-assessed health measures, standardized versus unstandardized results, Mexico, 1994.*

	Adults 20 and over only		All individuals	
Decile	Unstandardized	Standardized	Unstandardized	Standardized
1	2.0	1.90	1.79	1.74
2	2.11	1.91	1.87	1.75
3	1.99	1.91	1.89	1.76
4	1.97	1.90	1.81	1.77
5	1.90	1.90	1.81	1.78
6	1.90	1.90	1.77	1.78
7	1.90	1.91	1.80	1.79
8	1.86	1.91	1.76	1.81
9	1.77	1.91	1.69	1.81
10	1.65	1.92	1.60	1.82

*Standardized results use predicted probabilities from ordinary least squares (OLS) regressions.

ber of the household, due to either disease or accident, in the two weeks preceding the survey—shows a greater incidence among the adult population.
• The indicator "chronic diseases" also shows a higher incidence among the adult population.

Gender and Age Variations

In Tables 2 and 3, the information is presented in the form of standardized and unstandardized means of the health status of various income groups. The standardized results control only for gender and age groups. It is unfeasible for each income group to achieve the same health status level with different age and gender distributions. For instance, if older individuals have worse health status than younger individuals and if they are concentrated in lower-income deciles, unstandardized inequity indicators will tend to make inequality (favoring the rich) look worse than is actually the case.

With respect to self-assessed health, unstandardized measures of health and health status show that improvements are related to increases in income. The standardized measures show the opposite. Similarly, the unstandardized health measure of individuals reporting illness in the previous two weeks shows some evidence of pro-rich inequalities for the sample of adults, although these trends are less evident for the sample of all individuals. The standardized results for reported illnesses are similar to those based on self-assessed health measures, in which richer groups are more likely to have age and sex characteristics (they tend to be older and include more female members) that make them more likely to report illness than poorer groups.

For the indicator "chronic conditions" in Table 4, the unstandardized results are somewhat different. They show an increasing probability of illness with rising income. The standardized indicators are similar, although they show less of a tendency in this regard, and differences appear to favor the poor. Unlike the other health measures, chronic illnesses appear to affect the rich much more frequently or to be reported more frequently by them. It is possible that, because these illnesses strike later in life, the poor are less likely to suffer from them, because they tend to die earlier from other causes, such as infectious diseases. Mexico's epidemiologic transition is characterized by higher mortality from infectious diseases among poorer groups and higher mortality from non-contagious diseases among richer groups. Most of the latter diseases (diabetes, hypertension, etc.) require consultation with a physician and medical tests to be diagnosed. Even when the poorer groups suffer from these diseases, they are less likely to be diagnosed because there are fewer medical and diagnostic services in poor rural areas of Mexico.

The inequality index (Annex Tables A4 and A5) is negative, showing pro-rich inequalities for both the self-assessed health index and the probability of being sick. Nevertheless, for the chronic illness indicator, the inequalities in health are pro-poor. This may be because, as explained above, this health indicator reflects diseases that are more likely to strike the rich, but it is probable that the poor are just as likely to suffer from these diseases as the rich, but they are less likely to be aware of them.

In general, the results show greater inequality in health conditions in Mexico than in Jamaica and Ecuador. This is not surprising, because Mexico has a much larger degree of income disparity between upper- and lower-income groups than do Jamaica and Ecuador. At the same time, the level of inequality is less than in the United States and is similar to that reported by European countries such as the Netherlands and Finland. In drawing such comparisons, however, it is necessary to take account of cultural differences, which influence perceptions of illness and the action taken in response (e.g., visiting a physician in the case of those with adequate health coverage).

HEALTH CARE EXPENDITURES AND FINANCING

National Health Expenditures Accounts

Although some information can be shown, it should be said that no figures for national health expenditures are fully authoritative.[3] For example, it can be stated that in 1994 Mexico spent approximately US$ 21,000 million on health care, and per capita spending was US$ 223, or 5.6% of GDP. This is well below both Organization for Economic Cooperation and Development and Latin American standards. Other Latin American countries with lower per capita income, such as Venezuela and Colombia, spend in excess of 7% of GDP on health. Health care

TABLE 4. Percentage of individuals with chronic sickness or disease, standardized versus unstandardized results, Mexico, 1994.

| Decile | Adults 20 and over | |
	Unstandardized	Standardized
1	0.057	0.089
2	0.073	0.094
3	0.096	0.092
4	0.099	0.093
5	0.110	0.090
6	0.109	0.090
7	0.126	0.095
8	0.129	0.095
9	0.110	0.095
10	0.112	0.098

[3] Data are often unreliable and available information on health expenditure accounts is limited. There are three potential sources: (1) budgetary data from public institutions obtained through the SSA statistics office and the Ministry of Finance budget report; (2) information from the system of national accounts, produced according to international standards by the national statistics office; and (3) national income and expenditure and household health surveys.

expenditure is evenly distributed between the public and private sectors.

Public Sector Expenditures and Financing

Public sector institutions are financed mainly from two sources of revenue: federal budget appropriations and payroll tax contributions. The social security institutes account for a combined 43% of total public spending on health. The IMSS, the largest single provider, accounts for more than half that amount, spending approximately US$ 5,500 million on health care each year. The IMSS draws its resources from employer/employee contributions (approximately 70%), which are complemented by a federal subsidy calculated according to a legally established formula. IMSS spending per registered beneficiary amounts to approximately US$ 210 per year.

Social security health benefits for civil servants, oil workers, and members of the armed forces are also financed through employee/employer contributions, with the federal government contributing the largest share in its dual role as employer and subsidizer. Per capita spending for the ISSSTE was approximately US$54 in 1997. The better-funded PEMEX spent US$ 293 per beneficiary during the same year.

The principal health care providers for the uninsured, the SSA and the IMSS-Solidaridad program, receive their funds from yearly federal budget appropriations.[4] The share of total health care funds allocated to providers who serve the uninsured amounts to 13%. It is estimated that the SSA spends approximately US$ 28 per beneficiary, whereas IMSS-Solidaridad reports a per-beneficiary expenditure of US$ 18.

Private Sector Financing

Total private health care expenditure was estimated at US$ 8,600 million during 1997. Most of this spending consists of out-of-pocket payments to private providers. The burden traditionally has been disproportionately weighted against the poor. A small component of private health care financing is money spent directly on health insurance (mostly indemnity-type policies). The insurance industry provides partial coverage to approximately three to four million people and accounts for only 2% of total health care spending. Private health insurance is geographically concentrated in the northern

urban centers and among the top income decile of the population.

Inequalities in Health Financing

The study of inequalities in health financing in Mexico is complicated for a number of reasons. First, health expenditures are financed in a variety of ways, including the following:

- several coexisting social security systems that provide benefits out of taxes and contributions collected from insured workers;
- a separate SSA system that provides benefits to all workers (but is principally oriented toward those with no other health coverage), financed out of general tax funds; and
- private expenditures.

Second, assessing inequalities in the portion of health financing derived from general tax funds requires an understanding of the complexities of the Mexican tax code, which includes, among other features, 10 different income tax rates. It also includes a national sales tax, with four levels that apply to different categories of goods, and taxes on gasoline. Third, actual taxes paid—through sales tax or individual income tax—bear little relation to the taxes officially levied on individuals and groups, because tax evasion is widespread, especially among workers and consumers in the informal sector. Finally, information about the fiscal incidence of the various taxes is not readily available.

To derive useful estimates on inequality in financing, the National Income and Expenditures Survey of 1996 was used. This survey facilitated direct calculations of monetary expenditures on health care. However, because there is no information on taxes paid, for each household it was necessary to estimate the amount of tax that went toward health care by prorating health expenditure according to its share in overall financing.[5]

The principal results are shown in Table 5. Clearly, the Gini coefficient for inequality in pretax income is quite high—just over 0.500. Nevertheless, it is surprising to note that private health spending appears to be progressive

---

[4]In the case of the SSA, nominal user fees are charged at the point of service. These fees are adjusted for the income level of the recipient and do not represent a major source of funding for the SSA.

[5]An interesting area for future research in this regard is the change in the Mexican Social Security Law with regard to health financing of the IMSS. In July 1997, a change was introduced that replaced the high proportional tax formerly levied on workers' earnings with a fixed fee for workers who earn less than three times the minimum wage and a low proportional tax on earnings of workers who make more than three times the minimum wage. Additionally, federal contributions were increased significantly—from about 5% of total IMSS health financing to about 30%.

TABLE 5. Inequities in health care financing in Mexico.

	Total household adult equivalent income	Private spending on health	Direct taxes	Indirect taxes	Social security	Total health financing
% of total health taxes	...	42.7%	13.4%	8.6%	35.3%	100%
Gini	0.513	0.558	0.534	0.474	0.441	0.511
Kakwani inequity index	...	0.045	0.022	–0.114	–0.072	–0.02

... = not available.

TABLE 6. Utilization indicators in Mexican National Health Survey, 1994.

Indicator	Definition	Mean, all individuals	Mean, individuals over the age of 20
Hospitalization	During the past year have you been hospitalized?	0.033	0.049
Preventive health care	In the past two weeks, have you received services in any of the following areas: immunization, child health checkup, family planning, prenatal care, rehabilitation, Pap smear, dental visit, attention from mobile health clinic, or have you attended health talks?	0.017	0.015
Curative health care	(If the respondent reported suffering a health problem in the previous two weeks) Did you seek care in the past two weeks? If so, where?	0.508	0.474

compared with income levels. This contradicts earlier findings, which show that out-of-pocket health costs are normally higher as a percentage of total income for lower-income groups (Parker and Wong, 1997). It is possible that the severe economic crisis of 1995 led households to reduce their expenditures on health care, and the poorest groups reduced their expenditures the most.

Both social security taxes and indirect taxes appear to be somewhat more regressive than the distribution of pretax income, whereas direct taxes are more or less neutral with respect to pretax income.[6] Overall, the distribution of payments/taxes for health care is approximately neutral, which suggests that taxes/private payments for health care neither improve nor make worse the initial distribution of income in Mexico.

INEQUALITIES IN ACCESS TO AND UTILIZATION OF HEALTH CARE

The methods for measuring utilization patterns are similar to those for measuring health status. The three indicators of health care utilization in Table 6 are based on

[6]We believe the results concerning pretax income may be misleading, however, as we have used the actual tax law to estimate the tax burden, but it is probable that underreporting of income, nonreporting of informal sector activities, and deductions make the distribution of direct taxes more regressive than appears to be the case.

reported hospitalization and curative and preventive care visits. Although reported hospitalizations were 1.3 times higher for those over the age of 20 than for the entire population, there were a relatively higher number of preventive and curative visits for the entire population.

However, what emerges in the inequality indices in Tables 7 and 8 is that inequalities favor the rich. The indices show that inequalities in hospitalization (0.95), in preventive health care (0.90), and in curative care (0.80) are all highly pro-rich. Although wealthier income groups tend to receive more preventive care than poorer groups, standardizing for need reveals that the need for preventive and curative care is fairly constant across income groups and that children apparently suffer the greatest inequality with respect to preventive care.

The levels of inequality in curative care are much higher in Mexico than in Jamaica. Compared with Ecuador, inequalities in preventive care and curative care are slightly

TABLE 7. Concentration indices for health utilization variables: all individuals.

	Hospitalization	Preventive care	Curative care
C	0.130	0.122	0.082
Se(C)	0.00125	0.0179	0.0077
t test: C	10.4	6.81	10.7
HI	0.099	0.125	0.086
Se(HI)	0.0123	0.018	0.0076
t test: HI	7.99	7.01	11.2

TABLE 8. Concentration indices for health utilization variables: all individuals over the age of 20.

	Hospitalization	Preventive care	Curative care
C	0.067	0.0873	0.078
Se(C)	0.0141	0.0259	0.0102
t test: C	4.79	3.37	7.64
HI	0.086	0.098	0.077
Se(HI)	0.0139	0.0257	0.0102
t test: HI	6.17	3.81	7.51

higher. Health care utilization is much more unequal in Mexico than it is in Europe and the United States. In Finland and the Netherlands, only outpatient specialist visits show a degree of inequality approaching the level found in Mexico.

CONCLUSIONS

This chapter provides evidence of substantial inequities in both health status and utilization of health services in Mexico, and it is possible that the figures presented actually underestimate the levels of inequality in both areas. It has been shown that poor groups tend to report a lower incidence of illness than richer groups, but illness is more likely to be underreported for poorer groups than for richer groups. If this is the case, the inequity indices reported here would be even more pro-rich.

Perhaps the best that can be said on the issue of inequities in health in Mexico is that the financing system appears to be neutral. This is a recent development resulting, apparently, from a change in the distribution of private expenditures. The likely explanation is that, in the years between 1989 and 1996, the period for which data were examined, the tax structure became more regressive. There is need for further study of the health tax/payment burden and of the extent to which the tax structure adequately reflects the actual incidence of taxes used to finance health care.

REFERENCES

Parker S, Wong R. *Household Health Expenditures in Mexico.* Washington, DC: Paper Presented at the Meeting of the Population Association of America; 1997.

Wagstaff A, van Doorslaer E. *Inequalities in Health: Methods and Results for Jamaica.* Paper prepared for the Human Development Department of the World Bank. Washington, DC: World Bank; 1998a.

Wagstaff A, van Doorslaer E. *Equity in the Finance and Delivery of Health Care: A Review of the ECuity Project Findings.* Paper prepared for the Human Development Department of the World Bank. Washington, DC: World Bank; 1998b.

ANNEX

METHODOLOGICAL ISSUES

The principal empirical analysis of inequities within the Mexican health sector followed the methods suggested by van Doorslaer and Wagstaff (1998a), who divide the potential inequities in health systems into three groups: financing of the system, health outcomes, and utilization based on need and assessed in terms of health status.

Two types of data sets were used. One was the National Survey of Income and Expenditures (1996) to examine financing issues. It provides detailed data on all types of expenditures and income for a nationally representative sample of Mexican households. For the evaluation of inequities in health status and health utilization, two surveys were used. The first is the National Health Survey (ENSA) carried out in 1994. ENSA is the only nationally representative survey with information on health outcomes, and it provides fairly detailed information on recent health problems and utilization patterns of the population. However, it asks only one question about total family income. The solution to this problem is to impute family income levels with another survey containing similar socioeconomic information (i.e., education levels, etc.) but better information on income: the National Survey of Household Income and Expenditure (ENIGH) for 1994.[7]

ENIGH provides expenditure measures, which generally are preferred to income as measures of well-being. They are thought to be better measures of permanent income or consumption that is subject to less variation than income. It is well known that the assumption of adult

equivalence scales can drastically alter conclusions about poverty and inequality within a population. In this case, the assumption of adult equivalent scales is important as it can alter the distribution of households along the income distribution. Per capita income measures tend to overstate the poverty (income) of families with small children as they weight the needs of children to the same degree as those of adults. Using adult equivalence scales is generally justified by the need to weight children to a lesser degree than adults. Nevertheless, the problem of which set of weights to use then arises. The appropriate weights are likely country specific, and unfortunately in our case there are no studies in Mexico that might guide us in identifying them. In the absence of such studies, we have decided to use those used by Wagstaff and van Doorslaer (1998a):

$$e_h = (A_h + \Phi K_h)^\theta,$$

where e_h is the equivalence factor for household h, A_h is the number of adults in household h, and K_h is the number of children. We have set the two parameters Φ and θ equal to 0.75 and defined children as those under 14 years of age.

We began with the self-assessed health indicator and we experimented with two alternative specifications. In one case, a dummy variable was defined in which individuals in good and very good health were classified in one category and all those who rated their health as less than good were placed in the other category.[8] In the other case, we left this variable as a continuous measure. The problem with our self-assessed health measure, however, is that it is ordinal—that is, it runs from 1 to 5. Using simple averages or OLS regressions might be inappropriate as they assume that the difference between, say, 1 and 2 (very good and good health) is the same as the difference between 2 and 3 (good health and fair health), but there is no logical basis for believing this is true.

---

[7]Given the deficiencies of the data in ENSA, we also used another survey, the National Aging Survey. This nationally representative survey was applied to a sample of households in which at least one member was over 60 years of age. The survey contains excellent health and utilization information for elderly household members and thus is a good source of information with which to supplement our analysis. Of course, the results cannot be generalized to apply to inequities in health status for the entire population, but they may be revealing nonetheless. Its principal defect is that the income information is asked only of elderly members so that no total household income information is available. Again, we turned to the 1994 ENIGH to impute household income. These results will be included in the final version of this report.

---

[8]So that all our health measures would be higher with worse health, we classified those with good or very good health as 0 and all others as 1.

One solution to this problem was to create a bivariate variable, for instance by creating a dummy variable in which individuals who report having good or very good health are classified as 0 and individuals reporting worse health are classified as 1. We provide one set of estimations using this classification. Nevertheless, this reclassification is clearly arbitrary and loses some information. Therefore, we also experimented with a continuous variable estimation using ordered probits, which are designed precisely for cases in which the order of the values is the important factor. From our ordered probits we were able to estimate the predicted probability of each outcome and hence the expected value of the ordinal indicator.[9] However, these results were almost identical to the OLS results, so for our present purposes the OLS results are included.

UTILIZATION MEASURES

To construct the measure of health care needs, we carried out a probit regression of the determinants of each of the three indicators described above, controlling for age, sex, and health indicators for each individual. We used dummy variables for the following age groups: 0–4, 5–9, 10–14, 15–19, 20–44, 45–64, 65–75, and 75 years old and over. The health indicators are those used in the previous section (illness in the previous two weeks, self-assessed health, and chronic conditions).

The inequality index is represented in two ways. Tables A4 and A5 show the unstandardized index (C). In Table 7 the relevant indicator of health inequity is I, which represents the difference between the unstandardized index of health inequality and the standardized index.

TABLE A1. Probit determinants of hospitalization during previous year: regression results of utilization of health care.

Age group	Adults 18 and over only	All individuals
0–4		−0.014
		(−0.19)
5–9		−0.305
		(−3.95)
10–14		−0.359
		(−4.59)
15–19		−0.130
		(−1.75)
20–34	0.279	0.326
	(4.16)	(4.87)
35–44	−0.039	0.077
	(−0.55)	(1.10)
45–64	−0.044	−0.027
	(−0.647)	(−0.39)
65–74	0.070	0.071
	(0.87)	(0.89)
Gender (1 = female)	0.418	0.275
	(16.0)	(13.5)
Reported health problem in past two weeks	0.323	0.358
	(8.90)	(11.7)
SAH: Very good health	−0.573	−0.622
	(−4.27)	(−5.61)
SAH: Good health	−0.640	−0.621
	(−4.44)	(−5.24)
SAH: Fair health	−0.416	−0.458
	(−3.11)	(−4.14)
SAH: Poor health	−0.089	−0.091
	(−0.65)	(−0.78)
Chronic condition or disease	0.375	0.441
	(10.2)	(12.9)
Constant	−2.09	−1.87
	(−14.0)	(−14.6)
N	32,144	60,101

SAH = self-assessed health status.

[9] The ordered probit model can be expressed in the following manner: $y^* = \beta + \varepsilon$ where y^* is unobserved and $y = 0$ if $y^* \leq 0$; $y = 1$ if $0 < y^* < \mu_1$; $y = 2$ if $\mu_1 < y^* < \mu_2$; ...; $y = J$ if $\mu_{J-1} < y^*$. The threshold parameters (μ_j) are estimated in the model.

TABLE A2. Probit determinants of preventive care visit during past 2 weeks.

Age group	Adults 18 and over only	All individuals
0–4		1.11
		(6.87)
5–9		0.678
		(4.14)
10–14		0.515
		(3.11)
15–19		0.455
		(2.73)
20–34	0.715	0.721
	(4.46)	(4.48)
35–44	0.587	0.604
	(3.61)	(3.70)
45–64	0.358	0.367
	(2.20)	(2.24)
65–74	0.500	0.498
	(2.86)	(2.82)
Gender (1 = female)	0.428	0.190
	(10.5)	(13.9)
Reported health problem in past 2 weeks	0.546	0.597
	(10.9)	(16.7)
SAH: Very good health	–0.338	–0.125
	(–1.68)	(–0.754)
SAH: Good health	–0.348	–0.027
	(–1.63)	(–0.156)
SAH: Fair health	–0.302	–0.170
	(–1.51)	(–1.02)
SAH: Poor health	–0.374	–0.182
	(–1.76)	(–1.03)
Chronic condition or disease	0.210	0.242
	(3.57)	(4.49)
Constant	–3.26	–3.07
	(–12.7)	(–13.4)
N	32,311	60,465

SAH = self-assessed health status.

TABLE A3. Percentage of individuals receiving curative care during past 2 weeks, conditional on having an illness/injury during the preceding 2 weeks.

Age group	Adults 18 and over only	All individuals
0–4		0.076
		(0.62)
5–9		0.029
		(0.22)
10–14		–0.266
		(–2.04)
15–19		–0.253
		(–1.93)
20–34	–0.334	–0.328
	(–2.87)	(–2.85)
35–44	–0.228	–0.221
	(–1.89)	(–1.84)
45–64	–0.116	–0.114
	(–1.008)	(–0.992)
65–74	–0.104	–0.107
	(–0.76)	(–0.790)
Gender (1 = female)	0.068	0.044
	(1.31)	(1.06)
Reported health problem in past 2 weeks		
SAH: Very good health	–0.341	–0.157
	(–1.57)	(–0.947)
SAH: Good health	–0.087	0.180
	(–0.319)	(0.834)
SAH: Fair health	–0.233	–0.058
	(–1.08)	(–0.36)
SAH: Poor health	–0.206	–0.0002
	(–0.936)	(–0.001)
Chronic condition or disease	0.152	0.176
	(2.15)	(2.65)
Constant	1.17	1.02
	(4.78)	(5.12)
N	3,141	5,010

SAH = self-assessed health status.

TABLE A4. Concentration indices for health status variables: all individuals.

	SAH: dummy variable for good or very good health	SAH: continuous variable	Sick within past 2 weeks	Chronic condition or disease
C	–0.074	–0.0212	0.00144	0.166
$Se(C)$	0.0032	0.0013	0.007	0.009
t test: C	–22.7	–0.161	0.195	17.9
$I*$	–0.091	–0.0097	–0.0185	0.0889
$Se(I*)$	0.0032	0.00137	0.00735	0.0088
t test: I	–28.9	–7.04	–2.511	10.1

TABLE A5. Concentration indices for health status variables: all individuals over the age of 20.

	SAH: dummy variable	SAH: continuous variable	Sick within past 2 weeks	Chronic condition or disease
C	–0.093	–0.0367	–0.568	0.096
$Se(C)$	0.0040	0.0018	0.009	0.009
t test: C	–23.2	–0.196	–6.28	10.01
$I*$	–0.096	–0.0397	–0.063	0.0868
$Se(I*)$	0.0038	0.0018	0.0089	0.0092
t test: I	–25.2	–20.9	–7.02	9.40

HEALTH SECTOR INEQUALITIES AND POVERTY IN PERU

Margarita Petrera and Luis Cordero

BACKGROUND

In 1997 Peru had a population of 24.4 million, with 71.7% living in urban areas. The annual population growth rate is 1.7%.

The performance of Peru's economy has varied considerably during recent years. The depression of 1988–1992 was followed by a 52% expansion of national output between 1993 and 1997. In 1998 the economy grew only 1%, however, and modest growth is expected for 1999. Moreover, the period of high growth produced only modest reductions in unemployment and poverty.

In 1998, 8% of the economically active population was unemployed and 44% was underemployed. These high rates are difficult to reduce because the Peruvian workforce is growing at an annual rate of 3.5% and the ratio of employment to gross growth in Peru is 0.5 (World Bank, 1998a). This means that in order to absorb all new workers, the economy has to grow 7% or more annually.

As Table 1 shows, poverty decreased from 57% to 51% between 1991 and 1997, and extreme poverty dropped from 27% to 15%.[1] In 1997 the number of urban poor (6.7 million) was greater than the number of rural poor (5.6 million), but the proportion of poor people in rural areas (64%) was significantly higher than in Lima (36%) and other urban areas (49%). Extreme poverty is concentrated in rural areas.

The public sector reform that began in 1995 seeks to increase the impact of spending on poverty reduction and to direct State activities toward financing, regulating, and controlling social services, leaving their delivery in the hands of private and community agents.

According to a World Bank study,[2] the population's access to basic social services increased between 1994 and 1997. As a result, several social indicators improved: the rate of child malnutrition declined from 30% to 23.8%; illiteracy decreased from 13% to 10%; access to drinking water increased from 65% to 73%; and visits to public health care facilities increased from 21% to 36%.

The same study concluded, however, that inequalities increased during the same period. The Gini coefficient for income rose from 0.469 to 0.484 and the Gini coefficient for wealth increased from 0.695 to 0.726. One of the factors behind this outcome is the urban bias in public spending. Most improvements in the areas of education, health, and infrastructure (water, sewerage, and electricity) occurred in cities. Rural and indigenous communities were largely excluded. Between 1994 and 1997, the probability of being poor for an indigenous household rose from 24% to 29%.

HEALTH CARE SYSTEM

Within the public sector, health services are provided by the Ministry of Health (Ministerio de Salud; MINSA), the social security health care program (Seguro Social de Salud; ESSALUD),[3] and various hospitals operated by the armed forces.

The Ministry of Health provides centralized services through hospitals, national institutes of health, and health bureaus; the latter supervise the operation of departmental hospitals, health centers, and health posts. ESSALUD covers workers in the formal sector[4] and their immediate families; it operates through 24 departmental management units (gerencias departamentales). The armed forces hospitals serve military personnel and their immediate families.

---

[1]Poor households were defined as those whose expenditures could not cover the cost of a basic basket of food and other goods and services. Extremely poor households were defined as those whose expenditures could not cover the cost of a basket of food that satisfies minimal nutritional requirements.

[2] World Bank (1998b).

---

[3]Formally called *Instituto Peruano de Seguridad Social* (Peruvian Social Security Institute).

[4]In 1997, 94% of the workers insured by ESSALUD were formal-sector employees; only 6% were self-employed workers covered under the "voluntary affiliation" regime.

TABLE 1. Evolution of poverty, Peru, 1991, 1994, and 1997.

Levels of poverty	1991		1994		1997	
	Number	(%)	Number	(%)	Number	(%)
Extremely poor	5,886,507	26.8	4,326,950	19.0	3,564,498	14.7
Metropolitan Lima	633,738	10.1	360,342	5.5	1,867,259	2.4
Other urban	1,649,809	20.7	1,076,955	13.0	658,292	7.5
Rural	3,602,960	46.8	2,889,653	36.2	2,743,947	31.9
Poor	12,607,673	57.4	12,660,050	53.4	12,324,161	50.7
Metropolitan Lima	2,996,653	47.6	2,767,733	42.4	2,466,981	35.5
Other urban	4,160,388	52.2	4,162,973	50.4	4,279,640	48.8
Rural	5,450,632	70.8	5,249,944	65.6	5,577,539	64.8

Source: Cuánto SA. Based on the living standards measurement surveys (LSMS) for 1991, 1994, and 1997.

Private health services are provided by clinics, physicians, and, to a lesser degree, nongovernmental organizations (NGOs). They are concentrated in the country's main cities.

Figure 1 shows the level of utilization of health services, based on information on reported illness, symptoms of illness, and accidents in the 1997 Living Standards Measurement Survey (LSMS). Approximately 36% of the respondents said they had experienced illness or symptoms of illness or had an accident during the four weeks preceding the survey. Of this group, 73.5% considered it advisable to consult a health professional, and the remaining 26.5% did not. Among those who wished to consult a health professional, 19.5% were unable to do so. Of the 54% who were able to consult, 10.5% received noninstitutional help (mostly in pharmacies), and 43.5% obtained institutional care. Within this group, 25% received care in a facility operated by the Ministry of Health (which has the broadest network of health care establishments), 9.5% received care in an ESSALUD facility, 8% received care from private sector providers, and 1% received care at hospitals of the armed forces.

INEQUALITIES IN HEALTH CONDITIONS

Health Needs

Health needs in Peru were estimated through the proxy variable infant mortality rate (IMR).[5] IMR expresses the risk of a child dying at birth or before his/her first birthday. The greatest threat to the life of the newborn is disease, especially infectious disease. Diseases are difficult to avoid, especially in infants, but generally they do not have to cause death. The death of infants in countries with a high IMR, such as Peru, tends to be related to incorrect perceptions about the severity of certain diseases (and thus of health needs) and/or lack of access to health services. Misperception of disease leads to misperception of health needs and to death from diseases that are both preventable and treatable.

IMR was estimated for each of the 188 provinces of Peru on the basis of the information provided by the national census of 1993. Each child under the age of 1 at the time of the 1997 LSMS[6] was assigned a probability of death equal to the IMR of the province where he or she resided in 1997. Family income tended to be significantly lower in provinces with high IMR.

To calculate the distribution curve and the Gini coefficient,[7] the average IMR of each income decile was multiplied by the number of children under the age of 1. In this manner, the total number of deaths was obtained, as was the structure by deciles (Figure 2). The distribution of IMR by income decile is inequitable. The Gini coefficient is 0.0464, which indicates a higher death rate among the poor.

The analysis also revealed that provinces with high IMR tended to have large proportions of rural and indigenous population,[8] high illiteracy rates, and low percentages of housing with running water.

---

[5]Household surveys do not always provide adequate information about health needs because people's perceptions vary according to factors such as their educational level and place of residence. These factors can distort survey information, especially in societies with high social and economic heterogeneity, such as the Peruvian society. Estimations of the National Institute of Statistics and Information Science.

[6]The LSMS obtained data from a nationally representative sample of 3,843 households, stratified according to geographic divisions. The survey was developed and conducted by the How Much Institute Inc., with technical assistance from the World Bank.

[7]The Gini coefficient takes values from zero to one. Zero indicates total equity and one indicates the total absence of equity.

[8]Defined as people who speak Quechua, Aymara, and other Amerindian languages.

FIGURE 1. Levels of utilization of health services based on reported illness, symptoms of illness, and accidents,* Peru, 1997.

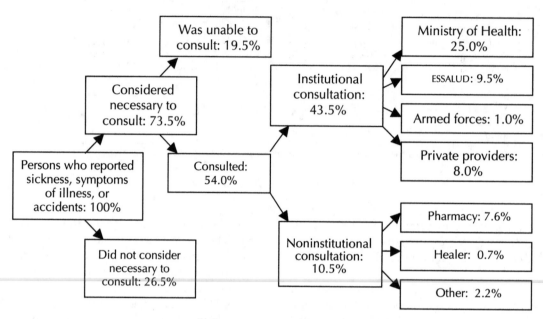

Source: LSMS, 1997.
*Utilization of services by people who reported illness or symptoms of illness or accidents during the four weeks preceding the 1997 LSMS.

FIGURE 2. Distribution of infant mortality rate (IMR) by level of income, Peru, 1996–1997.

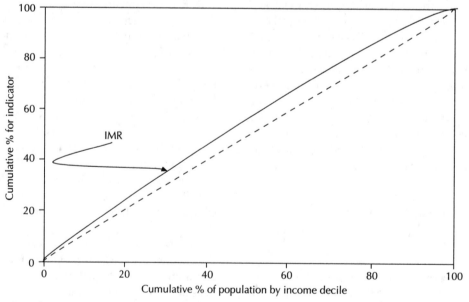

Sources: LSMS, 1997 and National Census, 1993.

Reported Illness, Symptoms of Illness, and Accidents

The 1997 LSMS provided information on reported illness, symptoms of illness, and accidents. During the four weeks before the survey, 11.6% of those interviewed experienced illness, whereas 23.9% perceived symptoms of illness and 0.5% had accidents.

As Table 2 shows, reports of illness, symptoms of illness, and accidents increased with income. In all cases, the distribution across income groups displays a pattern

TABLE 2. Reported illness, symptoms of illness, and accidents by income group, Peru, 1997.

Income decile	Illness	Symptoms of illness	Accident	No health problem	Total (%)
1	11.9	21.0	0.5	66.7	100
2	10.8	21.2	0.4	67.5	100
3	11.2	21.9	0.5	66.4	100
4	11.9	22.3	0.5	65.3	100
5	10.7	23.4	0.4	65.5	100
6	10.6	26.4	0.5	62.5	100
7	11.5	26.2	0.6	61.8	100
8	12.9	22.1	0.5	64.5	100
9	12.1	25.4	0.8	61.7	100
10	12.2	29.4	0.6	57.8	100

Source: LSMS, 1997. Decile 1 is the poorest.

that is only slightly inequitable, with a Gini coefficient of 0.00455 for illness, 0.0626 for symptoms of illness, and 0.078 for accidents.

Women reported more illness and symptoms of illness than did men, especially during the second half of the life cycle (Figure 3A and 3B).

The perception of illness and symptoms of illness differ across some socioeconomic categories. Perception of illness tends to be greater among the indigenous population and among families without access to basic sanitation services. On the other hand, perception of symptoms of illness tends to be greater among the nonindigenous

population and among families without access to basic sanitation.

HEALTH CARE EXPENDITURES AND FINANCING

Health Care Expenditures

Peru's health care expenditures in 1996 represented approximately 4.0% of gross domestic product, which is below the Latin American average. Per capita expenditure was US$ 121. The Ministry of Health spent an aver-

FIGURE 3A. Report of illness by age and gender, Peru, 1997.

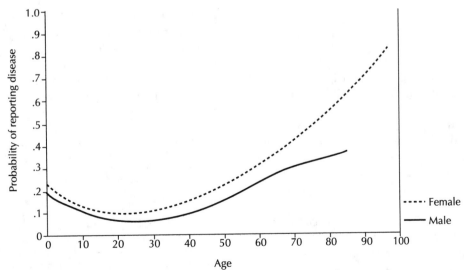

Source: LSMS, 1997.

FIGURE 3B. Report of symptoms of illness by age and sex, Peru, 1997.

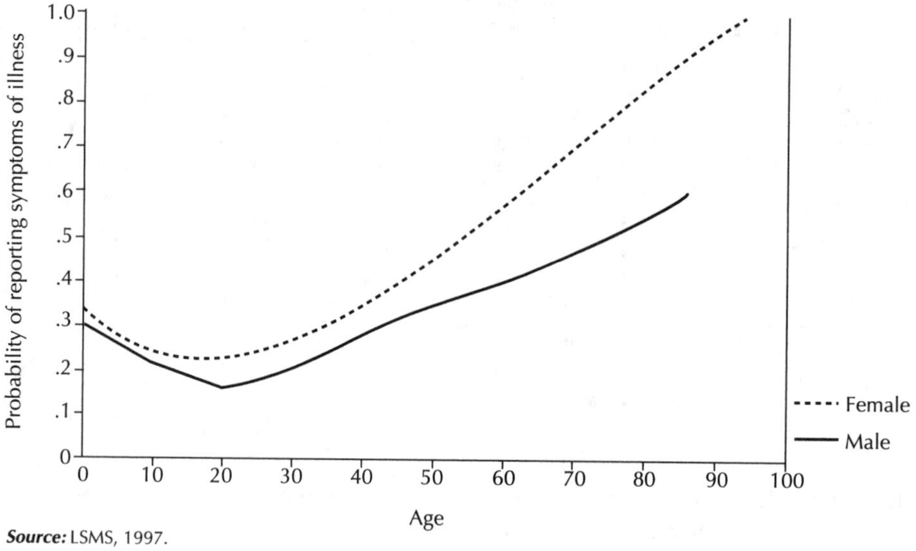

Source: LSMS, 1997.

age of US$ 91 per patient, and private health service providers spent US$ 174 (Grupo Técnico Interinstitucional, 1997).

Health Service Providers and Sources of Financing

Health service providers can be grouped into four categories: those who fall within the Ministry of Health network, those affiliated with ESSALUD, private sector providers, and NGOs. Table 3 shows the sources of financing for each of these categories.

Financial Flows

Figure 4 shows the financial flows between sources of financing, intermediate funders (i.e., insurance systems), and service providers. The government, households, and private companies account for 38%, 32%, and 29%, respectively, of health care financing. Government funds are channeled to the Ministry of Health and the health bureaus. Household financial resources are used to buy medicines in pharmacies, cover the fees charged by Ministry of Health health care facilities, and pay for private services. Few households make voluntary contributions to ESSALUD or purchase private insurance. Private companies make obligatory payments to ESSALUD to insure their workers, and some also purchase private insurance. ESSALUD and private insurance companies operate as financial intermediaries. Purchases in pharmacies account

for 27% of total health expenditures, a fact that suggests that self-medication is common and possibly ineffective.

Progressivity of Ministry of Health Subsidization

Public expenditures on health were defined as those of the health establishments of the Ministry of Health (hospitals, health centers, and health posts). The expenditures of ESSALUD were not considered because its source of funding is not the public sector but obligatory private contributions.

The public subsidy for the health sector was defined as the expenditures of the Ministry of Health minus the expenditures of its central administration and minus the revenue generated by user fees. The distribution of the subsidy was calculated on the basis of information on (a) geographic location of hospitals, health centers, and health posts and (b) the salaries of the health professionals in the different types of establishments.[9] Tables 4A and 4B show the distribution of expenditures by quintiles,

---

[9]Information on health expenditures classified by type of health establishment (health centers, health posts, and hospitals) is not available. Salary information was utilized to distinguish between expenditures for health centers and posts, on the one hand, and hospitals, on the other. It was assumed that the composition of the salaries of health workers in health centers/posts and in hospitals was the same as the composition of the subsidy for these categories of establishments. It was also assumed that the structure of the expenditure by income decile within each category (health center/post and hospital) was determined by the structure of the consultation. Finally, it was assumed that spending on children (persons under the age of 15 years) was equivalent to 0.75 of the spending on adults.

TABLE 3. Sources of financing and health service providers, Peru, 1998.

| | Sources of financing | | | | |
Health service providers	Central government*	Contributions to social security[†]	Voluntary private insurance	Out-of-pocket expenditures	International donors[‡]
Minister of Health	x		x	x	
ESSALUD		x			
Private for-profit			x	x	
NGOs				x	x

*Primarily tax revenue. There are no specific taxes earmarked for health.
[†]Employer contributions account for 94% of ESSALUD revenues. The remaining 6% come from employee contributions.
[‡]Includes loans and grants.

and Figure 5 shows the distribution of the public subsidy of the Ministry of Health and the utilization of health services by income quintile. The Gini coefficient is 0.1655, which indicates that the distribution of income is regressive. The degree of inequity is greater than that found in the case of service utilization (Gini coefficient = 0.1043).

Figure 6 shows the distribution of the public subsidy of the Ministry of Health, distinguishing between service provider (hospital and health centers/posts) and region (urban and rural). The subsidy for the first level of care (health centers/posts) in urban areas is progressive. In contrast, the subsidy for hospital care is regressive for rural residents, because hospitals are not available in rural areas. Their utilization by rural residents involves transportation and accommodation costs that poor families often are unable to cover.

INEQUALITIES IN ACCESS TO AND UTILIZATION OF HEALTH SERVICES

Distribution of the Utilization of Health Services

The utilization of health services in Peru increases with income. As Table 5 indicates, only 36% of individuals in the first income decile consulted health service providers during illness. The figure rises to 66% for individuals in the tenth income decile. The utilization of health services in Peru is inequitable (Gini coefficient = 0.1043) when no distinction is made between service providers (public or private), level of complexity of the services, and degree of user satisfaction.

Figure 7 shows the pattern of health service utilization (U) by income group, compared with the distribution of

FIGURE 4. Financial flows in health care, Peru, 1996.

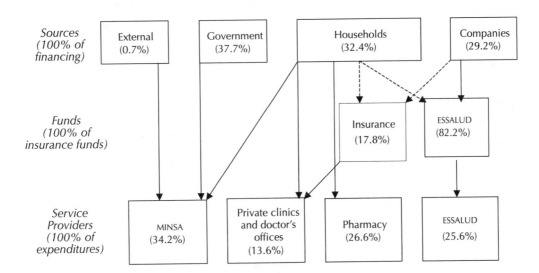

Sources: Reyes and Ventocilla (1997) and Grupo Técnico Interinstitucional (1997).
Note: Arrows with dotted lines indicate minor flows.

TABLE 4A. Distribution of the Ministry of Health subsidy by income quintiles, Peru, 1997 (figures expressed in Peruvian currency—thousands of new soles).

Quintile	Urban			Rural		
	Hospitals	MINSA health centers/posts	Total	Hospitals	MINSA health centers/posts	Total
1	127,254	104,541	231,795	21,295	27,617	27,638
2	144,413	96,499	240,911	36,782	25,664	25,701
3	138,693	92,478	231,171	67,756	38,775	38,843
4	148,702	90,066	238,768	112,282	27,059	27,171
5	144,412	45,837	190,249	114,218	35,707	35,821
Total	703,474	429,421	1,132,894	352,333	154,822	155,174

Sources: Portocarrero (1998) and LSMS, 1997.

TABLE 4B. Distribution of the Ministry of Health subsidy by income quintiles, Peru, 1997 (percentages).

Quintile	Urban		Rural		
	Hospitals	MINSA health centers/posts	Hospitals	MINSA health centers/posts	Total
1	18.09	24.34	6.04	17.84	20.10
2	20.53	22.47	10.44	16.58	20.70
3	19.72	21.54	19.23	25.05	21.00
4	21.14	20.97	31.87	17.48	20.60
5	20.53	10.67	32.42	23.06	17.60
Total	100.00	100.00	100.00	100.00	100.00

Sources: Portocarrero (1998) and LSMS, 1997.

FIGURE 5. Distribution of the Ministry of Health subsidy and utilization of health services, Peru, 1997.

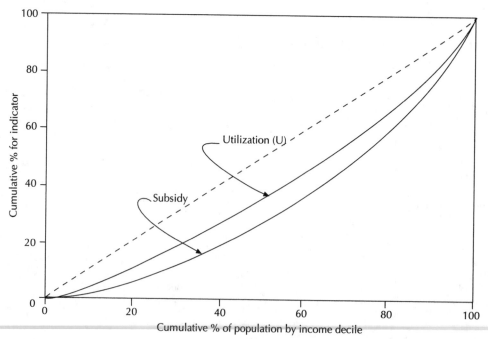

Source: LSMS, 1997.

FIGURE 6. Distribution of the Ministry of Health subsidy by service provider (hospital and health centers/posts) and region (urban and rural), Peru, 1997.

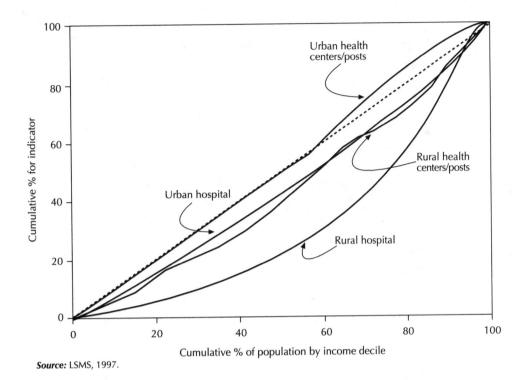

Source: LSMS, 1997.

TABLE 5. Reported health service utilization by income decile, Peru, 1997.

Income decile	Number of persons who reported illness	Percentage of individuals who utilized health services
1	233	36.1
2	283	44.1
3	283	43.0
4	324	48.2
5	357	53.0
6	426	58.6
7	436	58.4
8	444	64.3
9	464	61.6
10	563	66.1

Source: LSMS, 1997.

IMR, as a proxy variable of health need (N) and perception of health need (P).

Barriers to Health Care Utilization

Individuals who experience illness face several barriers to access to health care services. Table 6 shows that lack of financial resources is by far the most common obstacle to obtaining health services. Physical inaccessibility (due to excessive distance between potential user and provider) follows in importance. The perception that the services are of low quality is also an important barrier, especially for people who have health insurance.

Gender Differences

The pattern of health service utilization varies by gender. In general, women use health services more than do men. The difference reflects the greater use by women of private health care services and of those provided by the Ministry of Health, especially in Metropolitan Lima (Table 7). The differences between males and females are more marked as income grows (Table 8).

Access to Different Types of Health Care Services

Utilization of services can be analyzed according to type of provider, level of complexity of the services, and the quality attributed to them. Providers can be categorized

FIGURE 7. Distribution of health needs, perception of health needs, and utilization of health services by income group, Peru, 1997.

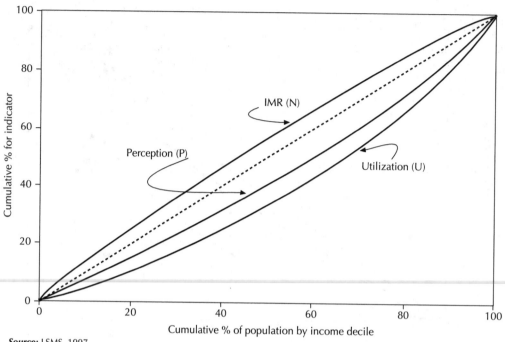

Source: LSMS, 1997.

TABLE 6. Reasons for not consulting a health professional, Peru, 1997.

	Lack of medicine	Insufficient service	Lack of money	Health service is not available	Long distance to health service	Service is not good	Other	Total (%)
Income quintile								
1	0.17	1.41	84.82	0.71	6.71	2.47	3.71	100
2	0.22	1.79	79.90	2.68	4.68	2.01	8.71	100
3	0.52	1.03	75.20	1.80	6.71	6.71	8.01	100
4	NA	1.86	66.29	1.86	10.01	7.05	12.97	100
5	NA	2.08	57.86	0.81	9.51	10.75	19.00	100
Poverty								
Poor (extreme)	0.18	1.98	79.82	2.34	9.18	2.16	4.33	100
Poor (nonextreme)	0.29	1.54	81.14	0.85	5.21	3.38	7.61	100
Nonpoor	0.15	1.24	66.25	1.71	7.25	8.93	14.49	100
Area of residence								
Metropolitan Lima	NA	1.32	76.73	NA	2.33	1.67	17.95	100
Urban	0.37	1.11	81.48	NA	0.74	7.52	8.81	100
Rural	0.18	1.87	72.47	2.82	11.62	4.49	6.56	100
Geographic region								
Coast	NA	1.10	75.55	2.50	4.06	4.67	12.14	100
Highlands	0.56	2.43	70.68	1.44	12.45	6.15	6.29	100
Amazon Region	NA	1.04	82.04	0.69	3.84	3.66	8.73	100
Gender								
Men	0.36	2.23	74.56	1.64	6.68	4.80	9.74	100
Women	0.09	1.03	76.62	1.51	7.35	4.99	8.39	100
Health insurance								
Yes	0.55	3.79	38.38	NA	10.28	17.31	29.74	100
No	0.17	1.33	79.69	1.73	6.70	3.59	6.77	100
Total	0.21	1.57	75.72	1.57	7.06	4.91	8.98	100

Source: LSMS, 1997.
NA = not applicable.

TABLE 7. Utilization of health services by provider, gender, and area, Peru, 1997.

Place of service	Metropolitan Lima		Other urban		Rural	
	Men	Women	Men	Women	Men	Women
ESSALUD	12.1	11.2	14.6	14.1	2.7	2.0
Private	9.6	13.0	7.4	8.9	4.0	4.4
Ministry of Health	19.2	23.6	21.7	23.5	25.1	27.7
Armed forces	2.5	1.7	1.1	0.9	0.2	0.1
Noninstitutional	12.5	10.5	11.7	9.4	9.6	7.9
Did not seek service	44.1	40.0	43.5	43.3	58.5	57.7
Total (%)	100.0	100.0	100.0	100.0	100.0	100.0
χ^2	Significant at 99%		Significant at 75%		Significant at 95%	

Source: LSMS, 1997.

TABLE 8. Utilization of health services by provider, gender, and income quintile, Peru, 1997.

Place of service	Quintile 1		Quintile 2		Quintile 3		Quintile 4		Quintile 5	
	Men	Women	Men	Women	Men	Women	Men	Women	Men	Women
ESSALUD	4.9	3.9	6.1	6.4	10.2	7.9	13.4	11.8	11.4	12.5
Private	1.7	2.3	3.6	5.2	5.2	5.6	7.1	9.2	14.4	17.0
Ministry of Health	26.3	23.4	21.6	26.3	23.6	28.4	22.0	26.3	18.5	21.6
Armed forces	...	0.1	10.0	0.5	1.9	1.1	1.2	1.7	1.6	0.5
Noninstitutional	8.4	6.9	10.5	7.6	11.5	10.6	12.4	10.2	12.8	9.9
Did not seek service	58.7	63.3	57.8	54.1	47.6	46.4	44.0	40.8	41.3	38.4
Total (%)	100.0	100.0	100.0	100.0	100.0	100.0	100.0	100.0	100.0	100.0
χ^2	Significant at 63%		Significant at 88%		Significant at 80%		Significant at 88%		Significant at 98%	

Source: LSMS, 1997.

as institutional (health professionals) and noninstitutional (traditional healers, pharmacists, family members). The level of complexity ranges from relatively simple services provided by health centers and posts to the relatively complex services provided by hospitals. The level of user satisfaction varies among service providers and according to the degree of complexity of the service.

Utilization of Institutional and Noninstitutional Services

No significant differences were found between the distribution of institutional and noninstitutional services by income group (Figure 8). The utilization of both types of services is inequitable across income groups, with a marked pro-rich pattern. The Gini coefficient is 0.1043 for institutional services and 0.1019 for noninstitutional services.

Utilization of Public and Private Services

Utilization of private services is more inequitable than use of public services. Among the latter, the services of the Ministry of Health are more equitable than those of

ESSALUD (Figure 9). This pattern reflects the higher cost of obtaining services from private providers and the fact that ESSALUD covers formal sector workers only. The Gini coefficient is 0.0447 for the Ministry of Health, 0.158 for ESSALUD, and 0.259 for private providers.

Utilization of Services with Different Level of Complexity

Utilization of first-level establishments (health centers and posts) shows the distribution that comes closest to being equitable (Gini = 0.020), and hospitals are at the opposite extreme (Gini = 0.086). The high cost of hospital services and their location in urban areas limit the ability of the poor to use them. As Figure 10 shows, the services of the Ministry of Health are less inequitable than those of ESSALUD and private providers. This reflects the public subsidization of first-level services.

Service Utilization According to Attributed Quality

Attributed quality is measured by the degree of reported user satisfaction with health services. In both the institutional and noninstitutional services, satisfaction has a pro-

FIGURE 8. Distribution of health service utilization: institutional and noninstitutional services, Peru, 1997.

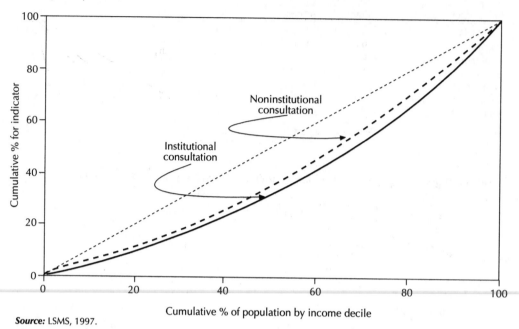

Source: LSMS, 1997.

FIGURE 9. Distribution of health service utilization: Ministry of Health, ESSALUD, and private, Peru, 1997.

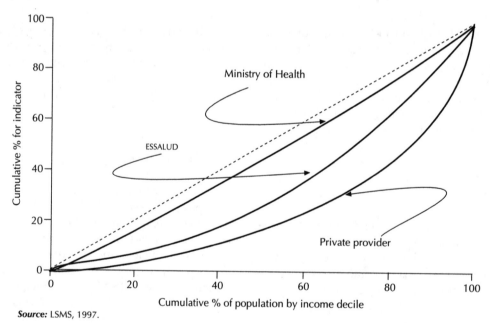

Source: LSMS, 1997.

rich distribution (Gini = 0.1043, 0.1019). Satisfaction is lower among the poor (Figure 11).

Table 9 shows the degree of satisfaction by area (rural, urban, and Metropolitan Lima), sex, and type of provider for each income quintile. In all quintiles, there is more satisfaction with private services. Care at the first level (centers/health posts) is the most satisfactory among public services in all the quintiles, which reflects increases in government expenditure at this level.

FIGURE 10. Distribution of utilization by level of complexity, Peru, 1997.

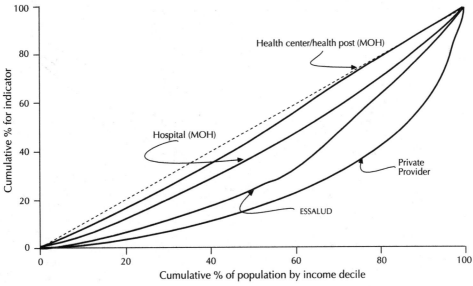

Source: LSMS, 1997.

FIGURE 11. Distribution of satisfaction with institutional and noninstitutional care, Peru, 1997.

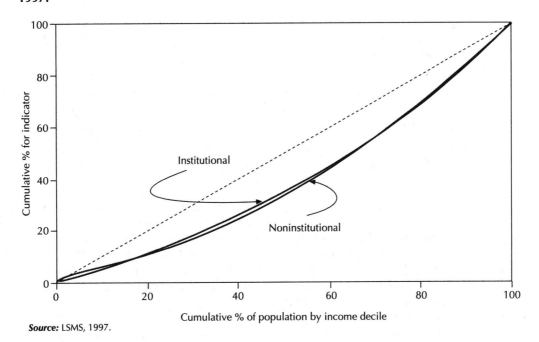

Source: LSMS, 1997.

The degree of satisfaction with ESSALUD services is the lowest for all income categories. The rural population tends to be less satisfied than the urban population. Both women and men (except women in the poorest quintile) reported greater satisfaction with the services of health centers and posts operated by the Ministry of Health than with the services provided by the Ministry's hospitals.

TABLE 9. Degree of satisfaction with institutional services, Peru, 1997 (percentage of satisfied users).

Income quintile	MINSA hospitals	MINSA health centers/posts	ESSALUD	Private
Quintile 1				
Metropolitan Lima	86	78	61	100
Urban	73	95	74	82
Rural	64	75	75	83
Men	72	85	61	91
Women	82	74	78	88
Total	77	80	69	89
Quintile 2				
Metropolitan Lima	73	75	46	91
Urban	67	86	70	100
Rural	79	85	67	73
Men	70	85	63	91
Women	71	80	63	90
Total	71	82	63	90
Quintile 3				
Metropolitan Lima	75	70	59	97
Urban	71	79	49	82
Rural	74	85	78	94
Men	72	84	54	86
Women	73	76	53	93
Total	73	79	54	90
Quintile 4				
Metropolitan Lima	63	70	69	91
Urban	65	79	55	90
Rural	67	85	65	90
Men	61	84	58	88
Women	68	76	66	92
Total	65	79	62	90
Quintile 5				
Metropolitan Lima	72	95	62	93
Urban	66	68	59	94
Rural	58	75	66	75
Men	61	79	54	92
Women	66	74	66	89
Total	64	76	61	90

Quantification of Inequities

To quantify inequity,[10] the variables health need, perception of health needs, and health service utilization were standardized following the methodology proposed by van Doorslaer and Wagstaff (1997), which is explained in the chapter titled "Inequity in the Delivery of Health Care: Methods and Results for Jamaica." Inequity in the distribution of the public subsidy to health services was quantified following the methodology developed by Selowsky (1979).

Figure 12 shows the distribution of the standardized variables across income categories: IMR (as a proxy for the variable need N^*), perception of health needs (P^*), utilization of health services (U^*), and the Ministry of Health subsidy (S^*). If the three gaps in equity are added, the result is a Kakwani index ($N^* - S^*$) of 0.243.

CONCLUSIONS AND POLICY RECOMMENDATIONS

Conclusions

Health needs in Peru (estimated on the basis of the proxy variable infant mortality rate) are greater among the poor, rural residents; the illiterate; and those who speak indigenous languages. These characteristics are also associated

---

[10]Horizontal inequity in access to health services is defined as a situation in which each individual receives care according to his or her needs, regardless of ability to pay.

FIGURE 12. Distribution of health need (*N**), perception (*P**), utilization of services (*U**), and Ministry of Health subsidy (*S**) (standardized).

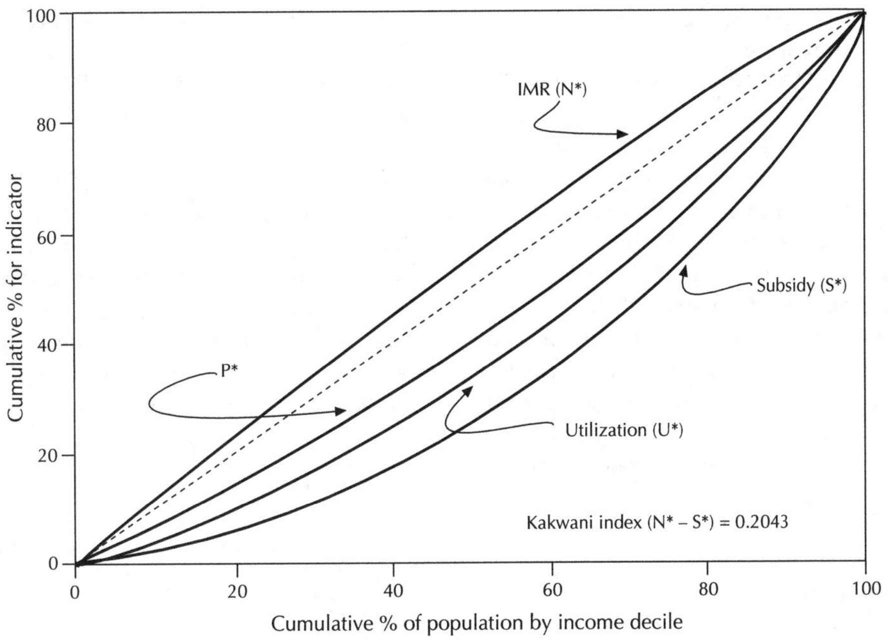

Source: LSMS, 1997.

with a lack of access to basic social services and socioeconomic marginalization.

The perception of symptoms of illness tends to increase with income; reported illness and accidents, on the other hand, do not vary significantly across income groups.

Reports of illness, symptoms of illness, and accidents vary considerably according to age and gender. Women report more illness, especially in the second half of the life cycle.

Although health needs are clearly greater among the poor, distribution of the utilization of health services favors the wealthy. When health services are classified by type and location, the only ones that show a nonregressive pattern of utilization are the health centers and posts operated by the Ministry of Health in urban areas. Private services display the most regressive pattern (only 4% of the population in the poorest income quintile utilizes private services). The pattern of utilization of ESSALUD services is also skewed toward the rich but less so than for private services. Utilization of the services of the Ministry of Health is the least regressive, but even in this case utilization of hospitals increases with income.

Users reported greater satisfaction with private services than with public services, and the satisfaction gap grew

with income. Users reported higher satisfaction with the services of the Ministry of Health than with the services of ESSALUD. Among the services of the Ministry of Health, those provided by health centers/posts were the most satisfactory for all the income categories. The increase in public spending at this level of care helps to explain this finding.

Public subsidies in the health sector (defined as the expenditure of the Ministry of Health less user fees and administrative costs at the central level) are regressive in nature, except the subsidy to the first level of care (health centers and posts) in urban areas. The progressivity of the latter reflects the important and sustained increase in governmental spending on the first level of care. However, the financing of first-level services in rural areas is regressive.

Public expenditure for hospital care reaches a very small proportion of the poor population. Access to hospital services is particularly limited among the rural poor. This reflects (a) the absence of an effective system to transfer patients from rural health services/posts to hospitals, and (b) the difficulties the rural poor have in covering the costs involved (hospital charges and travel expenses).

Utilization of health care services decreases among people with low educational levels and among the indigenous population. This is particularly true in the case of hospital services. The rural population reported less satisfaction with health care services than the urban population, reflecting the fact that the quality of the services tends to be lower in rural areas.

Distribution of the public subsidy to health care services was found to be inequitable. The degree of inequity was greater when health needs were measured through a proxy variable (infant mortality rates) than when they were measured through reports of disease and symptoms of illness. The Kakwani index increased from 0.1454 when the first measure was applied to 0.243 when the second measure was used. In spite of the inequity found, health care in Peru has a significant redistributive effect. This can be deduced by comparing the distribution of income (Gini coefficient = 0.48) with the distribution of health care service utilization (Gini coefficient = 0.1043) and the distribution of the public subsidy to health care (Gini coefficient = 0.1655).

Policy Recommendations

Reducing the gap between the health needs of the poor and their perception of illness requires intensive educational campaigns directed toward the rural and indigenous populations. The goal of these campaigns should be to translate health needs into greater demand for health care. There also should be an effort to redesign preventive health systems in order to identify health needs that are difficult to perceive, such as malnutrition.

Reducing the gap between health needs and utilization of services should focus on accessibility and effectiveness of care. To this end, three different types of interventions should be considered: (a) interventions aimed at increasing efficient use of resources in both the public and private sectors, encouraging competition among pro-

viders, and integrating private and public services; (b) interventions aimed at strengthening the response capacity of service providers by establishing networks that permit an expeditious mobilization of resources and patients; and (c) high-impact interventions targeted to the poor, such as national campaigns to reduce maternal mortality and spatially defined actions to combat diseases like malaria and dengue fever.

To increase the impact of public expenditures on the poor, three types of policies can be identified: (a) policies that create payment systems that provide positive incentives for providers; (b) policies aimed at modernizing administrative procedures in order to reduce expenditures and increase the effectiveness of interventions in poor areas; and (c) policies that mobilize resources based on the needs of specific populations and localities.

REFERENCES

Grupo Técnico Interinstitucional. *El sector salud en el Perú*. Informe preliminar no. 1. Lima: Grupo Técnico Interinstitucional; October 1997.

Portocarrero A. *Equidad en el gasto en público en salud Perú: 1997*. Lima: Informe de Consultoría Organización Panamericana de la Salud-Perú; October 1998.

Reyes C, Ventocilla M. *Revisión y actualización del financiamiento del sector salud 1995–1996*. Lima: Ministerio de Salud; August 1997.

Selowsky M. *Who Benefits from Government Expenditure?* Discussion Paper. Washington, DC: World Bank; June 1979.

van Doorslaer E, Wagstaff A. *Equity in the Finance and Delivery of Health Care: A Review of the ECuity Project Findings*. Washington, DC: World Bank; September 1997.

World Bank. Comparaciones de pobreza 1994–97. Resumen del informe principal. In *Diálogo sobre experiencias y retos en la lucha contra la pobreza*. First Forum October 26–27 1998. Lima: Oficina Subregional 6, Región de América Latina y El Caribe; October 1998a.

World Bank. Reforma laboral y creación de empleo: la agenda incompleta de los países de América Latina y El Caribe. Washington, DC: World Bank; 1998b.

Inequity in the Delivery of Health Care: Methods and Results for Jamaica[1]

Eddy van Doorslaer and Adam Wagstaff

Introduction

Equity is widely recognized to be an important policy objective in the health care field. Indeed, some authors go so far as to suggest that, among the population at large, equity takes precedence over other objectives, such as efficiency. Equity concerns take two forms. The first is the impact of health care financing and delivery arrangements on the distribution of income. In the ECuity project, we call this "equity in health care finance." The other concern is the impact of health care financing and delivery arrangements on the distribution of health care utilization. We call this "equity in the delivery of health care." The latter concern is the subject of this paper.

The literature in this field seeks to assess not just how utilization is distributed but rather whether it is distributed fairly. This calls for a notion of fairness. In our work to date we have taken as our starting point the notion that an equitable distribution of health care is one in which health care is allocated according to need.[2] Our work has

focused on the horizontal version of this principle—the requirement that persons with equal need be treated the same—and we have focused exclusively on the extent to which violations of this principle are systematically related to income. That is, our work has explored the extent to which persons in equal need end up being treated the same regardless of where they happen to be in the income distribution. This chapter follows this tradition, as do similar studies for other countries in the World Bank's project on equity in health care finance and delivery.

Comparative research on this topic clearly is potentially useful. Cross-country comparisons or comparisons over time may help shed light on the issue of whether, on the whole, health care is distributed more equitably in one type of health care system than in another. Undertaking research along these lines clearly requires a means of measuring inequity. One cannot answer questions such as "Is health care allocated less equitably in, say, Colombia than it is in, say, Brazil?" or "Has health care been allocated more equitably in Colombia since the recent reforms?" without an index of inequity. One of the aims of this paper is to set out in some detail a relatively simple set of methods that can be used to measure inequity in the delivery of health care. These methods build on those that were developed and applied to a number of industrialized countries in a forerunner of the ECuity project.[3] The methods employed and applied in the ECuity project itself differ from those used in earlier work in that they use the indirect method of standardization to adjust for need differences rather than the direct method of standardization.[4] The method is far simpler to implement and

---

[1] Paper prepared for the Human Development Department of the World Bank. Second Version, June 1998.

[2] This notion is not uncontroversial. Wagstaff *et al.* (1989) explored the alternative ideological points of view on equity. One is the "libertarian" viewpoint (e.g., Maynard and Williams, 1984). This regards health care as part of society's reward system and sees nothing wrong with people using their income and wealth to purchase more and better quality health care than others with similar medical needs if they so wish. The other is the "egalitarian" viewpoint, which views "access to health care [as] a citizen's right . . . , which ought not to be influenced by income and wealth" (Maynard and Williams, 1984: p. 96). Some people are more attracted to one viewpoint; some to the other. Policy statements in most European countries and Canada suggest a greater degree of support for the egalitarian viewpoint. This is consistent with a number of different positions on how medical care ought to be allocated. Allocation according to need, rather than income, is one view, but typically little justification for adopting this allocation rule instead of another is offered. Culyer and Wagstaff (1993) argue that allocating medical care so as to reduce health inequalities is a more ethically defensible position for an egalitarian.

[3] See Wagstaff *et al.* (1991a) for methods. For results, see van Doorslaer *et al.* (1992, 1993).

[4] See Wagstaff and van Doorslaer (1993) for the new methods. For international comparisons obtained using them, see van Doorslaer *et al.* (1997a).

can be used on individual-level data. Therefore, it ought to be more accurate. In practice, it appears to produce broadly similar results for categories of utilization where inequity is statistically significant.[5]

The second aim of this work is to apply these methods to the 1989 Jamaican Survey of Living Conditions (SLC). Clearly, Jamaica is not typical of the developing world or even of Latin America and the Caribbean (LAC). It is perhaps typical in terms of per capita gross domestic product—Jamaica lies among the lower middle-income countries. However, Jamaica's life expectancy (73.1 years in 1990) and infant mortality rate (15 per 1,000 in 1991) are comparatively good [e.g., United Nations Development Program (1993)]. By LAC standards, its income distribution is also fairly equal (a Gini coefficient of 0.435, compared with an LAC average of 0.500), the proportions of people living in poverty (below US$ 60 per day in 1989) and in extreme poverty (below US$ 30 per day) are fairly low, and the corresponding aggregate poverty gaps are also fairly low (cf. Psacharopoulos et al., 1997). Jamaica's predominantly publicly financed centralized health care system ensures that all members of the population have access to relatively good quality health care, even if the better off privately insured are able to obtain better quality privately provided care (e.g., Gertler and Sturm, 1997). However, the relative richness of the SLC—compared with the standard living standards measurement surveys (LSMS)—makes Jamaica an interesting test case. In Jamaica's case, the traditional LSMS health module has been supplemented with additional health and medical care utilization questions, many of which are of the type encountered in health interview surveys in industrialized countries and some of which are to be found in the new-generation LSMS surveys (cf. Planning Institute of Jamaica, 1992).

This chapter is organized as follows. The second section outlines the methods used to assess the extent of any inequity in the delivery of health care. The third section describes the data used and the variable definitions employed. The fourth section contains the empirical results for Jamaica. In addition to measuring and testing for inequity in the utilization of curative and preventive care, we also explore the role of private insurance coverage. The final section contains our conclusions.

---

[5]See Wagstaff and van Doorslaer (1993) for comparative results on Dutch data with the two methods. The only appreciable difference is for hospital days, but in neither case is the inequity index significant. The results suggest that, regardless of which method of standardization is used, there is significant pro-rich inequity in outpatient care utilization in the Netherlands but no significant inequity in general practitioner care or inpatient care. Similar results are found for about half the countries studied by van Doorslaer (1997a and 1997b), even though the countries in question have widely differing health care delivery systems.

METHODS

This section begins with a discussion of the new method for measuring inequity in health care delivery—the so-called HI_{WV} index.[6] Then a simple-but-accurate regression-based method is set out by which the indirect standardization underlying this index can be implemented. The techniques that are available for computing the HI_{WV} index, including a simple-but-accurate convenient regression method, are discussed. The issue of statistical inference is addressed and a simple but inaccurate way to compute standard errors for the HI_{WV} index, as well as a more complex but accurate method, is presented. Then the methods are summarized.

Measuring Inequity

The idea underlying the HI_{WV} index is simple. It involves comparing the actual distribution of medical care across income groups with the distribution of need. Let m_i denote the amount of medical care received by individual i in a given period. The distribution of medical care by income is captured by the medical care concentration curve $L_M(s)$ in Figure 1, which graphs the cumulative proportion of medical care against the cumulative proportion of the sample ranked by income. The concentration index C_M corresponding to $L_M(s)$ indicates the degree of inequality in the distribution of medical care. In itself, this tells us something about the degree of inequity in the distribution of medical care only in the unlikely event that need for medical care does not vary with income.

The next step, therefore, is to take into account need differences, which we do by using the method of indirect standardization. This generates a figure for each individual indicating the amount of medical care she would have received if she had been treated in the same way as other people with the same need characteristics were, on average, treated. We interpret this as her need for medical care. In the case in which there are just two need categories, the need of individual i for medical care is simply m^1 if she is in need category 1 and m^2 otherwise. Or, if one is working with income groups, each income group's need is a weighted average (or sum) of the sample mean quantities of medical care for need categories 1 and 2, where the weights are the proportions (or numbers) of persons in the income group who are in need categories 1 and 2. Thus, the gth income group's need can be measured as follows:

$$m_g^* = f_g^1 m^1 + f_g^2 m^2 \tag{1}$$

where the terms are as defined above.

---

[6]This subsection and the others in this section draw heavily on Wagstaff and van Doorslaer (1993).

FIGURE 1. Concentration curves.

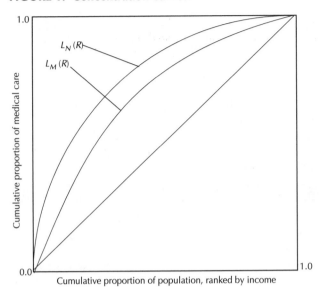

Each income group's share of need is then compared with its share of unstandardized medical care. If horizontal equity obtains, each group's medical care share will equal its share of need. Thus, for example, if there are just two income groups, the rich group's share of need is equal to

$$S_r^* = \frac{r\left(f_r^1 m^1 + f_r^2 m^2\right)}{p\left(f_p^1 m^1 + f_p^2 m^2\right) + r\left(f_r^1 m^1 + f_r^2 m^2\right)} \quad (2)$$

and its share of unstandardized medical care is equal to

$$S_r = \frac{r\left(f_r^1 m_r^1 + f_r^2 m_r^2\right)}{p\left(f_p^1 m_p^1 + f_p^2 m_p^2\right) + r\left(f_r^1 m_r^1 + f_r^2 m_r^2\right)} \quad (3)$$

If horizontal equity obtains, $m_r^1 = m_p^1 = m^1$ and $m_r^2 = m_p^2 = m^2$—i.e., people are treated alike in each need category regardless of whether they are rich or poor. In this case, we have $S_r^* = S_r$. If, by contrast, there is horizontal inequity favoring the rich, so that, within each need category, the better off receive more medical care, we have $S_r^* < S_r$.

In the more general case, in which there are more than two income groups and more than two need categories, it is useful to utilize the concept of a "need" concentration curve. This curve, labeled $L_N(s)$ in Figure 1, plots the cumulative proportion of the population—ranked by income—against the cumulative proportion of "need-expected" medical care utilization. The extent of horizontal inequity can then be assessed by comparing $L_M(s)$ with $L_N(s)$. If the latter lies above the former, there is horizon-

tal inequity favoring the better off; if the latter lies below the former, there is inequity favoring the worse off. The measure of horizontal inequity, HI_{WV}, is defined as twice the area between the need and medical care concentration curves:

$$HI_{WV} = 2\int_0^1 [L_N(p) - L_M(p)]dp = C_M - C_N \quad (4)$$

where C_N is the concentration index for need (i.e., indirectly standardized medical care). A positive value of HI_{WV} indicates horizontal inequity favoring the better off, a negative value indicates inequity favoring the worse off, and 0 indicates that the factor of proportionality (between medical care and need) is the same regardless of income.

Computation I: Standardization

The indirectly standardized medical care utilization m_i^* and the concentration index C_M can easily be computed by regression methods. The standardized values are simply the predicted values saved from the appropriately specified regression equation. Let x_i be a dummy variable taking a value of 1 if person i is in need category 2, and m_i is her use of medical care. Then we have

$$m_i = \alpha + \beta x_i + u_i \quad (5)$$

whereby

$$E[m_i \mid x_i = 0] = \alpha = m^1,$$
$$E[m_i \mid x_i = 1] = \alpha + \beta = m^2, \quad (6)$$

and hence

$$E[m_i \mid x_i] = \alpha + \beta x_i = m_i^* \quad (7)$$

Thus, the need of person i can be obtained simply by retaining the predicted value from Equation 5. This approach too is easily extended in cases in which a vector of need indicators is used. Thus, let x_i be a vector of need indicators together defining the various need categories, and let x be the vector of sample means of x_i. In this case, we have

$$E[m_i \mid \mathbf{x}_i] = \beta' \mathbf{x}_i = m_i^* \quad (8)$$

so that one simply runs a multiple regression of utilization on the vector of need variables and retains the predicted values. It is important to remember that, for the purpose of standardization, the vector x should contain only (proxy) indicators of need for medical care. As a result, Equation 8 is not to be interpreted as a behavioral model capturing all determinants of medical care utilization but rather as a sort of auxiliary equation used simply to obtain the means of the need categories. When measuring the degree of income-related inequity it is important not to include potential intermediary variables such as insurance status or area of residence. It is possible to include such variables later to see if their inclusion reduces the extent of any measured inequity. An example of this indirect approach to exploring the potential sources of inequity is given in another section of this paper.

The standardization should not necessarily be undertaken by using ordinary least squares (OLS). More appropriate methods are available for handling the special features of typical distributions of medical care consumption, such as the preponderance of zeroes, the tendency of many categories of use to be recorded as counts, and so on. One alternative to OLS is a count data model, such as a Poisson model or a negative binomial (or negbin) model. This is more appropriate when the utilization variable is a discrete number of (relatively few) counts, as is often the case for utilization data such as general practitioner visits, specialist visits, and inpatient days.[7] In the case of the negbin model, the indirectly standardized quantity of utilization is

$$E[m_i \mid \mathbf{x}_i] = \exp(\beta' \mathbf{x}_i) \qquad (9)$$

where β is the vector of estimated coefficients from the negbin estimation procedure (see, e.g., Greene, 1991). Another alternative to OLS is a two-part model.[8] This builds on the observation that

$$E[m_i \mid \mathbf{x}_i] = \Pr[m_i > 0 \mid \mathbf{x}_i] \cdot E[m_i \mid m_i > 0, \mathbf{x}_i] \qquad (10)$$

so that the expected amount of medical care utilization, conditional on a particular vector of demographic variables, is the product of the probability of positive utilization and the amount of utilization conditional on there being at least some. Candidates for the first part are the logit or probit models, and for the second part obvious choices are truncated OLS or a truncated Poisson model or negbin model.[9] In the case of a probit model, the standardized probability of a positive quantity of medical care in the indirect standardization is simply

$$\Pr[m_i > 0 \mid \mathbf{x}_i] = \Phi(\beta' \mathbf{x}_i) \qquad (11)$$

[7] Cameron and Trivedi (1986) have used the negative binomial model to analyze physician visits.

[8] See, for example, Manning et al. (1981, 1987) and Duan et al. (1983). A two-part model was also used in the standardizations undertaken as part of the comparative work on equity in health care delivery reported by van Doorslaer et al. (1992).

[9] Grootendorst (1995) and Pohlmeier and Ulrich (1995) use the negbin model in the context of a two-part model; Grootendorst used a probit for the first stage and Pohlmeier and Ulrich used a negative binomial for both stages. Greene (1991: pp. 542–555) provides details of the truncated negative binomial model.

where $\Phi(.)$ is the cumulative density function of the standard normal distribution and β is the estimated coefficient vector. Where the second part is modeled with a truncated negbin model (with the truncation at 0), the standardized quantity of utilization, conditional on utilization being positive, is

$$E[m_i \mid m_i > 0, x_i] = \exp(\beta' x_i) + \{\theta / [\theta + \exp(\beta' x_i)]\}^\theta \qquad (12)$$

where β is the estimated coefficient vector and $1/\theta$ is the variance of the exponential of the error term and hence reflects the degree of overdispersion in the data. The expected total utilization of the two-part models is then simply obtained from Equation 9. So, indirectly standardized values are obtained simply by saving the predicted probability of positive usage from the first-stage model and the predicted quantity of medical care utilization conditional on positive usage from the second-stage model, and then taking the product of the two to get m_i^*.

Computation II: Inequity Index

Turning to the computation of HI_{WV}, if m is the sample mean of m_i, C_M can be computed as

$$C_M = \frac{2}{N \cdot m} \sum_{i=1}^{N} m_i R_i - 1 \qquad (13)$$

where N is the sample size and R_i is the relative rank of the ith person. C_N can be calculated analogously, with m_i^* replacing m_i. Alternatively, C_M and C_N can be computed by means of "convenient" regressions. Thus, C_M can be computed by using

$$2\sigma_R^2[m_i/m] = \gamma_2 + \delta_2 R_i + u_i \qquad (14)$$

The OLS estimator of δ_2 is equal to

$$\hat{\delta}_2 = \frac{2}{N \cdot m} \sum_{i=1}^{N} (m_i - m)\left(R_i - \tfrac{1}{2}\right) \qquad (15)$$

which, from Equation 13, makes $\hat{\delta}_2$ equal to C_M. C_N can be calculated analogously, with m_i^* replacing m_i, and then HI_{WV} can be computed as the difference between C_M and C_N. Alternatively, HI_{WV} can be computed directly by using the following convenient regression:

$$2\sigma_R^2\left[\frac{m_i}{m} - \frac{m_i^*}{m^*}\right] = \gamma_2 + \delta_2 R_i + u_i \qquad (16)$$

where m^* is the mean of m_i^*. The OLS estimate of δ_2 will be equal to HI_{WV}.

Statistical Inference

Given that inequity indices are computed from samples, it is important to compute standard errors to assess the statistical significance of indices and of changes over time and differences among countries. Building on results obtained by Kakwani et al. (1997) we present estimators for the standard errors of both indices.

Application of OLS to Equation 14 automatically provides a standard error for C_M and, when using indirectly standardized values, for C_N. OLS applied to Equation 16 provides a standard error for HI_{WV}. However, in each case this method of obtaining standard errors overlooks the fact that the observations of Equations 14 and 16, being ranks, are not independent of one another. A more accurate estimator for the standard error of HI_{WV} that takes into account the serial correlation in u_i can be obtained as follows:

$$\text{var}(\hat{HI}_{WV}) = \frac{1}{N}\left[\frac{1}{N}\sum_{i=1}^{N}(a_i - a_i^*) - \hat{HI}_{WV}^2\right] \quad (17)$$

where a_i is defined as in Equation 18 below and a_i^* is defined analogously to a_i except that indirectly standardized values are used instead of actual values in its calculation.

$$a_i = \frac{m_i}{m}(2R_i - 1 - \hat{C}_M) + 2 - q_{i-1} - q_i \quad (18)$$

with

$$q_i = \frac{1}{m}\sum_{\gamma=1}^{i} m_\gamma f_\gamma \quad (19)$$

being the ordinate of $L_M(R)$, with $q_0 = 0$.

Summary of Methods

Our aim is to measure the extent to which persons in equal need are treated the same, regardless of their income. In this paper, we have used an index that is based on a comparison of two concentration curves. The first, labeled $L_M(s)$ in Figure 1, graphs the cumulative proportion of utilization against the cumulative proportion of the sample ranked by income. Comparing this with the diagonal, or "line of equality," shows the degree of inequality—across income groups—in the distribution of utilization. This says nothing about inequity in the sense of persons in equal need being treated unequally depending on their income, except in the unlikely case that need and income are uncorrelated. The relevant curve against which to compare $L_M(s)$ is not the diagonal but the curve labeled $L_N(s)$ in Figure 1, which graphs the cumulative proportion of need against the cumula-

tive proportion of the sample ranked, as before, by income. If $L_N(s)$ lies above $L_M(s)$, the implication is that need is distributed more unequally across income groups than is utilization and, hence, among persons in equal need, persons at the top end of the income distribution are being treated more favorably than those at the bottom. The HI_{WV} index is simply twice the area between these two concentration curves and therefore is equal to the difference between the corresponding concentration indices C_M and C_N. It is positive in the case of pro-rich inequity and negative in the case of pro-poor inequity [$L_N(s)$ lies below $L_M(s)$].

The indirect method of standardization is used to obtain the amount of medical care a person needs. This indicates the amount of medical care the person would have received if she had been treated as other people with the same need characteristics were, on average, treated. This can be computed simply by means of regression analysis, retaining the predicted values of a regression of utilization on the vector of variables capturing the person's need characteristics. Although OLS can be used for this regression, alternative methods may be better, such as a negbin model or a two-part model, with a probit model being used for the first part and either truncated OLS or a truncated negbin being used for the second part.

Once the standardized utilization (or need) values have been obtained for each individual, the values of C_M, C_N, and HI_{WV} can be obtained by means of convenient regression equations. In the case of C_M, for example, this involves regressing a simple transformation of the individual's utilization on the individual's relative rank in the income distribution. The same procedure can be used in the case of C_N, replacing the individual's utilization by his need. The slope coefficients in each case are equal to the relevant inequality index. The HI_{WV} index can be computed directly by regressing a transformation of the difference between the individual's utilization and his need on this relative rank. Although the convenient regression approach gives a standard error for C_M, C_N, and HI_{WV}, it is not entirely reliable because of the autocorrelation induced by the relative rank variable. Accurate estimators for the standard errors have been derived by building on the work of Kakwani et al. (1997) and are reproduced in the paper. These are used in the next section.

DATA AND VARIABLE DEFINITIONS

The survey used is the 1989–1992 Jamaican SLC. This shares features of the LSMS surveys used extensively in World Bank work, but it also contains some variables, notably in the health module, that are not contained in the typical LSMS. Our focus in this version of the paper is on adults (i.e., 16 and older); after deletion of cases with missing information, the sample size is 10,132 cases.

Socioeconomic Status

Our measure of socioeconomic status (i.e., our ranking variable) is household expenditure per equivalent adult. There seems to be a general preference among LSMS users for using household expenditure as a measure of a household's command over resources rather than income due to factors such as underreporting of income, assignment of monetary values to homegrown produce, and so on. Our equivalence scale is that proposed by Aronson et al. (1994),

$$e_h = (A_h + \Phi K_h)^\theta \qquad (20)$$

where e_h is the equivalence factor for household h, A_h is the number of adults in household h, and K_h is the number of children. We have set the two parameters Φ and θ equal to 0.75. This results in an equivalence scale that lies somewhere between the Rothbath and Engel scales discussed by Deaton and Muellbauer (1986).[10]

Medical Care Utilization

The amount of medical care received, m_i, was measured with four measures of medical care utilization: (a) the probability of reporting at least one curative visit in the last month before the survey, (b) the number of curative visits, (c) the probability of reporting at least one preventive care visit in the past 6 months, and (d) the number of preventive visits. As shown in Table 1, curative visits are defined as due to injury or illness, whereas preventive visits are defined as occurring besides injury or illness. We analyzed the probability of a visit and the number of visits separately to see whether any inequity differed

TABLE 1. Medical care utilization variables used.

Indicator	Definition
Number of curative visits	First question: Due to illness or injury, have you visited a doctor, nurse, pharmacist, midwife, healer, or any other health practitioner during the past four weeks?
	Second question: How many times did you visit this place?
Probability of curative visit	Dummy variable equals 1 if at least one curative visit was reported
Number of preventive visits	First question: Besides illness or injury did you seek health care within the past six months? Have you had prenatal checkups, preventive health checkups, family-planning services, or other?
	Second question: How many visits did you make in the past 6 months to health practitioners?
Probability of preventive visit	Dummy variable equals 1 if at least one preventive visit was reported

between the likelihood of use and the amount of health care usage.

The question about preventive visits is unconditional, but the question about curative visits is conditional on a positive reply to the question "Have you had any illness or injury during the past 4 weeks?" Only those with a positive response are then asked "Due to this illness or injury, have you visited a doctor, nurse, pharmacist, midwife, healer, or any other health practitioner during the past 4 weeks?" and "How many times did you visit this place?"[11] Both questions were repeated for those who also visited a second place during the past four weeks. We used the total number of visits reported in both questions as the rate of curative visits.

Need Indicators

The vector of variables used in the need standardization x_i always includes a vector of demographic characteristics consisting of a gender dummy and a vector of age dummies corresponding to the age categories 18–34, 35–44, 45–64, 65–74, and 75+ years old. The various additional health questions used as need indicators are listed in Table 2. Appropriate vectors of dummy variables were created in each case.

[10] The Engel scales reported by Deaton and Muellbauer (1986) for a couple, a couple with one child, and a couple with two children are 1.00, 1.41, 1.77 for Sri Lanka; 1.00, 1.45, 1.86 for Indonesia (children under 5); and 1.00, 1.58, 2.22 for Indonesia (children older than 5). Their Rothbath scales are lower: 1.00, 1.12, 1.21 for Sri Lanka; 1.00, 1.10, 1.16 for Indonesia (children under 5); and 1.00, 1.12, 1.22 for Indonesia (children over 5). They argue that "true costs are generally overstated by the Engel method and understated by the Rothbath method, but the latter unlike the former can provide a sensible starting point for cost measurement" (p. 720). The Aronson et al. (1994) scale, with the two parameters both set at 0.75, is 1.00, 1.27, and 1.52. On the basis of Deaton and Muellbauer's advice, the scale of Aronson et al. (0.75, 0.75) is a reasonably good one to use.

[11] The questionnaire further allows one to distinguish between the type of practitioner, public and private visits, etc.

TABLE 2. Additional need indicators used.

Indicator	Definition
Self-assessed health	In general, would you say your health is excellent, very good, good, fair, or poor?
Activity limitation	Does your health limit you *at all* in any of the following activities: (a) vigorous activities such as running, lifting heavy objects, participating in strenuous sports, doing hard labor; (b) moderate activities, such as moving a table or doing repairs; (c) walking uphill or climbing stairs; (d) bending, kneeling, or stooping; (e) walking more than a mile; (f) walking 100 yards; (g) eating, bathing, or using a toilet?
Illness or injury	Have you had any illness or injury during the past four weeks? For example, have you had a cold, diarrhea, injury due to an accident, or any other illness?
Illness days	For how many days during the past four weeks have you suffered from this illness or injury?
Restricted-activity days	For how many days during the past four weeks were you unable to carry on your usual activities because of this illness or injury?

RESULTS

Regression Results

The indirect standardization was undertaken with various combinations of need indicators to allow for future comparisons with results from LSMS surveys for other countries with less detailed health information than the Jamaican 1989 SLC. In Tables 3 and 4 we compare the basic OLS regression results for "at least one curative visit" and "number of visits" for one such specification with the results obtained using alternative model specifications. As an alternative to OLS for "at least one visit" we used a probit equation. We used a negbin model and a two-part model consisting of a probit equation for the first part and truncated OLS for the second part to model the number of visits.[12]

The prediction of any curative care utilization and of the number of visits is largely dominated by the very significant dummy for "illness or injury in the past four weeks." This is not surprising because reporting of any use is conditional on such illness or injury. When it is

---

[12] Because only about 7% of individuals in the sample report at least one curative visit (mean 0.11) and about 19% a preventive visit (mean 0.45), a two-part model may be more suitable to predict medical care utilization. We report only the results of the probit + truncated OLS model here because the truncated negbin model failed to converge for the curative visits model.

included in the equation, the adjusted R^2 dramatically increases, but few coefficients for other variables remain significant. Interestingly, neither age, sex, nor self-assessed health still has a significant and consistent effect on the utilization rate after controlling for reported illness. Only some of the functional limitations still show a significant effect. It can also be seen that there is little difference between the OLS and the non-OLS model specifications in terms of significance of explanatory variables. Interestingly, in the truncated OLS regression on positive users only the dummy "illness or injury" could not be included and none of the remaining explanatory variables remains significant. Therefore, it seems that most of the impact of the need indicators on utilization of curative care is through their influence on the decision whether to use rather than on the number of visits.

The regression results for preventive visits show a much more significant impact of age and self-assessed health both on the probability of usage and on the number of visits. The female dummy is very significant because of the importance of prenatal checkups. The large and significant estimate of α (=$1/\theta$) in the negbin model indicates that overdispersion in the data is an issue and that a negbin model is preferred over the simpler Poisson count model. However, because the results of the more sophisticated models do not differ dramatically from the simpler OLS models, we have used OLS regressions in the sensitivity analysis of the inequity indices with respect to different specifications.

Quintile Distributions and Inequity Indices

The next step is to compare the quintile distributions of actual and need-predicted utilization rates. These are presented in Table 5 for curative visits and in Table 6 for preventive visits.

The actual probability of someone in the first quintile reporting a contact with the health care system in the past four weeks appears to be a good deal lower than the probability that would be expected on the basis of a set of self-reported need indicators. The opposite is true for the top quintile. There is not a particular gradient but rather a U-shaped pattern in the distribution of the actual number of curative visits, with the middle quintile reporting the smallest share of visits. Only the first and third quintiles appear to be having fewer visits than expected; the opposite is true for all other quintiles.

These patterns are also reflected by the estimates of C_M, C_N, and HI_{WV}, which are presented at the bottom of the table. Both the "needed" visit probability and the "needed" visit rate show a negative concentration index, whereas the actual visit probability and visit rate show a

TABLE 3. Regression results for curative visits.

Variable	At least one visit		Number of visits		Log (posit visits)
	OLS	Probit	OLS	Negbin	Truncated OLS
Female	0.0061	0.1023	0.0091	0.0906	−0.0321
Age 35–44	0.0151*	0.2689*	0.0432*	0.4569*	0.0640
Age 45–64	−0.0018	0.0582	0.0030	0.1880	0.0081
Age 65–74	−0.0069	0.0005	−0.0116	0.1034	−0.0100
Age 75+	−0.0159	−0.0765	−0.0485	−0.0353	−0.1104
Illness last month	0.4900*	2.8482*	0.7674*	5.2679*	n.a.
SAH poor	0.0091	0.1157	0.0755*	0.2102	0.0945
SAH fair	0.0200*	0.2796*	0.0515*	0.2226	−0.0095
SAH good	0.0060	0.1519	−0.0069	−0.0187	−0.0591
SAH very good	−0.0049	−0.0379	−0.0177	−0.1455	−0.0901
Limitation in vigorous activities	−0.0011	−0.0222	−0.0075	−0.0674	−0.0562
Limitation in moderate activities	0.0340*	0.3143*	0.0634*	0.3000*	0.5067
Difficulty walking up stairs	−0.0394*	−0.3510*	0.0159	−0.0728	0.0031
Difficulty bending, kneeling, or stooping	0.0001	−0.0186	−0.1616*	−0.4816*	−0.1369
Difficulty walking 1 mile	0.0147	0.1518	0.0833	0.3273*	0.1437
Difficulty walking 100 yards	0.0375*	0.1910	0.0748	0.1604	0.0009
Difficulty eating, dressing, toilet	−0.0005	0.0471	−0.0083	−0.0056	−0.0190
Constant	−0.0073	−3.1297*	−0.0109	−5.8114*	0.3207*
1/θ				0.7358*	
Adjusted R^2	0.457		0.192		0.0062

SAH = self-assessed health.
* Asterisk denotes statistical significance at the 95% level. n.a. = not applicable.

TABLE 4. Regression results for preventive visits.

Variable	At least one visit		Number of visits		Log (posit visits)
	OLS	Probit	OLS	Negbin	Truncated OLS
Female	0.1370*	0.4602*	0.2681*	0.8420*	0.0950*
Age 35–44	−0.0032	0.0734	0.0096	0.0540*	−0.0971*
Age 45–64	0.0154	0.0375	−0.0286	0.0993	−0.1080*
Age 65–74	0.0859*	0.2552*	0.0786	0.1940	−0.1594*
Age 75+	0.1050*	0.2508*	0.0416	0.2947*	−0.1775*
SAH poor	0.0471	0.5491*	0.7774*	1.0677*	0.2320*
SAH fair	0.0012	0.4289*	0.4586*	0.8374*	0.2104*
SAH good	−0.1080*	0.1089*	0.0597	0.1729*	0.0408
SAH very good	−0.1280*	0.0291	−0.0133	−0.03801	−0.0359
Limitation in vigorous activities	0.0301*	0.1170	0.1470*	0.3842*	0.0406
Limitation in moderate activities	0.0041	0.0102	−0.0426	−0.0244	−0.0002
Difficulty walking up stairs	−0.0083	−0.0315	−0.0461	−0.1096	−0.0494
Difficulty bending, kneeling, or stooping	0.0941*	0.2590*	0.2302*	0.2750	0.0775
Difficulty walking 1 mile	0.0219	0.0592	0.1316	0.1381	0.0735
Difficulty walking 100 yards	−0.0115	−0.0361	0.0552	−0.0046	0.1122
Difficulty eating, dressing, toilet	−0.0700*	−0.1616*	−0.0701	−0.0280	−0.0068
Constant	0.2040*	−1.4351*	0.1388*	−1.8582*	0.4890
1/θ					
Adjusted R^2	0.075		0.068	4.669*	0.049

SAH = self-assessed health.
* Asterisk denotes statistical significance at the 95% level.

TABLE 5. Quintile distributions of actual and need-predicted curative visits.

Quintile	At least one visit			Number of visits			
	Actual	OLS	Probit	Actual	OLS	Negbin	Probit + OLS
1	0.071	0.080	0.080	0.121	0.129	0.129	0.107
2	0.064	0.066	0.065	0.112	0.106	0.106	0.087
3	0.065	0.070	0.071	0.097	0.112	0.114	0.094
4	0.078	0.070	0.079	0.117	0.110	0.111	0.093
5	0.077	0.069	0.067	0.120	0.110	0.108	0.089
C_M, C_N	0.0403	−0.0158	−0.018	0.0126	−0.0188	−0.0223	−0.0199
HI_{WV}	n.a.	0.056	0.0583	n.a.	0.0313	0.0349	0.0324
t value	n.a.	3.57	3.76	n.a.	0.95	1.07	0.99

Note: Need for curative visits estimated on the basis of regressions presented in Table 3; C_M and C_N computed using Equation 13, HI_{WV} index computed as the difference of the two, and standard error computed using Equations 17–19.
n.a. = not applicable.

TABLE 6. Quintile distributions of actual and need-predicted preventive visits.

Quintile	At least one visit			Number of visits			
	Actual	OLS	Probit	Actual	OLS	Negbin	Probit + OLS
1	0.227	0.265	0.212	0.345	0.526	0.568	0.411
2	0.250	0.259	0.196	0.427	0.474	0.500	0.371
3	0.236	0.250	0.192	0.463	0.462	0.489	0.362
4	0.242	0.237	0.176	0.453	0.416	0.429	0.326
5	0.290	0.233	0.174	0.593	0.403	0.418	0.319
C_M, C_N	0.047	−0.0274	−0.0274	0.1075	−0.0537	−0.064	−0.0526
HI_{WV}	n.a.	0.0744	0.0744	n.a.	0.1611	0.1715	0.1601
t value	n.a.	7.61	7.61	n.a.	9.1	9.58	9.05

Note: Need for preventive visits is estimated on the basis of regressions in Table 4; C_M and C_N are computed using Equation 13, HI_{WV} index computed as the difference of the two, and standard error computed using Equations 17–19.
n.a. = not applicable.

positive concentration index. As a result, both variables show a positive HI_{WV} index, but it is smaller in magnitude for the number of visits. Only the visit probability's inequity index is significant on the basis of the t test. Again, there are hardly any differences between the OLS and more sophisticated models. Therefore, it seems as if there is some inequity favoring the rich with respect to the probability of a contact but a clear pattern of inequity in the distribution of the number of visits does not emerge for Jamaica. We will explore the sensitivity of this result to different "need" specifications in the next section.

The picture is quite different for preventive visits. Both the probability and the number of actual visits show a clear upward-sloping gradient by income quintile: higher-income groups make more use of preventive services. In contrast, the opposite gradient emerges for the pattern of "needed" preventive care: lower-income groups seem to be in greater need of preventive care. Large positive values of C_M coupled with (in absolute value) large negative values of C_N generate significantly positive values of HI_{WV}. The index values for the number of visits are about twice the size of those for the visit probability but, again, they do not differ substantially between

the various regression models used in estimating the need for preventive care. Clearly, the utilization of preventive care is not distributed according to these measures of need and there is a strong indication of inequity favoring the richer groups.

Both curative care and preventive care are, on balance, pro-rich in their distribution. By contrast, the need for both types of care is concentrated among the poor. Regardless of the regression model used, both the probability and the number of curative and preventive visits show a positive HI_{WV} index, but the value is not statistically significant in the case of the number of curative visits.

The situation is illustrated in Figure 2, which graphs the corresponding concentration curves for numbers of visits. The number of curative visits and the need for curative visits are both fairly equally distributed on balance. As a result, both concentration curves are fairly close to each other and the area between the two curves is very small. By contrast, preventive visits are appreciably pro-rich in their distribution and their concentration curve is well below the diagonal, whereas the need for preventive visits is appreciably pro-poor in its distribution with a concentration curve well above the diagonal. Therefore,

FIGURE 2. Concentration curves for visits and need (need estimated using ordinary least squares (OLS), with "illness or injury in the past month" included in case of curative visits and full model in the case of preventive visits).

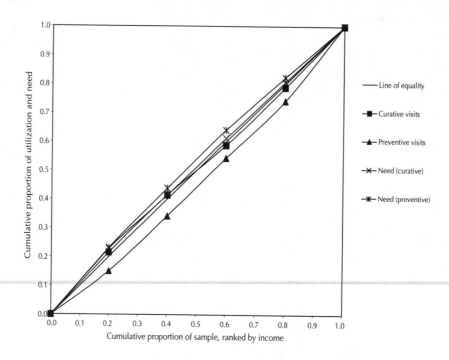

it is not surprising that the area between the two curves is significantly different from zero for preventive but not for curative visits.

Sensitivity Analysis

It is clear that the distribution of "need" depends crucially on the number and type of indicators included in the regression equation estimating need-expected utilization. In this section, we explore the sensitivity of our baseline results for changes in the set of variables used in the vector of need indicators. Because we did not observe substantial differences between the results obtained using the simpler OLS regressions or other techniques, we confine ourselves in the sensitivity analysis to OLS methods. In the selection of (combinations of) need indicators we were largely guided by the availability of variables in the LSMS-type surveys. Because the Jamaican SLC 1989–1992 is unusually rich in terms of health variables and because for most other LSMS surveys the choice of need indicators is substantially more limited, we have looked primarily at the impact on the inequity index of using more limited sets of need indicators. The results are presented in Table 7.

The table does not exhaust all possible combinations of indicators but serves to illustrate that most of the re-

sults are not dramatically sensitive to the selection of need indicators used. All indicators referring to the past four weeks could not be used as need indicators for preventive visits in the past six months. It might even be objected that an individual's need for preventive care does not, in fact, depend on his health, as we have assumed, but rather depends only on his age and gender. Table 7 shows that the "purely demographic" need model results in large positive and significant inequity indices. Inclusion of indicators of more permanent health status increases the HI_{WV} index values only slightly.

With regard to curative visits, only one variable has a large impact on the HI_{WV} index: inclusion of ILLIN (illness or injury in the past four weeks) substantially reduces both the index and the t values. In the case of the number of curative visits, it even reduces it below conventional levels of significance, as was the case in our baseline estimates in the preceding section. In all other specifications, inequity favoring the rich is significant for both types of utilization. Apparently, illness or restricted-activity days are more heavily concentrated among the poorer segments of the population than the illness or injury dummy. This may be an indication of greater severity of illness in lower-income groups that does not show up in the illness/injury prevalence. We can conclude that inequity favoring the rich emerges in all specifications and for all types of utilization, except when the illness/

TABLE 7. Inequity indices and *t* values for various need specifications.

Specification: age-sex variables plus	Dummy curative visit (four weeks)	Number of curative visits (four weeks)	Dummy preventive visit (six months)	Number of preventive visits (six months)
None	0.0762 (3.67)	0.0479 (1.32)	0.0652 (6.59)	0.1388 (7.75)
ILLIN	0.0496 (3.16)	0.0215 (0.65)	...	...
ILLIN + RADs	0.0617 (3.97)	0.0468 (1.43)	...	...
ILLIN + SAH	0.0543 (3.46)	0.0315 (0.95)	...	...
ILLIN + ACTLIM	0.0524 (3.34)	0.0254 (0.77)	...	...
ILLIN + RADs + SAH	0.0636 (4.10)	0.0506 (1.55)	...	...
ILLDAYS	0.0997 (5.66)	0.0747 (2.26)	...	...
ILLDAYS + SAH	0.1035 (5.91)	0.0799 (2.42)	...	...
ILLDAYS + ACTLIM	0.1049 (5.97)	0.0792 (2.39)	...	....
RADs	0.1071 (5.70)	0.0862 (2.54)	...	...
RADs + SAH	0.1162 (6.21)	0.0961 (2.83)	...	...
RADs + ACTLIM	0.1167 (6.21)	0.0952 (2.81)	...	...
SAH	0.1011 (4.92)	0.0774 (2.17)	0.0722 (7.37)	0.1567 (8.85)
SAH + ACTLIM	0.1071 (5.22)	0.0831 (2.33)	0.0744 (7.59)	0.1617 (9.16)
ACTLIM	0.0926 (4.48)	0.0652 (2.96)	0.0688 (6.95)	0.1512 (8.49)

Notes: Health indicators:
(1) Have you had an illness or injury during past four weeks (ILLIN)?
(2) How many days have you suffered from this illness or injury during the past four weeks (ILLDAYS)?
(3) How many days were you unable to carry on usual activities during the past four weeks (RAD)?
(4) How would you say in general your health is (SAH vector)?
(5) Does your health limit your activities (ACTLIM)?

injury dummy is included in the number of curative visits equation. The fact that this result is not very sensitive to the particular combination of need indicators used in the standardization is reassuring with regard to future comparisons with results from LSMS or other surveys from other countries.

Exploring Potential Causes of Inequity

Finally, it seems worth considering the question: "What might drive the inequity found for utilization of curative and preventive care in Jamaica?" Several possibilities in terms of system characteristics might be explored. One such possibility is differential insurance coverage among the rich and the poor. Although all Jamaicans have access to the public health care system, the higher-income groups, especially, take out supplementary insurance coverage, which gives them access to higher-priced and higher-quality private sector care. The proportions of respondents with private insurance coverage in each of our quintiles are 1.0%, 1.8%, 5.2%, 10.1%, and 24.0%, respectively.

Gertler and Sturm (1997), using the same data set,[13] showed that lower-income groups in Jamaica make relatively more use of the public sector than higher-income

individuals, whereas the opposite is true for the use of the private sector. They also show that this is largely due to the effect of health insurance being strongly positively associated with income and that the effect of insurance on the use of private care is particularly strong for preventive care visits.

To test indirectly whether the uneven distribution of private insurance coverage could account for (part of) the observed inequities, we reestimated the standardization regressions reported in Table 7 with a dummy variable for private insurance coverage among the regressors and then recalculated the HI_{WV} indices. The insurance dummy was never significant for the probability of a curative visit but was always positive and highly significant for the number of curative visits and for the probability and the number of preventive visits. Its inclusion also reduces the HI_{WV} index to below significance in the case of the number of curative visits but not in the case of preventive visits or the probability of curative visits. So, in all cases, including insurance coverage does somewhat reduce the significant pro-rich inequity in the expected direction, but it does not "explain away" the phenomenon—significant pro-rich inequity remains in most cases, even after "standardizing" for private insurance coverage. Consequently, the inequity we find is not merely a matter of unequal distribution of private insurance coverage across the income distribution. Other factors seem to be playing a role too.

---

[13]In fact, their sample is taken from the combined Jamaican SLC in 1989 and 1990 and is about twice as large as ours (*n* = 19,708).

Conclusions

This chapter describes how inequity in the delivery of health care can be measured and tested by the method of indirect standardization by comparing actual with "needed" utilization. We show how regression-based methods can be used to compute standardized values of health care utilization and to calculate a quantitative summary of the extent of inequity by means of an index. The paper also presents estimators for the standard error of this index.

The empirical part of the paper contains an analysis of inequity in Jamaica. The findings are fairly robust with respect to the set of need indicators used in the standardization procedure. Curative visits in the 4 weeks prior to the survey are distributed fairly randomly across the population, as is the need for these visits, as computed using a regression of utilization of visits on a vector of health indicators and demographic variables. There is evidence of significant inequity in the likelihood of reporting a curative visit over this short period, but the evidence is less clear for the total number of curative visits. However, it may well be that the four-week recall period for both illness and curative care visits is too short to capture systematic differences in utilization and need across income groups. This is worth remembering when designing the next generation of LSMS surveys. It may be worthwhile to consider, for example, extending the four week recall period for outpatient care to two or three months or, alternatively, supplementing the fairly detailed utilization questions for the four-week reference period with some less detailed questions for a longer recall period.

A different picture emerges for preventive visits. These are substantially pro-rich in their distribution, but the need for them appears to be concentrated among the lower income groups. Significant pro-rich inequity emerges whichever econometric technique is used to undertake the standardization and even if need is assessed simply on the basis of age and gender. The concentration of private insurance coverage among the higher-income groups contributes to this finding of pro-rich inequity, but it does not appear to be the sole factor responsible for this phenomenon.

References

Aronson JR, Johnson P, Lambert PJ. Redistributive effect and unequal tax treatment. *Economic Journal* 1994; 104:262–270.

Cameron AC, Trivedi PK. Econometric models based on count data: comparisons and applications of some estimators and tests. *Journal of Applied Econometrics* 1986; 1(1):29–53.

Culyer AJ, Wagstaff A. Equity and equality in health and health care. *Journal of Health Economics* 1993; 12:431–457.

Deaton A, Muellbauer J. On measuring child costs: with applications to poor countries. *Journal of Political Economy* 1986; 4:720–744.

Duan N, Manning WG, Morris CN, Newhouse JP. A comparison of alternative models for the demand for medical care. *Journal of Business and Economic Statistics* 1983; 1:115–126.

Gertler P, Sturm R. Private health insurance and public expenditures in Jamaica. *Journal of Econometrics* 1997; 77(1):237–258.

Greene WH. *LIMDEP Version 6 User's Manual and Reference Guide.* Bellport: Econometric Software, Inc.; 1991.

Grootendorst PV. A comparison of alternative models of prescription drug utilisation. *Health Economics* 1995; 4(3):183–198.

Kakwani N, Wagstaff A, van Doorslaer E. Socioeconomic inequalities in health: measurement, computation and statistical inference. *Journal of Econometrics* 1997; 77(1):87–104.

Manning WG, et al. A two-part model of the demand for medical care: preliminary results from the health insurance study. In: van der Gaag J, Perlman M (eds). *Health, Economics and Health Economics.* Amsterdam: North Holland; 1981, pp. 103–123.

Manning WG, Newhouse JP, Duan N, Keeler EB, Leivowitz A, Marquis MS. Health insurance and the demand for medical care: evidence from a randomized experiment. *American Economic Review* 1987; 77(3):251–277.

Maynard A, Williams A. Privatisation and the National Health Service. In: Le Grand J, Robinson R (eds). *Privatisation and the Welfare State.* London: Allen & Unwin; 1984.

Planning Institute of Jamaica. *Survey of Living Conditions.* Kingston: Planning Institute of Jamaica; 1992.

Polmeier W, Ulrich V. An econometric model of the two-part decisionmaking process in the demand for health care. *Journal of Human Resources* 1995; 30(2):339–361.

Psacharopoluos G, Morley SA, Fiszbein A, Lee H, Wood B. *Poverty and Income Distribution in Latin America.* Washington, DC: World Bank; 1997.

Rothman K. *Modern Epidemiology.* Boston: Little, Brown & Co.; 1986.

United Nations Development Program. *Human Development Report 1993.* New York: Oxford University Press; 1993.

van Doorslaer E, Wagstaff A. Equity in the delivery of health care: some international comparisons. *Journal of Health Economics* 1992; 11:389–411.

van Doorslaer E, Wagstaff A, Rutten F (eds.). *Equity in the Finance and Delivery of Health Care: An International Perspective.* Oxford: Oxford University Press; 1993.

van Doorslaer E, Wagstaff A, Bleichrodt H, *et al.* Income-related inequalities in health: some international comparisons. *Journal of Health Economics* 1997a; 16:93–112.

van Doorslaer E, Wagstaff A, *et al. Equity in the Delivery of Health Care: Further International Comparisons.* ECuity Project Working Paper 10. Rotterdam: Erasmus University; 1997b.

Wagstaff A, van Doorslaer E. Equity in the delivery of health care: methods and findings. In: van Doorslaer E, Wagstaff A, Rutten F (eds). *Equity in the Finance and Delivery of Health Care: An International Perspective.* Oxford: Oxford University Press; 1993, pp. 7–97.

Wagstaff A, van Doorslaer E, Paci P. Equity in the finance and delivery of health care: some tentative cross-country comparisons. *Oxford Review of Economic Policy* 1989; 5:89–112.

Wagstaff A, van Doorslaer E, Paci P. On the measurement of horizontal inequity in the delivery of health care. *Journal of Health Economics* 1991a; 10:169–205.

Health Policies, Health Inequalities, and Poverty Alleviation: Experiences from Outside Latin America and the Caribbean[1]

Margaret Whitehead

INTRODUCTION

The purpose of this work is to review selected experiences from outside Latin America and the Caribbean to identify the role of health policies and improved health in poverty alleviation and the reduction of inequalities in access to services. A companion paper assesses the extent of inequities in the health systems of Latin America and the Caribbean with special emphasis on the characteristics and the sources of inequities affecting the poorest 20% of the population.

To understand how health policies may help to alleviate poverty, however, it is first necessary to put the issue into context. What is included in the definition of poverty used here? What are the principal causes and consequences of poverty? How might these causes and consequences be reduced? It is then possible to consider where health policies fit in: What is the most effective contribution the health sector can make to the overall process of poverty alleviation and to the promotion of equity in health care?

This chapter aims to cover these questions and it is divided into two parts. The first part draws on the literature to identify the emerging consensus about what poverty is and what its main causes and consequences are for health. The second part focuses more specifically on equity in health care: on policies for improving access of low-income groups to health services and to allocate resources more equitably.

POVERTY: CAUSES AND CONSEQUENCES

What Is Poverty?

In the literature of both health and development, there is a concept of absolute poverty, equated with starvation, hunger, and destitution—insufficient income to survive in a physically fit condition. Although poverty by this definition is still widespread in some developing countries and demands attention, the concept has proved insufficient to encapsulate the state that many people find themselves in today. Human needs go beyond mere physical survival, and income is not the only resource that is important. In recent development literature, poverty is seen as an inadequacy of a range of resources needed to reach and maintain "well-being"—including health, knowledge, and education; environmental well-being; and income (Marga Institute, 1995).

There is also a relative element in the notion of poverty that is now in common usage. Relative poverty means poverty defined in relation to the living standards and expectations of the time and place in which a person lives. For example, Townsend's widely quoted definition, which emphasizes the relative aspect of poverty, states:

> Individuals, families and groups in the population can be said to be in poverty when they lack the resources to obtain the kinds of diet, participate in the activities and have the living conditions and amenities which are customary, or are at least widely encouraged and approved, in the societies to which they belong.... Their resources are so seriously below those commanded by the average individual or family that they are, in effect, excluded from ordinary living patterns, customs and activities (Townsend, 1979: 31).

The notion of exclusion from social participation is gaining a particularly strong emphasis in the European

[1]This is an excerpted version of a paper prepared for the Pan American Health Organization/United Nations Development Program/World Bank, Investment in Health, Equity, and Poverty in Latin America and the Caribbean Project 1998–1999. Revised 24 August 1999.

definition of poverty. The European Union, for example, which encompasses 15 affluent countries in Western Europe, states in its official documents:

> The poor shall be taken to mean persons, families and groups of persons whose resources (material, cultural and social) are so limited as to exclude them from the minimum acceptable way of life in the member states in which they live (Commission of the European Communities, 1993).

This shift to the notion of social exclusion is significant, because it introduces issues of social relations across society—how power is shared out and what society overall is doing to include or to marginalize sections of the population from their full participation. It requires an examination of what is happening in the whole of society and not just in the most disadvantaged groups within the population, leading to an emphasis on the right of all citizens to respect and dignity.

For management of poverty alleviation, the concept of poverty needs to be expressed in more operational terms, with measurable indicators. For operational purposes, Gross (1997) suggests that poverty exists when individuals or groups are not able to satisfy their basic needs adequately. Basic needs are considered in Gross's model to include food, social and cultural life, primary education, health, and favorable living and environmental conditions. Poverty occurs when individuals or groups are "too far" from essential resources, and the means, such as time and income, are not sufficient for adequate access to basic needs. Gross concludes that:

> Poverty consists of at least three dimensions that must be considered by poverty alleviation strategies: (a) the availability of essential resources for basic needs; (b) financial and other means of poor individuals and groups; and (c) the physical, intellectual, social and cultural status and position of poor individuals and groups. The severity of poverty is the collective gap between the availability of the essential resources (a) and the individual ability to meet basic needs (b) and (c). (Gross, 1997)

To this he adds a fourth dimension that must be considered in any analysis of policies—the political and cultural overall condition of a society, which has great influence on the nature of poverty experienced by the population.

Ill Health and Poverty: How Are They Linked?

Poverty and ill health are closely interrelated. Ill health can lead to poverty, but equally poverty can cause ill health. This means that people who are chronically sick or disabled can face a double jeopardy: their ill health puts them at greater risk of poverty, and their poverty is likely to further damage their health.

Disease, disability, and injuries are major causes of absence from work and greatly reduce opportunities to earn income through employment. Without work, the risks of financial poverty and also of social exclusion increase in many countries. From a national perspective, productivity lost through poor health is a hindrance to economic growth. It is important, however, to make a clear distinction between a focus on health as it relates to economic growth in general and a focus on the relationship between health and the poverty of different groups in the population, as discussed below.

The Relationship between Health and Economic Development

There are a number of studies by the World Bank and other international organizations on the issue of the positive relationship between improved health and economic development in general. For example, in a study of leprosy prevention it was calculated that if deformity had been eliminated in India's 654,000 lepers, then $130 million would have been added to the 1985 gross national product (GNP) of the country (World Bank, 1993). For many African countries, the human immunodeficiency virus (HIV)/AIDS epidemic is causing much suffering and is threatening productive capacity. In Tanzania, for example, it is estimated that because of HIV/AIDS, GDP is between 14% and 24% lower than it would have been without the epidemic (World Bank, 1993).

Malnutrition is another factor that takes a devastating toll on development. The loss of social productivity caused by four overlapping types of malnutrition—nutritional stunting and wasting, iodine deficiency disorders, and deficiencies of iron and vitamin A—amounted to almost 46 million years of productive, disability-free life in 1990 alone (World Bank, 1993). Studies of women tea planters and mill workers in China and Sri Lanka have shown reduced productivity due to anemia in most pregnant women. The United Nations Children's Fund (UNICEF) reports that vitamin and mineral deficiencies cost some countries the equivalent of more than 5% of their GNP. In Bangladesh and India, which are greatly affected by these deficiencies, the loss of GNP would amount to a total of US$ 18 billion in 1995 (United Nations Children's Fund, 1998).

A note of caution should be sounded at this point. The major problem with these types of studies is that they often focus on economic growth in general without any consideration of how the resources are distributed in society. In this macroeconomic perspective, there is a danger that the most efficient interventions may be judged to be those that secure or improve the health of "highly productive people," such as the well-educated with a "productive" job. When they get sick or die early, there is a greater loss in terms of economic growth than for illness and premature deaths among poor children and unemployed adults.

This has been recognized as an ethical problem among health economists for some time, and it is now almost routine to put the same "value" on everyone, regardless of economic status. From an equity perspective, however, this does not go far enough. One has to go one step further and ask how better health can improve the economic situation of poor families—that is, how it can contribute to poverty alleviation. At the same time it is of critical importance to analyze why poor health is a main cause of poverty in many countries.

The Relationship between Health and Poverty of Households

It is estimated that 200 million people with mental or physical disabilities are living in deep financial poverty (having a consumption power of less than US$ 1 per day); they represent one-sixth of the total population experiencing this level of poverty. Analyses to estimate the effects of different health conditions on the income of the affected individuals have been carried out. For example, leprosy is still a common disease in parts of Africa and South Asia. It causes serious deformities in 30% of those affected, which inhibits their ability to work. In a study of lepers in Tamil Nadu, India, it was estimated that the elimination of deformity would more than triple the expected earnings of those with jobs (World Bank, 1993).

Complications of pregnancy and childbirth are leading causes of death, disease, and disability in women of reproductive age in developing countries, accounting for between 25% and 33% of all deaths of women in many developing countries in this age group, and for 18% of the global burden of disease for women of reproductive age. The problem is particularly acute in Asia and sub-Saharan Africa: in parts of eastern and western Africa the lifetime risk of maternal death is 40 times higher than in the developed world (World Health Organization, 1996c). Poor maternal health also jeopardizes fetal survival and the newborn's health.

The social and economic costs of maternal morbidity and mortality are enormous, increasing a woman's own risks of poverty and reducing productivity, but also af-

fecting her household and children's life chances. In particular, household income for children's food, education, and health care is reduced when the mother is ill. A study of households in Tanzania where an adult woman had died within the previous year found that children spent half as much time in school as children from households where an adult woman had not died. Pregnancy-related health problems hinder women's ability to work and can lead families into debt. It has been estimated that the female labor force in India would be about 20% higher if women's health problems were addressed (World Health Organization, 1995).

Armed conflicts are a cause of physical handicap and subsequent poverty among civilians, even more so than among the military. One factor is the widespread existence of land mines: an estimated 65 to 100 million in the ground and a further 100 million in storage. In Angola, there are 50,000 amputees who are victims of land mine explosions, out of a population of 10 million; in Cambodia there are 100,000 persons in the same condition, out of a population of 8.5 million (Dahlgren, 1996).

Furthermore, access to many of the prerequisites for health is restricted by poverty. Malnutrition, for example, is widespread and can be both a cause and a consequence of poverty. As well as causing death and morbidity through starvation, inadequate nutrition weakens people's ability to fight off infections. It stunts children and hinders their capacity to learn in school. It interferes with physical development of young women so that they have high risks of complications in pregnancy and childbirth, and it weakens adults' ability to work productively. Discrimination and violence against women are major causes of malnutrition in some developing countries (United Nations Children's Fund, 1998). All these effects put people at greater risk of poverty and suffering. Access to other prerequisites for health—such as clean water and sanitation, shelter and education, social support, and participation—can be compromised by poverty and put health at risk in a downward spiral.

From the experiences in Africa and Asia, four possible health policy approaches to poverty alleviation have been advocated.

1. Identify specific diseases or health conditions prevalent among the poor and single them out for concerted effort. Examples include the near eradication of malaria in Sri Lanka between 1947 and 1977 and the accumulative gain in national income. Similar effects have resulted from programs to control river blindness in 11 northern and central African countries and international programs to control parasitic worms, which cause stunted growth, delayed puberty, and severe anemia in children.

2. Concentrate on some of the basic prerequisites for health such as food and nutrition and public health. This will tend to remove precarious living conditions in what is referred to as the strategy of support-led security. The case of Sri Lanka is identified as a benchmark of how good health can be achieved: (a) at a low cost through universal support and not by economic growth per se and (b) by the use of available resources to benefit all sections of the population.

3. Empower disadvantaged groups by promoting human rights. Carry out programs to increase the literacy rate, particularly female literacy, and to improve the social status of women. The benefits of these policies are illustrated in the experiences in the Indian state of Kerala and in 13 African states where a 10% increase in female literacy rates was associated with a 10% reduction in child mortality.

4. Widen eligibility and access to essential preventive and clinical services. This includes improving financial, geographic, and cultural access to challenge the common state of affairs in which health services are sparser and of poorer quality in areas serving disadvantaged populations.

It is important that health policies are seen as one essential element in a broader, intersectoral strategy for poverty alleviation.

Promoting Access, Utilization, and Quality of Health Care for All

The basic fact that poor people tend to be sicker raises fundamental issues for the organization of any health care system itself. It means that poor people, because of their greater morbidity and risk of mortality, have greater need for health care services. In addition, because of their deprivation they may find it more difficult to gain access to services. Even when they have gained access, poor people may not respond as well or as rapidly to treatment as their more affluent counterparts. This could be due to their poorer nutritional and immunological status and to disadvantaged living conditions, which make it harder to recover from illness. In spite of all these aspects of greater need, a common finding is that health services are sparser and of poorer quality in areas serving disadvantaged populations and access is more difficult. This phenomenon has become known as the "inverse care law"—that is, the provision of services is inversely related to the need for those services (Tudor Hart, 1971). There are several dimensions of access to which this "law" can be seen to apply:

- Financial access: Regulations on eligibility and entitlement may bar poorer groups from using the services; user charges may be prohibitive. High user fees not only reduce access and utilization of health services but also make people bypass medical personnel when in need of drugs. In countries where almost all drugs can be bought over the counter without prescription, this can lead to overconsumption of antibiotics and consequently resistance to treatment when needed. This worrying development is already under way in several countries.

- Geographic or physical access: There may be uneven distribution between urban and rural areas, for example, or concentration of the system on providing tertiary services serving relatively few, while primary care services, which benefit many, are neglected.

- Cultural access: Negative attitudes of health workers to poor people may discourage their utilization of services; there may be discrimination against girls and women for health care when resources are scarce; discrimination against ethnic minorities is also an important issue.

The following examples outline policies in both developing and developed countries that have been devised to challenge this state of affairs.

Promoting Reproductive Health Rights and Services

In the developing world, women use health services less than men do (World Health Organization, 1995). There is a particular problem of access to care for women because of a combination of cultural factors (outlined above in relation to "missing women") and the greater poverty suffered by women with all the added barriers that presents. The most pressing needs are for improvements in access and quality of maternal health services, and this is an area where clinical and preventive services can make an immense difference to the lives of many poor women. It is important to note that maternal deaths are experienced almost exclusively by poor women. Reduction of maternal deaths, therefore, has a very strong link to poverty alleviation.

Each year, over half a million women die from the complications of pregnancy and childbirth, predominantly in Asia and sub-Saharan Africa. This cause represents between 25% and 33% of all deaths of women of reproductive age in many developing countries (United Nations Children's Fund, 1996). In addition, half of all perinatal deaths (eight million) are estimated to be due primarily to inadequate maternal care during pregnancy and delivery (World Health Organization, 1996a). Moreover, up to 300 million women—more than one-quarter of all adult women now living in the developing world—suffer from short- or long-term illness related to pregnancy and childbirth (United Nations Children's Fund, 1996), accounting for 18% of the burden of disease among women of reproductive age in developing countries (World Health Organization, 1996a). When the causes of this morbidity and mortality are analyzed, the conclusion is that:

> Quality health care during and immediately after the critical period of labor and delivery is the single most important intervention for preventing maternal and new-born mortality and morbidity. (WHO, 1998)

Such health care provision has been shown to be a highly cost-effective investment in health. It has been estimated that to provide antenatal, postpartum, and delivery care, together with family planning, for women in low-income countries would cost between US$ 1 and US$ 3 per woman per year. The associated alleviation of poverty and increase in productivity are predicted to be considerable (World Health Organization, 1998).

However, the current picture reveals low access and utilization rates, with only 53% of deliveries in developing countries taking place with the assistance of a skilled birth attendant, fewer than 30% of women receiving postpartum care, and only 63% of women in Africa and 65% in Asia receiving antenatal care. When the reasons for low utilization rates are examined the causes reflect financial, geographic, and cultural barriers to access to care. These include long distances to travel to health services, particularly in rural areas; user fees and costs for transport, drugs, and supplies; poor quality of services, including the attitude of health providers to poor women, which can discourage them; multiple demands on women's time, including child care; and women's lack of decision-making power within the family (World Health Organization, 1996a). This last factor is illustrated by a study in Zaria, Nigeria, which found that women almost always needed their husbands' permission to seek health services, including life-saving care. If a woman went into labor while her husband was away from home, others often were unwilling to take the woman for care, even if the need was urgent.

A two-pronged strategy is recommended to address these problems:

- Ensuring access to maternal health services by tackling the barriers listed above. This needs analysis in each locality of what the specific barriers are for access to a service.
- Addressing gender inequalities and the poverty and discrimination women face. It has been proposed that

maternal mortality should be redefined as a "social injustice" rather than as a "health disadvantage." This would then provide stronger arguments for governments to ensure maternal health care for all women (World Health Organization, 1998).

Experiences in Africa and Asia show that improvements in access to maternal health services can be made with a concerted effort to identify the barriers and enlist community support in devising solutions. Box 1 lists some examples of the types of initiatives that have been developed that are showing promise.

Improving the quality of maternal health services also is of critical importance. Audits of maternal deaths highlight the role played by substandard care. A study in Egypt, for example, found that 92% of 718 maternal deaths could have been avoided if standard health care had been provided. Causes of poor quality include substandard care (due to staff being poorly supervised, underpaid, and/or overworked); supply shortages and infrastructure problems; delays in referrals; and insensitive treatment of women by providers. Box 2 lists some strategies that have proved successful in improving the quality of care in these services, even under conditions of severe resource constraints.

Protecting Equity in Universal Health Care Systems

Many developed countries are facing common problems of ensuring access to health services for people experiencing poverty. In the 20 years after World War II, all the countries in Western Europe greatly extended public support for health care, accepting that ensuring access to health care for all sections of the population was a collective responsibility. Most are compulsory insurance-based schemes for social security. Some systems, like those in the United Kingdom and Sweden, are based on general taxation. All are universal systems, although some are more comprehensive than others in the range of services they cover. Although in theory they all provide extensive access to health care for the whole population, including poor and vulnerable groups, continual vigilance is required to ensure that access is equitable in practice.

The issue of maintaining equitable systems has become more pressing in Europe since the early 1980s, as many have been facing common problems: economic recession and rising unemployment, which have pushed more people into poverty and ill health (Whitehead, 1992), coupled with retrenchment and cost containment in health systems in response to the economic climate, as well as the introduction of market-oriented reforms. The need for health care for poorer groups is greater than ever,

BOX 1: STRATEGIES TO IMPROVE ACCESS TO MATERNAL HEALTH SERVICES IN DEVELOPING COUNTRIES

Reducing the barriers of distance and lack of transport by:

- Assigning health workers trained in midwifery to the village health post level, backed up by a functioning referral system (e.g., put in place in Matlab in Bangladesh, in Sri Lanka, and in Cuba).
- Upgrading local health facilities to provide additional services such as obstetric first aid.
- Decentralizing care to the lowest level of the health care system that is able to provide it adequately (e.g., Mozambique, nurses trained to perform cesarean sections).
- Setting up systems for emergency transport and referral of complications (e.g., Uganda—the "rescuer" project ensures that trained birth assistants have radio communication to call for help and that local transport can be obtained at short notice).
- Establishing maternity waiting homes close to formal health facilities to bridge the gap between women and the health system (e.g., Cuba, Ethiopia, and Mongolia).

Tackling cost barriers, including ensuring access for poor women through government action:

- Providing maternal and infant heath services for free (e.g., South Africa, Bangladesh, Sri Lanka).
- Instituting fee structures to make services affordable—such as flat fees that cover routine prenatal and delivery care, including complications.
- Promoting insurance schemes that are affordable for poor women and their families, plus government subsidies to ensure access.
- When fees are charged, retaining at least some of the funds locally and using them to improve the quality of services.

Overcoming cultural barriers:

- Improving attitude and response of providers through training in patient care, counseling, and interpersonal skills; improving working conditions for providers.
- Community education and mobilization.
- Increasing women's status and power, by education of women and girls, and by raising awareness of the critical importance of women's health to children and families.

Source: Adapted from the World Health Organization (1998).

BOX 2: STRATEGIES FOR IMPROVING THE QUALITY OF MATERNAL HEALTH SERVICES IN LOW-INCOME COUNTRIES

- Decentralize services—to make them available close to homes (e.g., in Bangladesh, a mentoring program links 11 district hospitals with the obstetric and gynecology departments of 11 medical colleges. The program emphasizes decentralizing obstetric care by upgrading skills and facilities, developing clinical protocols, and mobilizing communities).
- Set standards and ensure supervision.
- Develop and use protocols for managing obstetric complications (e.g., in Ghana).
- Improve training and upgrade provider skills (e.g., South Africa).
- Improve infrastructure and upgrade facilities.
- Establish referral systems (e.g., China).
- Establish and strengthen mechanisms to evaluate the quality of services, including both client and provider perspectives (e.g., Malaysia), and introduce tools to improve quality including home-based maternal records, maternal deaths case reviews, and audits.

Source: World Health Organization (1998).

yet some of the cost-containment and market-oriented policies have a tendency to work against access for poorer groups if they are not tightly regulated (Whitehead, 1994). Currently, a pressing task for Western European systems is to maintain the access that has been achieved for all sections of the population, including poorer groups, in the face of mounting forces working against this aim. More intense focus has been put on devising mechanisms for:

- More equitable resource allocation for purchasing health care, by using assessments of need for care based not only on a given population's size and age structure, but also according to disease burden and socioeconomic characteristics of that population;
- Equity audit of the provision of care; and
- Tackling the identified barriers to access to care for different groups in the population.

In addition, several countries are reviewing the evidence on the most effective ways to improve access to marginalized groups, including the needs of minority ethnic populations (Arblaster et al., 1995; Gepkens and Gunning-Shepers, 1993).

Methods of Resource Allocation

Against this background there has been renewed interest in devising methods of resource allocation that take into account the differential need for care in different populations. This involves taking into consideration the identified social inequalities in mortality and morbidity that exist and that indicate differential levels of need in different places and for different groups of people. If insufficient account is taken of the differential need for care, then some health service providers will be underfunded for the individuals they are contracted to serve and quality may suffer, while others will make windfall profits.

The United Kingdom and Sweden, for example, have National Health Services (NHS) with universal coverage funded from general taxation. Funds are allocated on a geographic basis to official health authorities to cover the health care needs of the residents in each administrative area. A certain amount is allocated to the authorities per person per year. But if full account is not taken of heavier need and use of services in more disadvantaged populations, then access and quality may deteriorate in the areas with poorer communities. Both countries have developed resource allocation formulas to allocate public funds to local health authorities for purchase of hospital care based on weighted capitation to try to overcome this problem (Diderichsen et al., 1997). Both have used the extensive routine data available on social inequalities in health and use of services to identify the best indicators of increased need for care in poorer groups. Box 3 shows the variables chosen in the latest formulas to take into account increased need in poorer communities—both countries have selected lack of employment and living alone as important indicators of increased need for health care resources. Sweden has added indicators of poorer housing, and the United Kingdom has taken into account the proportion of households with single parents as well as direct health indicators (Carr-Hill et al., 1994).

BOX 3: NEED INDICATORS USED IN ALLOCATING RESOURCES TO HEALTH SERVICE PURCHASERS IN THE UNITED KINGDOM AND SWEDISH NHS

United Kingdom: The York formula—area-based need indicators

- All-cause standardized mortality ratio
- Proportion of people of pensionable age living alone
- Proportion of dependents living in households with only one career
- Standardized limiting long-standing illness ration
- Proportion of economically active persons unemployed (Carr-Hill et al., 1994)

Sweden: The Stockholm model

The Swedish approach does not use direct health indicators but concentrates entirely on socioeconomic characteristics of individuals:

- Age
- Socioeconomic group based on occupation and employment
- Cohabitation and marital status
- Housing conditions based on tenure and size of dwelling (Diderichsen et al., 1997)

There is continual adjustment and refinement of such resource allocation models, but the need to adjust for deprivation is well accepted in both countries. This principle forms the basis of continuing efforts to find equitable allocation methods not just for hospital care but recently also for primary and community health services. Similar issues arise for other countries introducing reforms in which the function of purchase of services is separated from the provision of care—the so-called purchaser-provider splits.

Equity Audits

There is increasing recognition that equitable resource allocation is a necessary, but not sufficient, requirement for achieving equity of access for all social groups. The way the resources are deployed is also influential in determining the quality of care received and any barriers to access faced by people living in poverty. Tools for equity audit are being developed in some European systems in response to this need. Audit in its medical sense is a cyclical process for the review and improvement of health care, involving standard setting, collection of baseline data, comparison against standards, identification of required change, implementation of change, and evaluation. An equity audit introduces the concept of equity as the basis for the standards against which services are reviewed (Johnstone et al., 1996). For example, an equity audit undertaken in a health authority in northern England led to discussions among all the providers and purchasers of health care in the area about fairer distribution of community nursing and primary medical services in response to the excess need identified in the poorer localities (Johnstone et al., 1996).

In the United Kingdom, authorities responsible for purchasing services for their resident populations are now being required by the NHS to carry out equity audits of the services under their control (Department of Health, 1995, 1997). As a way to ensure that responsibility for providing equitable access to services is taken seriously, assessment of fair access is being built into the statutory management performance review in the NHS. This supplements the narrower concentration on monitoring financial efficiency, which characterized the early years of market-oriented reforms in the country (Goddard and Smith, 1998). This includes cultural sensitivity training of professionals, increasing access to female doctors and nurses for communities where this is a sensitive issue, providing link workers and health advocates for people whose first language is not English, and providing outreach preventive and health promotion services to take the services closer to where people live instead of waiting for them to come to the services.

The Ethics of Resource Allocation in Developing Countries

The question of how to allocate resources in the health sector is also an important policy issue for most developing countries, although the challenge for policy makers is clearly more pressing and severe. In many low-income countries, universal and comprehensive health systems are not available. The quality of the public services in some tends to be low and important segments of the poor do not have access to them. There is a tendency under such conditions for the rich and the middle classes to rely increasingly on private services and insurers, and investment in the public sector may fall still further. Under such conditions, far from alleviating poverty, some health care policy choices run the risk of causing greater poverty in the population. The possibility of such an outcome has already been mentioned in Part I, where it was suggested that introduction of a policy based on very high direct user charges, with the intention of raising more finances for public services, may have a disproportionately greater effect on the poorer and sicker members of the population, deepening their poverty and ill health.

Given these circumstances, some analysts (Dahlgren, 1994) are advocating the adoption of conceptual frameworks for analyzing the policy options that make the ethical values and equity objectives explicit and at the forefront of the development of any strategy.

CONCLUSION

This review emphasizes that poverty is not only related to inadequate income but also encompasses the experience of social exclusion and inadequate access to education and to the prerequisites for health. The close interrelationship between poverty and ill health has been stressed: ill health leads to poverty, but poverty is also a cause of ill health. This means that action to improve health needs to be an integral part of any strategy to alleviate poverty.

Policy discussions in Europe have been developing along the same lines. In some European countries facing severe pressures to contain costs, national debates on how to set priorities for health care that maintain the principle of equitable access have been initiated. National commissions have been set up in the Netherlands, Finland, and Sweden, with extensive consultation to try to reach a consensus on the principles of fair allocation of available health care resources. The emphasis is on establishing the underlying ethical and moral values in those societies concerning rights of citizens to health and health care—before devising the practical mechanisms for any priority setting or rationing of services.

When considering what contribution health policies and improved health can make to the overall strategy of poverty reduction, four main entry points can be distinguished: a focus on specific diseases or health conditions, direct public support across a broad front to raise the standard of living and quality of life, empowerment and promotion of human rights, and widening eligibility and access to essential health care services. Each has advantages and disadvantages, but experiences cited from around the world indicate that health policies in all four areas have much to offer.

Three concluding points from this review need to be stressed. First, there is a need for the health sector to get more involved in issues of poverty alleviation. There is much still to do to increase understanding of the many ways poor health causes poverty and how poverty causes ill health. Second, there are some dangers to avoid in this line of inquiry. If too much stress is put on how health can improve productivity and the national economy, then "human development is [...] reduced to a tool for economic growth" (Dahlgren, 1993). The goal of promoting equity must be kept firmly in sight. The ultimate goals of development must be expressed in terms of human development and not economic growth per se.

Third, there are promising lines of health policy development, but policy makers themselves need to be made more aware of the evidence and the urgency of the situation—the need to take action. Being aware of the problem is of course only the first step in a process of change. This process also must include development of realistic strategies and methods to implement policies and the political will and capacity (power) to do so.

REFERENCES

Arblaster L, Entwistle V, Lambert M, Forster M, Sheldon T, Watt I. *Review of Research on the Effectiveness of Health Service Interventions to Reduce Variations in Health*. CRD Report No. 3. York: NHS Centre for Reviews and Dissemination, University of York; 1995.

Carr-Hill R, Sheldon T, Smith P, Martin S, Peacock S, Hardman G. Allocating resources to health authorities: development of methods for small area analysis and use of inpatient services. *British Medical Journal* 1994; 309:1046–1049.

Commission of the European Communities. *Background Report on Social Exclusion—Poverty and Other Social Problems in the European Community*. Brussels: Commission of the European Communities; 6 April 1993.

Dahlgren G. Economic analyses of health development. *NU News on Health Care in Developing Countries* 1993; 7(2):4–7.

Dahlgren G. The political economy of health financing strategies in Kenya. In: Chen L, Kleinman A, Ware N (eds). *Health and Social Change in International Perspective*. Boston: Harvard University Press; 1994.

Dahlgren G. Sectoral approaches to poverty reduction: health. In: Swedish International Development Agency. *Promoting Sustain-*

able Livelihoods: A Report from the Task Force on Poverty Reduction. Stockholm: Swedish International Development Agency; 1996.

Department of Health. *Variations in Health: What Can the Department of Health and the NHS Do?* London: Department of Health; 1995.

Department of Health. *The New NHS White Paper*. London: The Stationery Office; 1997.

Diderichsen F, Varde E, Whitehead M. Allocating resources to health authorities: the quest for an equitable formula in Britain and Sweden. *British Medical Journal* 1997; 315:875–878.

Dunning A (Chairman). *Choices in Health Care: A Report by the Government Committee on Choices in Health Care*. Ryjwijk: Ministry of Welfare, Health, and Cultural Affairs of the Netherlands; 1992.

Finnish National Research and Development Centre for Welfare and Health. *From Values to Choices: Report of a Working Group on Prioritisation in Health Care*. Helsinki: Finnish National Research and Development Centre for Welfare and Health; 1995.

Gepkens A, Gunning-Schepers L. *Interventions for Addressing Socioeconomic Inequalities in Health*. Amsterdam: Institute of Social Medicine, University of Amsterdam; 1993.

Goddard M, Smith P. *A Review of Equity of Access to Health Care in the English National Health Service*. York: NHS Centre for Reviews and Dissemination, University of York; 1998.

Gross R. Nutrition and the alleviation of absolute poverty in communities: concept and measurement. In: *ACC/SCN Nutrition and Poverty Symposium Report*. Nutrition Policy Paper 16, November 1997. Vietnam: Subcommittee on Nutrition; 1997.

Johnstone F, Lucy J, Scott-Samuel A, Whitehead M. *Deprivation and Health in North Cheshire: An Equity Audit of Health Services*. Liverpool: Liverpool Public Health Observatory; 1996.

Marga Institute. *Poverty Alleviation Strategies to Reach and Mobilize the Poorer Section of the Population: The Sri Lanka Experience*. Study commissioned by Swedish International Development Agency Task Force on Poverty Reduction. Colombo: Marga Institute; 1995.

Townsend P. *Poverty in the UK*. Harmondsworth: Penguin; 1979.

Tudor Hart J. The inverse care law. *Lancet* 1971; i:405–412.

United Nations Children's Fund. *The Progress of Nations 1996*. Oxford: Oxford University Press; 1996.

United Nations Children's Fund. *The State of the World's Children 1998*. Oxford: Oxford University Press; 1998.

Whitehead M. The health divide. In: Townsend P, Whitehead M, Davidson N (eds). *Inequalities in Health: The Black Report and the Health Divide*, 2nd Ed. London: Penguin; 1992.

Whitehead M. Is it fair? Evaluating the equity implications of the NHS reforms. In: Robinson R, Le Grand J (eds). *Evaluating the NHS Reforms*. London: King's Fund; 1994.

World Bank. *Investing in Health. World Development Report for 1993*. Oxford: Oxford University Press; 1993.

World Health Organization. *Women's Health: Improve Our Health, Improve the World*. Geneva: World Health Organization; 1995.

World Health Organization. *Safe Motherhood Progress Report 1993–1995*. Geneva: World Health Organization; 1996a.

World Health Organization. *Maternity Waiting Homes: A Review of Experiences*. Geneva: World Health Organization; 1996b.

World Health Organization. *Revised 1990 Estimates of Maternal Mortality: A New Approach by WHO and UNICEF*. Geneva: World Health Organization; 1996c.

World Health Organization. *Report of the Technical Consultation on Safe Motherhood, 18–23 October 1997, Sri Lanka*. Geneva: World Health Organization; 1998.

Policy Implications of a Health Equity Focus for Latin America[1]

William D. Savedoff

In recent decades, international assistance to Latin America in the health sector has been largely oriented toward improving the health conditions of the poor. Within this broad objective, however, a range of different policies have been promoted and tried. In the 1980s, efforts were focused on increasing access, largely through the expansion of primary health clinics to previously unserved areas. In the 1990s, the World Bank's 1993 *World Development Report* outlined a complementary, but not identical, approach to increase the efficiency of public health spending by directing it toward cost-effective activities. Also in the 1990s, programs to "modernize the state" began to influence policy in the health sector, with significant changes occurring in countries as diverse as Argentina, Venezuela, Jamaica, and Mexico with regard to forms of insurance, financing, coverage, and payments in the health sector. Such programs hold the promise of addressing the health conditions of the poor by changing the structure of incentives in a way that would lead resources to be allocated more effectively to policies and programs that address the health problems of the poor.

A large part of the political debate about the health sector since the 1980s has been focused on the problem of equity. A great deal of this attention has been generated by dissatisfaction with how state reforms have affected the health sector—the structural reforms of the 1980s in Latin America or, in the case of Britain, the Thatcher reforms of the same decade. Studies of the equity of health in Europe have advanced quite steadily over the past few decades, with a substantial literature on the wide variation in health status across socioeconomic classes.[2] In examining this literature and applying modern techniques of distributional analysis to household surveys in Europe, van Doorslaer et al. (1993) found inequities in different countries in the Organization for Economic Cooperation and Development that could be related to the structures of their health systems.[3] More recently, this approach has been applied with World Bank and Pan American Health Organization (PAHO) funding to Latin American countries under the EquiLAC project, whose papers are presented here. PAHO's involvement in the project is understandable, given the prominent attention that has been given to equity in most of PAHO's deliberative bodies since at least the mid-1980s.

A key difficulty in most studies of equity, whether of health status or anything else, hinges on choosing the appropriate definition of equity. This choice is not merely an issue of choosing the right technical instruments for measurement. Rather, it has a critical impact on the interpretation of results and implications for policy. In these comments, I question the particular definitions of "health equity" that are commonly used in political debates in Latin America by demonstrating that they can lead to policies that result in less equitable rather than more equitable health systems. This paradox occurs because the most common definitions focus attention on measures of inequality that overlook behavioral responses to policies in terms of (a) individual choices about utilization of public or private care, (b) performance of public providers, and (c) the effectiveness of tax enforcement. As a result of these behavioral responses, appropriate public policies—those aimed at improving the conditions of the poor—will have to accept, and sometimes even encourage, apparent "inequities" in the health system as a whole.

[1] I would like to thank Ruben Suarez and Adam Wagstaff for their invitation to comment on the papers prepared under the EquiLAC project at the World Bank, and for various formative conversations and ideas. Philip Musgrove provided valuable comments on an earlier version of these comments and provided continuing inspiration. I would also like to thank Norberto Dachs for introducing me to a broad literature on this subject. The views and interpretations in this document are mine and should not be attributed to the Inter-American Development Bank. Any remaining errors are clearly my responsibility as well.

[2] See, for example, Wilkinson (1996) and Whitehead (1990, 1992).
[3] See van Doorslaer *et al.* (1993) and Wagstaff and van Doorslaer (in press).

Addressing health inequities through the policies that Latin America tried in the past—namely, seeking to deliver the same care to everyone free of charge—has been ineffective and counterproductive. Countries must adopt policies that aim to make their health systems efficient so that they can become effective instruments for raising the health conditions of the poorest.

These comments cannot attempt a complete review of the literature or discussion of health equity, which is extensive. Rather, I begin by reviewing some evidence that, in some cases, health conditions and utilization of services are distributed much more equitably than other social measures. I then evaluate the implications of some of the most common definitions of equity and follow with a discussion of some misconceptions about equity in health financing. Finally, I conclude with a discussion of the policy implications for the health systems of Latin America.

DISTRIBUTION OF HEALTH IN PERSPECTIVE

How much inequity is a lot? Is a Gini index of 0.06 for child mortality or self-assessed health status a lot of inequity or a little? Rather than establish an arbitrary level, van Doorslaer et al. (1993) wisely sought to address this question by comparing countries. Finding out that a country is as equitable as Sweden or as inequitable as the United States has more meaning than a single index number. Although this is a significant advance, the index numbers also need to be put in perspective relative to other distributional outcomes in society—certainly income, if not also other indicators of social status or well-being. In this regard, given the high income elasticity of health expenditures and the association of higher income with higher education (with all its attendant benefits for an individual's health through behavior modifications), one expects health outcomes to be more inequitably distributed than income.[4] From another perspective, income has no relevant upper limit, whereas health status is capped, relatively speaking, by good health. Therefore, health status is expected to be better distributed than income. In fact, by almost any measure, the latter is a more accurate characterization. Health outcomes appear to be distributed more equitably than income. This fact is not presented by way of apology but rather to indicate that the standard against which public policy affects the distribution of health conditions matters for the conclusions we draw.

An example can be used to illustrate this point. Brazil is among the most inequitable countries in the world, as measured by the distribution of income. The Gini index for income is about 0.59, with the bottom quintile receiving about 2.5% of national income and the top quintile receiving 63% (see Figure 1).[5] The distribution of education is also one of the most inequitable in the world. It is highly skewed: for heads of household between the ages of 25 and 65 in 1995, the bottom quintile had an average educational attainment of about 2.4 years compared with an average of 8.5 years for the top quintile of this age group. As shown in Figure 1, this represents a skewed distribution but one that is somewhat more equitably distributed than income, particularly for the lowest income groups.[6]

Comparing the distribution of health service utilization, we find that it is much more equitably distributed than education. Campino et al. (1999) calculated the number of visits for supervision of a chronic problem by income quintile. These range from about 10% of individuals in the lowest quintile seeking care to about 14% in the highest quintile.[7] It is obvious that the utilization by income class is substantially more equitably distributed than income and perhaps even better distributed than education. The findings for preventive and curative care are similar, with concentration indices on the order of 0.1 to 0.2. When adjustments are made for age, sex, and self-assessed health status, the distributions are much better, with concentration indices below 0.10.[8] Even when attention is shifted toward the distribution of need for chronic and curative care, the concentration indices hover close to 0 (0.04 and –0.04, respectively).

Peru offers another instructive example (Ministerio de Salud [MINSA], 1998) (Figure 2). Here also the distribution of income is highly unequal, with a Gini index of 0.46. Again, the utilization of services is much more eq-

[4]Clearly, this also assumes that health expenditures have a positive impact on health, which is always true.

[5]The figures on inequality are taken from Inter-American Development Bank (1998).

[6]These estimates of the educational distribution curve are actually a lower bound because they are based on an average for the quintile, which should shift each of the points on the curve some amount to the right (i.e., toward greater equality). The estimates also need to be qualified as possibly underestimating the degree of inequality for two reasons: (a) the quality of each school year received by poorer students is likely to be lower than the quality for richer ones, and (b) the "value" of each school year may be different (i.e., higher returns per year at higher levels of schooling; see Inter-American Development Bank, 1998). On the other hand, looking at an alternative measure would demonstrate much greater equality: the average 18 year old from families in the bottom quintile had a little more than 4 years of education in 1995, compared with 8.8 years for those from families in the top quintile. This is much more equitably distributed than for the population heads of household or for the population as a whole, and it indicates that public policy and/or social behavior has offset the country's huge income inequities to a strong (although still insufficient) extent.

[7]The unadjusted rates range from 12% to 17%.

[8]Note that self-assessed health status is not necessarily independent of income and education, although the impact appears to vary by country and study.

FIGURE 1. Distribution of income, health, and education, Brazil.

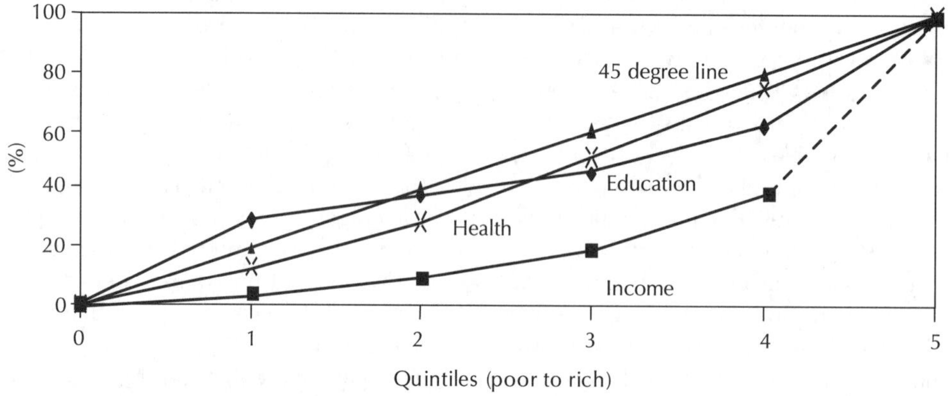

Note: Education is the average educational attainment for heads of household between 25 and 65 years of age (Brazil's National Household Sample Survey [PNAD], 1995); income is per capita household income (Inter-American Development Bank, 1998); and health services are the "need predicted chronic visits" as reported by Campino et al. (1999).

uitably distributed, with a concentration index of 0.17. However, when services are differentiated between MINSA, the Social Security Institute (IPSS), and the private sector, the distributions are quite different. Private sector consultations are distributed quite close to the inequitable distribution of income; consultations with IPSS (which largely serves formal sector workers) by income quintile are more equitably distributed; and MINSA services are distributed quite equitably. It is also apparent that public health care utilization is more equitably distributed than education.

As the MINSA study points out, the main issue of equity in its broader sense for Peru is that particular diseases and causes of mortality that are relatively easy to prevent are highly concentrated among the poor. Infant

and maternal mortality rates are indicators of this. The study estimates that the concentration index for the infant mortality rate in Peru is about –0.05—that is, infant mortality is overrepresented among the poor. As for the allocation of public resources, it appears that MINSA actually does reach the poor more than one would predict based on income alone, but the poor continue to experience certain illnesses that are relatively simple to prevent and cure.

So, if health service utilization and outcomes are compared with income distribution or other social services, they do not look quite as bad as one would expect. This is not to belittle or minimize the impact of the remaining inequities on the people whose lives are affected, but it does provide a standard against which to evaluate how

FIGURE 2. Distribution of income, education, and health, Peru.

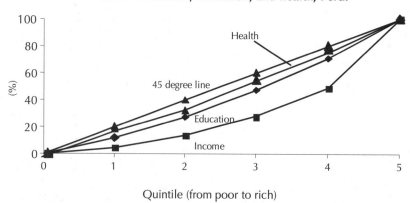

Note: Education is the average educational attainment for heads of household between 25 and 65 years of age (PNAD, 1995); income is per capita household income (Inter-American Development Bank, 1998); and health services are estimated from utilization curves in Figure 12 of MINSA (1998).

"unfair" the utilization rates are in Latin America, and it provides some perspective for policy. This is only a first step. We know that poorer individuals tend to receive poorer quality medical attention and that they have more illness. We also know that all illnesses are not alike—some are life threatening and some are temporary or mild. A proper evaluation of the distribution of health status requires that these factors be taken into account. The presentation of the distribution of infant mortality in Peru is one step in this direction and may be representative to the degree that infant mortality is a proxy for the distribution of other health status indicators. Nevertheless, the relatively equitable distribution of utilization shown here does contradict common beliefs about the equity of Latin American health systems and demonstrates the need for good data to properly evaluate the political debate.

HEALTH EQUITY

What is an appropriate definition of equity? Various definitions can be found in the literature and appear to be intuitive. An explicit statement of a very strong definition of equity is a situation in which a person's health status is independent of his or her income. This clearly involves a maximal level of policy interventions to equalize not only the utilization of services and knowledge but also behaviors. A somewhat more modest definition is a system in which those with equal need receive equal treatment. This sets a standard for public policy to ensure that everyone gets the services they need, and it is implicit in the policy of offering health care services free of charge either universally or for those with insufficient means. A third definition, almost identical to the second, is a health system in which a person's utilization of health services is independent of his or her income. This standard is slightly weaker than the previous one because it sets a standard only of ensuring that everyone who seeks care receives it; the equity standard is based on the demand for services rather than some objective measure of need.

The primary difficulty encountered by these and similar definitions is that they are unattainable unless you are willing to give everyone the same level of insurance as Donald Trump and Bill Gates. This is fundamentally true because richer people are prepared to pay more for, and thereby receive more, health services than the poor or the middle class. The only way to keep the upper income classes from obtaining more or better quality health services is to make private health services illegal—and even then the rich will opt out by flying to Miami, the Hague, or Toronto.

Instead of getting angry and frustrated by the wide-open options of the rich, we can move toward another definition of equity that sets a better standard for public policy and not by lowering our sights. If, instead of defining health equity against an independent standard, we judge public policies by whether they are equity increasing, then we can state that any health policy that improves the health conditions of the least well off is equitable. This definition is attractive because it is feasible in the context of feedback responses within the limit of the production frontier and it provides a more useful guide to designing policies that really improve the health conditions of the lower socioeconomic classes.

The problem with the earlier three definitions is that they measure equity in ways that provide positive value to a decline in the service utilization or health status of the rich even if there is no associated gain for the poor. These are all equity measures that can be considered egalitarian in the sense that they value the equality among individuals independent of the consequences for the distance from society's total production of services or health status. Utilitarian measures of equity are only slightly better. Although a reduction in service utilization or health status of the rich has to be offset by a gain for the poor, the utilitarian standard also could lead to solutions in which more services are provided to the rich when their potential health gain is greater than for the poor. The equity-increasing definition provided above is closer to the maximin solution advocated by John Rawls in his *Theory of Justice*. The maximin solution seeks to improve the condition of the least well off. This standard can accept some degree of inequality whenever it is justified by net gains to society. The health sector represents a case in which this could not be more critical.

To understand this point, it is useful to consider the standard equity-versus-efficiency argument. Figure 3 shows a standard production possibility frontier, which can be interpreted as the production of services or health status, distributed between rich and poor. Point X represents a situation that is producing efficiently but not equitably—i.e., the rich get more services or enjoy better health than the poor. The situation is inequitable whether measured by an egalitarian standard (represented by the line) or a maximin standard (represented by the L shape).[9] The usual argument is that society is better off by redistributing from the rich toward the poor, even if this means producing services or health status inefficiently (indicated by point Y being inside the production possibility frontier). Being unable to reach the egalitarian point on the

---

[9] The maximin solution is a gross simplification of a standard established by Rawls in his *Theory of Justice* in which society seeks to improve the condition of the least well off. In this simple figure, the optimal allocation under a utilitarian standard coincides with the egalitarian and maximin solutions. This discussion and the figures are drawn from Olsen (1997).

FIGURE 3.

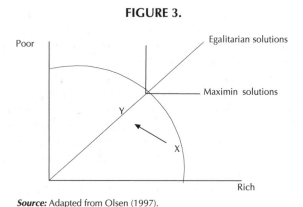

Source: Adapted from Olsen (1997).

FIGURE 4.

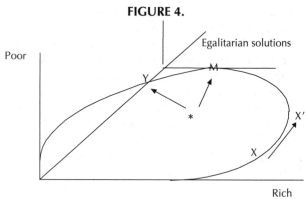

Source: Adapted from Olsen (1997).

production frontier can be due to a variety of complex (e.g., incentive effects) or simple (e.g., administrative costs) reasons.

Nevertheless, Figure 3 grossly simplifies behavioral responses that alter the likely shape of the production frontier. Figure 4 shows a situation in which production is on the frontier (point X), but the production frontier is upward sloping over various ranges. For example, the rich might be better off if they privately purchase services that maximize their health status (moving from X to X′), but these services could have externalities that incidentally improve the health of the poor (e.g., installing sanitation and drainage). In this case, there is no efficiency/equity tradeoff. An alternative example is redirecting funds spent on curing the rich of contagious diseases that could have been avoided if cost-effective basic services (vaccinations, screening) had been provided to the poor.[10]

This kind of argument is not consistent with the presumption that society is probably far from the efficiency indicated by the production frontier. In fact, an internal point (such as that marked by the asterisk) is more likely to reflect the actual situation. In such a case, how do we move toward a more equitable situation? Note that, because of the slope of the production frontier, the egalitarian and maximin solutions diverge. Moving toward an egalitarian solution (point Y) represents accepting lower utilization or health status for both rich and poor. Moving from point Y to point M can represent net benefits for all for a variety of reasons. Externalities of increased health services for the rich can improve the health services of the poor, as in the case of sanitation or economies of scale in production of new medications. More relevant to the case in Latin America, when rich people opt out of public systems, they can be left with the potential for applying more resources to the health needs

of the poor. Competition from private providers can induce more efficient and better production of health services in the public sector for the poor, or public systems that are more effective at reaching the poor may enjoy greater public support. All these reasons, which begin to consider the relationship between consumer and producer behavior, force a change in the shape of production possibilities that cause the egalitarian solution to diverge from the maximin solution. It is important to recognize the implications: an equity-increasing policy (moving from * to M) does not necessarily reduce the gap between rich and poor, but it does reduce the gap between the current and potential health status of the poor.[11]

HEALTH EQUITY AND HEALTH SERVICE PROVISION

The complexity of the notion of equity leads to numerous difficulties in the Latin American debates about improving health in the region. One of the key problems in the debate about health equity is that perfectly reasonable goals, coupled with some knowledge, can be a dangerous thing. Most countries have adopted laudable goals: universal coverage and equitable access. Most people are aware that publicly funded systems (e.g., Sweden) tend to be more equitable than those that rely largely on private spending (e.g., the United States).[12] The political process in most Latin American countries puts a high premium on equity (in rhetoric if not in practice) and leaps from these positions to aim for public provision of free health services. This has even been enshrined in several constitutions.

Difficulties arise when we recognize that people in society respond to public policy in ways that undermine

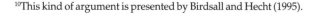

[10]This kind of argument is presented by Birdsall and Hecht (1995).

[11]Note that this argument glosses over the definition of least well off. For a discussion of the potential contradiction between treating those with the most severe illnesses and treating those who can be helped most by treatment, see Musgrove (1999).

[12]For more information see Wagstaff and van Doorslaer (in press).

the original goals. In particular, two such processes are common in Latin America. First, unless public services are of high quality, the upper income classes opt for private services that compete for medical personnel and drive up public sector costs.[13] They also seek to evade taxes earmarked for services they do not utilize. Along with this, it is not uncommon for governments to finance (or provide) high-quality care for particularly costly interventions. Upper income groups then have the opportunity to reduce their insurance premiums by agreeing to exclude such coverage and resort to the public sector for these costly events.

The second process derives from an agency problem when the public sector finances or provides medical services. Accountability within public agencies that purchase or provide medical services is very difficult and frequently is constrained by civil service provisions and political interference. This is compounded by the political-economic difficulties of establishing sustained collective action around public health programs that are either underfunded or ineffectively promoted.

For both these reasons, the advantage of public financing (or provision of services) in terms of increased equity as demonstrated by European countries can be radically offset by reasonable responses of wealthier individuals and public sector personnel. In many Latin American countries, these disadvantages have been large enough to undermine the goals of universal equitable coverage. Only policies that fully recognize these behavioral responses can be expected to redress inequities.

Attempting to equalize utilization or health expenditure at this time runs against these two processes. Pursuing equity under these conditions, when it is defined as equal care for equal need, equal utilization independent of income, or equal health status independent of income, is simply unattainable because of the opportunities of private spending and provision. They can be reached only by some kind of leveling. By contrast, improving the health conditions of the least well off is equitable in the sense of being fair or desirable even when it may, strictly speaking, increase the gap in health status, utilization, or care between rich and poor.

In essence, public policy should aim to establish a minimum service guarantee (e.g., something like a basic heath service package oriented toward diseases concentrated among the poor) coupled with efforts to improve the quality of care financed by the public sector. An example of the first part of this prescription can be found in the MINSA study analysis of the provision of rural health posts. Expanding access to rural areas may thin out public resources in the urban areas, encouraging more households to opt out of the public system and evade tax or social security payments; it may further exacerbate poor public service quality because it is difficult to attract qualified personnel to those areas. Nevertheless, the net impact on health status may be more equitable, even if those health posts are of worse quality than urban ones and even if health service consumption in the private sector increased more than proportionally. An example of improving the quality of provision can be found in Costa Rica where, despite its difficulties, the public sector is sufficiently good to reduce demand for private sector services.[14]

FINANCE AND HEALTH EQUITY

Up to this point, the source of funding for health services or health-promoting actions has not been addressed. This is not an accident. Another part of the general debate argues that not only should health services be equitably distributed but they also should be paid for according to ability to pay. Just as in the case of the distribution of services or health status, most of the discussion of financing health services fails to recognize that the form of raising funds affects the total volume of resources available. This section argues that in some cases health status of the poor is best served by raising taxes proportionally and in some cases even regressively.

We can begin by asking what is an appropriate definition of equitable financing for health services? The answer to this question has been made difficult by the use of two different standards against which the progressivity of taxation and expenditures are measured. In common parlance, a tax is considered progressive relative to the income distribution curve. It is considered progressive if the rich pay a larger share of their income than the poor and it is regressive in the opposite instance. By contrast, expenditures are judged against per capita spending and not income. Consequently, expenditures are considered progressive if a larger amount per person goes to the poor than to the rich and regressive if the poor receive less per person.

As a result of these definitions, it is entirely possible to have a regressive tax policy and a regressive expenditure policy that nevertheless redistribute resources from the rich to the poor.[15] Consider Figure 5. The tax curve

---

[13]Costs can be driven up by raising salaries or, more commonly, by absenteeism in public facilities.

[14]For a discussion of the relationship between the private and public health sectors, see Inter-American Bank (1996), Maceira (1996, 1998), and Musgrove (1996). Costa Rica cannot be considered a paragon of public service provision either. Costa Rica spends a very high share of national income on its services, which have been demonstrated to be very inefficient. One study estimated that absenteeism in Costa Rican public facilities was as high as 30%.

[15]A more complete discussion of this can be found in a report by the Inter-American Development Bank (1998), from which it is derived.

FIGURE 5.   Regressive policies that redistribute resources.

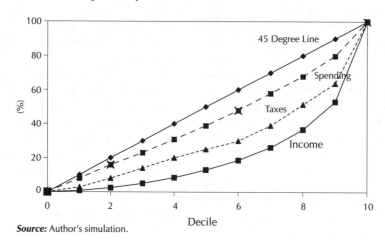

Source: Author's simulation.

lies above the income curve representing a regressive tax policy: in the example, the bottom quintile receives 3% of the nation's income but pays 8% of the taxes. The expenditure curve lies below the 45-degree line, indicating a regressive expenditure policy: in the example, the bottom quintile represents 20% of the population but it receives only 16% of the spending. Nevertheless, there is a net redistribution from the rich to the poor represented by subtracting the area between the tax and income curve from the area between the expenditure and income curve. A numeric example is also shown in Table 1.

This is not an idle curiosity. In Latin America, much of health spending is closer to the 45-degree line than to the income curve and the countries that have the most progressive impact are those that spend more. Therefore, the key problem in Latin American countries is to have tax policies that are effective in raising revenue more than being progressive. Essentially, a country that raises a lot of revenues through a value added tax and spends them roughly in proportion to the population in each quintile (e.g., Argentina) can have a much more redistributive impact than a country that raises very little revenue through a highly progressive income tax and spends very little (e.g., Guatemala).

Theodore et al. (1998) demonstrate this clearly for Jamaica. The authors find a very equitable public health

system, with resources coming from general revenues and going to the population in roughly equal shares—except for the upper class, which is underrepresented. Effectively, the rich opt out of the public system, but their taxes (through general revenues) continue to support it. Ironically, a country like Costa Rica, whose public sector health services are utilized by a broader share of the population, may have an apparently regressive spending structure simply because the middle and upper middle classes actually use the services their taxes are supporting! Yet, the Costa Rican health system is still, at least anecdotally, preferable to what currently exists in Jamaica.

The Chilean health system, which is regularly criticized as being inequitable, may be the most progressive health system in the world in terms of the distribution of public spending by income quintile. Milanovic (1995) showed that the concentration curve for public health spending in Chile is significantly above the 45-degree line, indicating highly progressive spending. By contrast, British health spending is close to but above the 45-degree line and Hungarian spending lies below. A more recent study by Bitrán (1998) also shows that the top income classes (those who are enrolled in private insurance companies called ISAPRES) receive only 2.5% of public health subsidies, whereas the rest of the income classes redistribute resources toward the least well off. The reputation Chile has for being inequitable may be the result of the rapid expansion of higher quality private care available to middle and upper income groups since the health reform of the early 1980s. Yet, it may be precisely because richer families can opt out of the system that the remaining public spending is so progressive. In other words, large inequities can exist in health systems that are strongly redistributive.

TABLE 1.   Example to demonstrate the impact of hypothetical regressive policies.

	Initial income	Minus taxes	Plus subsidies	Total
Poor	20	15% = 3	5	22
Rich	80	10% = 8	6	78
Total	100	11	11	100

The key issues for the equity of health finance then are not whether taxation and expenditures are progressive. Instead, there are three primary implications for policy. First, what is the best way to ensure funding for health services? This is a difficult question because of the political-economic context that makes every solution imperfect. Earmarked taxes have been tried in many countries (including a tax on financial transactions that funds a large part of Brazilian health services today). This solution is imperfect, however, if the middle and upper classes find ways to evade the tax (because they do not believe they receive any benefits from it). Financing health services from general revenues may be more equitable, but it is not always assured because it must compete with other important public demands. Lasprilla et al. (1998) showed that the social security program in Ecuador for a particular group of peasants is quite progressive. It is tempting to look at such a program as a model for other countries. However, it is questionable whether such a scheme could be replicated in a different context, where the peasants are less well organized and the central authorities are under pressure to use their limited resources elsewhere. It is also attractive to think of redirecting private spending on health through the public health system channels, but this is an illusory source of funding. Private spending is high precisely because those who do it receive direct and immediate benefits from it, whereas a tax or public insurance premium is not clearly directed toward individual benefit.

The second issue in financing health services is the effectiveness of the tax system. This is much more important than the progressivity of taxes, as discussed above, because without tax revenues, there can be no redistribution. The third issue is to make public spending on health services gradually more progressive. This cannot be done by offering services free of charge to everyone. The Brazilian experience with the 1988 Constitution, which guarantees free health care for everyone, effectively allowed the wealthier classes to begin raiding federal revenues to pay for health services they previously paid for themselves. As a consequence, public spending on health has become more inequitable in the past 10 years, and out-of-pocket expenditures have become more regressive.[16] Health spending can be made more progressive (a) by ensuring basic minimum services that address the health problems most concentrated among the poor, and (b) by improving the quality of health services provided with public funding so that the floor of health service quality in the country is gradually but steadily raised.

---

[16]Medici (1998).

SUMMARY

Attention to equity in health care is important but full of pitfalls. The benchmark against which equity is measured, and the choice of definition, can confuse the policy debates by holding up the health system to an unattainable standard. The studies done as part of the EquiLAC project demonstrate that health conditions are generally worse among the poor and that services are also utilized unevenly across income classes. Nevertheless, the inequalities detected in the distribution of public health services and public health spending are generally small relative to the inequitable distribution of income that prevails in most of these countries.

Given that families of means will always spend on what they perceive to be the highest quality of care attainable, equity measured as the distribution of services and spending may be an unhelpful measure. Rather, equity measured by access to basic services among the poor may be an attainable and effective policy—even if it has a minimal impact on the overall distribution of spending or services.

In the case of equity in health care financing, the progressivity of taxes or even spending is not of great importance relative to three other issues. The first issue is how to ensure funding for the health sector, taking into account politics, tax evasion, and flight. The second issue is how to effectively raise revenues, even if in equal proportion to income across the income scale, rather than enacting progressive taxes that generate little money for redistributive programs. Finally, spending needs to be made progressive in the sense of ensuring access to basic cost-effective services while steadily improving the quality of services provided with the backing of public funds.

REFERENCES

Birdsall N, Hecht R. *Swimming Against the Tide: Strategies for Improving Equity in Health.* Working Paper Series 305. Washington, DC: Office of the Chief Economist, Inter-American Development Bank; 1995.

Bitrán R. *Equity in the Financing of Social Security for Health in Chile.* Bethesda, MD: Partnerships for Health Reform, Abt Associates; 1998.

Campino A, Coelho C, Diaz DM, Paulani LM, de Oliveira RG, Piola S, Nunes A. Equity in health in LAC–Brazil. Presented at the World Bank/United Nations Development Program/Pan American Health Organization/World Health Organization Technical Project Workshop *Investment in Health, Equity, and Poverty in Latin America and the Caribbean,* January 22, 1999. Washington, DC; 1999.

Inter-American Development Bank. *Making Social Services Work, Economic and Social Progress in Latin America, 1996 Report.* Baltimore: Johns Hopkins University Press; 1996.

Inter-American Development Bank. *Facing up to Inequality in Latin America, Economic and Social Progress in Latin America, 1998–1999 Report*. Baltimore: Johns Hopkins University Press; 1998.

Maceira D. *Fragmentación e incentivos en los sistemas de atención de la salud en América Latina y el Caribe*. WP-335. Washington, DC: Office of the Chief Economist, Inter-American Development Bank; 1996.

Lasprilla E, Granda J, Obando C, Lasprilla C. Equity in health in LAC, country studies: Ecuador. Presented at the World Bank/United Nations Development Program/Pan American Health Organization/World Health Organization Technical Project Workshop *Investment in Health, Equity, and Poverty in Latin America and the Caribbean*, January 22, 1999. Washington, DC; November 1998.

Maceira D. *Income Distribution and the Public-Private Mix in Health Care Provision: The Latin American Case*. WP-391. Washington, DC: Office of the Chief Economist, Inter-American Development Bank; 1998. http://www.iadb.org/oce/324a.cfm?CODE=WP-391.

Medici A. *O SUS e a política 'Hood Robin' de saude*. Washington, DC: 1998. Mimeograph.

Milanovic B. The distributional impact of cash and in-kind transfers. In: Van de Walle D, Nead K (eds). *Public Spending and the Poor: Theory and Evidence*. Washington, DC: World Bank; 1995.

Ministerio de Salud. Equidad en la atención de salud, Perú 1997. Informe final preliminar, December, Oficina General de Planificación del Ministerio de Salud, Peru. Presented at the World Bank/United Nations Development Program/Pan American Health Organization/World Health Organization Technical Project Workshop *Investment in Health, Equity, and Poverty in Latin America and the Caribbean*, January 22, 1999. Washington, DC; 1998.

Musgrove P. Un faundamento conceptual para el rol público y privado en salud. *Revista de Analisis Económico* 1996; 11(November):2. Also available in English as a World Bank Discussion Paper.

Musgrove P. *Public Spending on Health Care: How Are Different Criteria Related?* Washington, DC: World Bank Institute, World Bank; 1999.

Olsen JA. Theories of justice and their implications for priority setting in health care. *Journal of Health Economics* 1997; 16:625–639.

Theodore K, Stoddard D, Yearwood A, Thomas W. Health and equity in Jamaica. Presented at the World Bank/United Nations Development Program/Pan American Health Organization/World Health Organization Technical Project Workshop *Investment in Health, Equity, and Poverty in Latin America and the Caribbean*, January 22, 1999. Health Economics Unit, University of the West Indies; December 1998. Washington, DC; 1998.

van Doorslaer E, Wagstaff A, Rutten F. *Equity in the Finance and Delivery of Health Care: An International Perspective*. Commission of the European Communities, Health Services Research Series, No. 8. Oxford: Oxford Medical Publications; 1993.

Wagstaff A, van Doorslaer E. Equity in health care finance and delivery. In: Culyer AJ, Newhouse JP (eds), Chapter 40. *North Holland Handbook of Heath Economics*. Amsterdam: North Holland Press; in press.

Whitehead M. *The Concepts and Principles of Equity and Health*. Copenhagen: World Health Organization, Regional Office for Europe; 1990.

Whitehead M. *Inequalities in Health*. London: Penguin; 1992.

Wilkinson RG. *Unhealthy Societies: The Afflictions of Inequality*. London: Routledge; 1996.

World Bank. *World Development Report*. Washington, DC: World Bank; 1993.

APPENDIX

High-Level Meeting of Experts in Economics, Social Development, and Health on

IMPACT OF THE INVESTMENT IN HEALTH ON ECONOMIC GROWTH, HOUSEHOLD PRODUCTIVITY, AND POVERTY REDUCTION

Health and Economic Growth[1]

George A. O. Alleyne
Director, Pan American Sanitary Bureau

This meeting will deal with a topic that is of great interest to me, and I wish to give you some background on this interest and also explain how it will be relevant to PAHO's work in the immediate future. I will also indicate my expectations in terms of the results of this meeting.

My interest in health and economic growth perhaps can be traced to the time when I was a practicing physician and Professor of Medicine at the University of the West Indies. I saw the need to expand my thinking beyond the care of the problems of individual patients and wrote a paper entitled "Health and Development," which I submitted to our *Journal of Social and Economic Research*. It was rejected, and I still recall the reviewer's comment, which was that the paper "contained an interesting germ of an idea."

When I came to PAHO in 1981, there was more sympathy for this line of thinking, and the paper was published in the then-*PAHO Bulletin*. As I read the paper now I appreciate that it was not a brilliant piece of work, in that my ideas about the issue were still quite primitive. But even at that time I appreciated that the indicators of social progress were not very good. I believed that at the turn of the last century the indicators of social progress included consideration of such variables as health and housing, and there was not the exclusive focus on measures of national wealth such as the gross domestic product. So, about 15 years ago I telephoned Sir Arthur Lewis, who was then at Princeton University, and asked if he could think of ways one might relate social indicators, such as health, to some markers of development. He listened to me carefully and in typical fashion said "I know nothing of this subject, but I suggest you speak to someone like Burton Weisbrod." That rang a bell, because Weisbrod had written a book in the early 1970s on the eradication of schistosomiasis from Saint Lucia. His thesis was that if you could eradicate schistosomiasis, the economic performance of Saint Lucia would improve. I read Weisbrod's book again, and one of the factors that complicated his analysis was the high level of unemployment. If my memory serves me correctly now, one of his observations was that there was some relationship between sex and the cure of the disease.

Weisbrod's book caused me to look again at some of the work of earlier economists such as Marshall, who had stated that the health and strength of the population are the basis of industrial wealth. I could find several references to the effect

[1] Inaugural speech delivered at the opening of the "High-level Meeting of Experts in Economics, Social Development, and Health on Impact of Investment in Health on Economic Growth, Household Productivity, and Poverty Reduction," held at PAHO Headquarters, Washington, DC, 5–6 October 1999.

that the eradication of specific diseases had on productivity, but little reference to health in the aggregate. For example, in a speech Dr. Eric Williams gave at the University of the West Indies, he made the point that if hookworm were eliminated from Caroni, the productivity of the workers would increase.

And there were other examples from the Caribbean. Dr. George Giglioli was one of the most famous investigators to work in that part of the world. When he worked in the mines in McKenzie, in what was then British Guyana, he discovered a very high hookworm infestation rate among miners. He treated them with tetrachloroethylene, which, parenthetically, is hepatotoxic, but it did get rid of the hookworms. He then showed that workers could shovel considerably more ore after treatment.

There are many other studies of this nature. Viteri showed that productivity of sugar cane cutters improved after treatment for anemia. Ram and Schultz, showed increased productivity after malaria control and, of course, I must mention the PAHO-supported study carried out by Gladys Conley in Paraguay on the economic impact of malaria.

It appeared to me at the time that it was obvious, as Marshall had said, that health was important for national economic growth, but I could not find any clear formulation of a general mechanism. Then I came across Theodore Schultz's papers, in which he advanced the thesis that human capital was an essential factor in estimating national economic performance. I have sometimes offended certain sensibilities by alluding to human capital, but that is not significant. Partly as a result of reading Schultz's work, I found much comfort in the work of Sir William Petty—a physician and a fellow of my college, the Royal College of Physicians—who was perhaps the first to express the view that human capital was important. In putting forward the idea of the worth of human lives, he went as far as to calculate the economic value of a life. Indeed, William Petty's work made me bolder in my discussions with my economist friends, as I could point out that their profession was born out of the accurate observation of a good physician. I am not sure that this endeared me to them.

I wondered why economists were not more concerned with the possibility that health would stimulate economic growth, and came to think that perhaps most health economists, certainly in this country, were much more interested in the cost and efficiency of health care. By the mid to late 1980's it was clear to me that we in PAHO should be looking at the impact of health on economic growth and also the contribution of health to enhancing the impact of education on economic growth. Many of you will be familiar with George Psacharopoulos' work on education and I wondered why we did not have a Psacharopoulos in health. Why did health not receive the same treatment as education?

I frequently tell a story of an acquaintance of mine who was close to the government in one of the Caribbean countries. The story perhaps is a caricature of the truth. When ministers sat around the Cabinet table discussing the budget, the minister of transport would say that if they invested so much in roads then produce would reach the ports more quickly. The minister of mines would say that investment in that sector would increase productivity and, therefore, increase the gross domestic product. Then the minister of health would fold his arms and say that health is a basic human right. To whom do you think the money went?

I began to wonder if we at PAHO were not being deficient in not producing the data for our ministers that would allow them to make a better case for investing in health. It was also apparent that the two approaches to health should be centered around health as a desideratum that had its own intrinsic merits and health as being instrumental for development.

At that time I became fascinated by Mahbub Ul Haq's *Human Development Report* and the idea that health was one of the critical life options. When we read Arthur Lewis we find that he points out that we value the essentials of human development as being important for all human beings. We wish to be healthy in order to enjoy the best of what life has to offer. These are what Amartya Sen refers to, perhaps in a different formulation, as the "basic freedoms." The idea that health could be important in itself as well as being instrumental in securing the other life options was very attractive to me. Health is an important aspect of human development, but it is also important in ensuring that those other life options are available. Health is important in ensuring that there will be economic growth. It is important for optimizing education. It is important in ensuring that we enjoy the essential political freedoms and rights.

That is the background to my decision to stimulate this area of work at PAHO. Perhaps we can still find a Psacharopoulos for health. We are now involved in examining the mechanism by which health can lead to wealth. At the 1998 Santiago, Chile, Meeting of Heads of State I said that the health of nations was the wealth of nations and thought it was original, but I believe it was Will Durant who first used the expression. Our thinking in this area has also been supported by the work of the economic historian Fogel, who points out that much of the economic growth of Europe in about the last one and one-half centuries was due to improvements in health and nutrition.

I had many fruitful discussions with Antonio Campino, when he was here, on the relationship between measures of wealth and health. He convinced me that one had to look not only at wealth, but at the distribution of both wealth and health. One had to look at the distribution of those factors that are thought to be determinants of health. One of my regrets is that we did not pursue this and publish our data on the effect of income distribution on health before this became popular and has been now shown in numerous settings.

I have come to the conclusion that this move to consider distributional characteristics of the determinants of health is one of the major shifts of the last 20 years. Much of the former work stratified groups in terms of what is known as socioeconomic status and related these groupings to health status. The tendency has been to apply the risk factor approach to individual characteristics. Campino and I agreed that measures such as income inequality represented fundamental characteristics of our social structures, and that examining the distribution of characteristics would be a significant conceptual advance.

I am currently intrigued by the possibility that income inequality is just another marker of what is called social incongruence. Dressler, who worked with Fernando Viteri while he was at PAHO, has published data on the effect of social incongruence on some aspects of health. Blood pressure, for example, is higher in those societies with a high degree of social incongruence. If we go back 100 years, we will find that Durkheim said the same thing. These social differences that produce what he called "anomie" may result in severe stresses that provoke suicide, for example.

Let me now explain PAHO's current and future interest in this area. I believe that institutions and organizations such as ours have a responsibility to find new forms of conceptualizing the importance of health and its place in the social agenda.

Of course, the political agenda is a part of the social agenda. This must be done without causing damage to the very laudable appreciation of health from the moral and humanitarian point of view. Let me be clear. I am not disputing the advantage of good health or the attention to providing services to the population. We are adding another dimension to the debate. We cannot ignore the effect of health on poverty. The standard approach is that the poor are unhealthy and one must first alleviate poverty. We now believe that we should also consider income inequality in addition to poverty, and health may be instrumental in alleviating both.

When I became Director, I said that there were two principles that would guide our Organization. One of them is equity. As many of you know, income distribution in the Americas is the worst in the world, and I am concerned that I do not see major efforts in terms of improving that situation. The standard mode of economic organization in our part of the world virtually predicates a worsening of income distribution in the coming years. Does that mean that we in health should throw up our hands in despair? I do not believe so. If we can demonstrate that we can reduce inequalities in social spheres such as health perhaps this may contribute to reducing income inequalities.

I am going to support work on the inequalities in health outcomes, because they are important for determining where inequities lie, as you can only speak of inequity if the disparities or inequalities are socially unjust. Of course, the notion of what is fair or just is one that has exercised philosophers for a long time.

But we think that it is our task as an organization to help countries demonstrate what are the inequalities and where they lie, as well as what are the distribution characteristics of the health indicators that we normally measure as averages. As I have said on various occasions, my reluctance to remain only with averages is based on my own inclination towards egalitarianism. We have concentrated attention on health and its relation to economic growth, but I wish to see us becoming involved in the relation between health and education as well as between health and the other essential life options.

We cannot do all this alone, and that is why I am delighted to see so many other agencies here and so many persons from disciplines related to the social sciences. But our field is very much one of the social sciences. I refer often to one of the quotes of one of my heroes—Rudolf Virchow—who said about 150 years ago "medicine is a social science and politics is nothing more than medicine on a grand scale." We really do seek partnerships with other agencies and disciplines.

But let me share with you one of my concerns or deficiencies in relation to your discipline of economics. I abhor the mathematical formulations, but I take comfort in what Arthur Lewis once said to me, "if it is not written in plain English, do not read it." Most of these strange formulations are for the cognoscenti in the discipline and are their means of communicating with one another. So I hope that the further work in this area will be in plain English, Spanish, Portuguese, or French. Mathematics is not one of the official languages of the Organization.

What do I expect of this meeting? I expect that some of the studies we have promoted and developed will come in for scrutiny and debate. I hope that at the end, my bias is confirmed or refuted and perhaps you will show why it is important that we go deeper into the problem of the manner by which health investment contributes to the enhancement of other life options.

This meeting has taken a long time to be developed, but it has been worthwhile waiting to have a group of experts examine the work we are promoting. I have only alluded in passing to the problem of poverty, even though its relationship with health is clear. Luckily, in the Americas there has been a slowing of the increase in poverty. But that is cold comfort because there are still 200 million persons living in poverty. This presents a challenge in terms of providing health services. We must note here the work of Birdsall and Londoño, who have shown that inequality in access to assets like land and those that produce human capital contribute to poverty. We are interested in this line of work because if we can reduce inequalities in health this may reduce poverty, in the sense that health is a major contributor to human capital formation.

So, once more, let me welcome you and indicate how enthusiastic I am about this meeting. I hope that the work that has gone into its preparation will be rewarded by the intensity of your participation and the final outcome.

Thank you.

Summary of Meeting Proceedings

Objectives

1) To submit for the consideration of high-level experts in economics, social development, and health the findings of the following research projects:

- "Investment in Health and Economic Growth" (IDB, ECLAC, PAHO)
- "Investment in Health and Household Productivity" (IDB, ECLAC, PAHO)
- "Investment in Health and Poverty Reduction" (UNDP, the World Bank, PAHO)

2) To collect participants' recommendations regarding monitoring the economic and social impact of investing in health; the policies to strengthen the mutually beneficial relationships among investment in health, economic growth, and poverty reduction; and the new research designed to fill the gaps remaining after the aforementioned projects.

Issues and challenges

Discussions about the technical, policy, and general aspects of the research led to the identification of research gaps and of general suggestions from the institutions to promote and develop this research agenda.

Technical and Methodological Findings

Discussions revolved around issues related to the information used, the interpretation of results, and the points to consider for further analysis.

Data/Information Issues

- There is a need to combine quantitative and qualitative data.
- Future research may benefit more from combining data sources and improving the overall quality of data. The amount of data is not a problem for Latin America and the Caribbean—there are more than 100 household surveys on living conditions and health, mainly Living Standards Measurement Study (LSMS) household surveys and demographic and health surveys (DHS). In addition, there are many surveys on household income and expenditures.
- The methodology must be standardized before useful comparisons can be made. Definitions, concepts, and variables must be reviewed, and before any compari-

son is drawn, it is important to identify the questions the research wants to answer and the type of information being used.

- The inclusion of revenue periodicity in the analysis of income may enrich the analysis, because the timing of the earnings is often an important determinant of utilization.

Result Interpretation

- The interpretation of results should be done carefully. It is important not to assume more than what the results offer.[1]
- The assessment of health needs is not clear cut among the studies. A point that is important for developing policies is the assessment of the difference between estimated health care needs and the observed utilization of health care.
- The terms "equity" and "inequality" could be better applied. They should adequately represent whether a national health system is pursuing equity per se, whether it can be proven that health systems are driving towards equity, or whether there is a trade off between equity and efficiency.
- Research recommendations should also be practical. It is impractical to advocate a given idea without thinking through all the aspects required to make it work. If more investment in health is advocated, consideration should be given to where the funds would come from.

Points to be Considered for Future Analysis

- Considering the "dynamics" of the utilization of health services may offer a richer picture than the more static one offered by income inequality versus health utilization. This approach could be introduced into the analysis of the patterns of disease and sick absences to understand the dynamics of maladies on income.
- Considering such elements as geographical differences, mortality indicators for different age groups, and comprehensive health care needs might enrich the assessment of inequality.
- Considering the analysis of the supply side of the equation, like the normative criteria, is important for deciding what is a need for health care and the circularity of multiple factors that can enabling or hinder the population's use of services.
- The models could benefit from the incorporation of institutional specifications. However, this should be done with care, considering that health institutions in Latin America and the Caribbean have undergone profound structural changes.

---

[1] For example, in asserting that "hospitalization that benefits the rich is related to some corruption," it is important to keep in mind that other factors may play an important role among the poor, such as the extra cost that being hospitalized represents to them. Therefore, it is important to consider not only corruption, but also any self-selection pattern that may have occurred because the additional costs prevented poor families from staying in hospital.

Policy Applicability

- Communicating and disseminating results should be considered part of the researchers' responsibility; they should seek ways to easily present their results to policy makers.
- Research utilization may be more easily promoted when the research topic emerges out of a national health policy issue. Researchers must propitiate the interaction with policy makers.
- Suggestions for policy makers should lead health systems toward means of solidarity and equitable funding.
- The "political culture" should be taken into consideration—policy makers, as a rule, are not accustomed to the use of research information in formulating policies. To offset this, the involvement of every institution must be sought.

General Comments

- A review of similar research conducted outside the Region would greatly benefit this exercise.
- The three research projects reviewed here only begin to scratch the surface of the problem; they should be considered as the initial step in the learning process. There are still not enough elements in hand to be able to advise ministers of health, of finance, or of economy about what they should do with these results.
- The whole area of the relationship between health and inequities, although fairly old by now in some parts of the developed world, is still relatively new to many countries in this Region.
- PAHO should take the lead and quickly work to organize the data. Participants commended PAHO for calling for research in health, economic growth, and poverty reduction in Latin America and the Caribbean.
- There have been examples of how economic development policies sometimes are inequitable, with investments going to unique areas or regions, and not being distributed where people might get healthier.[2]
- Interdisciplinary work is necessary.

Research Gaps

The research agenda for the future should build on existing knowledge regarding how the research is conducted. Some of the gaps are:

- Understanding the pathways and the specific mechanisms that lead to inequity and inequalities.
- Understanding the determinants of health and the perception and the meaning of illnesses for different population groups, including age, gender, and ethnic groups.
- Understanding how much people are willing to pay for health care, the reasons for differential use, the best way to measure illnesses, and the real value of self-reporting in predicting such indicators as actual morbidity and mortality.

---

[2] The case of Mongolia, for example.

- Understanding the institutional setup of health systems, their organization, regulation, financing, payment systems, and these factors' impact on different population groups.
- Understanding inequities in the distribution of different services.
- Understanding the role of health in the labor market.
- Understanding the role that enterprises and professional organizations play in health and economic growth.

Instrumental Issues

- It is important to be able to produce research that addresses comparative issues between countries or within countries, or both simultaneously.
- Sets of variables and their pathways in health financing, health sector organization, and health service delivery should be identified, as should issues involving supply and demand of health services.
- Strictly quantitative research has left many unanswered questions. The time has come to integrate qualitative tools in the analysis and incorporate the insights, theories, and approaches of disciplines such as history, sociology, and political science. It is relevant to use past examples from Latin America and the Caribbean, such as the poverty assessment surveys conducted in the eastern Caribbean, which carried out in-depth interviews in households.

Statements

- Few relationships have been proved wrong elsewhere in the world, such as that increased official health care expenditure would lead to greater equity in health care utilization, or that greater national income would lead to greater equity.
- Healthier countries tend to grow faster, but not always—there are extraordinary exceptions, such as Cuba. There is a missing link here. At what point people or countries get healthier growth isn't understood automatically. A qualitative analysis or a better understanding of the labor market once people get healthier probably are necessary.

General Suggestions

- To develop sound partnerships among institutions, so that each one will bring its comparative advantage to this research agenda.
- To develop a strategy for disseminating research results and discussing them with policy makers.

INTERVENTIONS ON BEHALF OF INSTITUTIONS

After briefly introducing their respective organizations, participants discuss how the meeting's topic would fit in their area of cooperation and/or the possibilities integration or contribution in the future for this line of work. (The list of participants follows this section.)

United Kingdom Cooperation

The Department for International Development (DFID) is a British Government cooperation organization that works through resource centers. These centers, which pursue various areas of interest, include the Institute for Health Sector Development and the Center of Resources for Sectoral Reform. The topics discussed during the meeting are extremely well suited to the cooperation strategy of the British Government. Equity and poverty are completely interwoven. Moreover, this topic of research and collaboration should be discussed and presented to the European Region as a whole. There are many countries that want to collaborate with Latin America and the Caribbean in different ways, and this could become one way to channel that cooperation.

Great Britain has supported health sector programs in Bolivia, Peru, Brazil, Mexico, and the Central American region in three areas: health sector reform, reproductive health, and disease control and surveillance. These areas are believed to complement the main objective of Great Britain's cooperation in Latin America, the Caribbean, and other regions—poverty elimination.

However, DFID still needs to answer specific questions to the ministries or the person who represents some continuity at the government level, such as "how should financing options be organized" and "which is the best option with the organization." The answer should not begin with "depends" or "maybe," because this lack of specificity may generate more inequity than it solves. Clearer answers must be sought.

DFID considers it convenient to disseminate research results with more in-depth discussions on fundamental issues germane to a given country. This could become a strategy for the dissemination of publications at the country level.

Rockefeller Foundation

The new strategy of the Rockefeller Foundation's Health Sciences Division includes a very strong health equity program. Through this program, the Foundation is working to strengthen the global knowledge base and its application for health equity. The Rockefeller Foundation is open to form partnerships and to be a part of further discussions.

The institution has been undergoing a major transition. Upon reviewing efforts in the health sciences, the Foundation has embraced a new framework that entails looking at the root causes of health outcomes. Of the three areas that the Foundation has chosen to focus on, one ties into this meeting's discussions—the strengthening of global leadership. This component will support leaders who are working to develop actions that effectively enhance equity. In addition, a "Global Health Watch" component will bring transparency and accountability to key global institutions in their effort to prevent health threats.

To pursue this goal the Rockefeller Foundation would participate in the creation of more powerful and effective coalitions, networks, and public and private partnerships; it also will invest in human and technological resource development.

The mechanisms whereby the Foundation hopes to support this work would be through fostering research, developing tools to enable policy makers to address health equity, and by ensuring that key institutional actors are monitored and kept transparent and accountable through health watch efforts.

The Global Health Equity Initiative—which the Rockefeller Foundation has co-sponsored with the Swedish International Development Agency (SIDA)—includes a network of more than 100 researchers conducting health equity research in 13 countries. The researchers have uncovered three shared key findings: i) data disaggregated by social group is needed to uncover inequities, ii) many health sector reform policies fuel rather than address inequities, and iii) social policies also are powerful determinants of health equity.

Two case studies offer interesting parallels—Chile and Bangladesh. Chile's study found that during the study period, per capita GDP had increased and life expectancy at birth had risen dramatically. However, the gap between rich and the poor in health had continued to widen. A striking finding is that overall growth has been coupled with an actual backsliding: men who were at the lower level of life expectancy at birth actually declined over the past decade, so their life expectancy, in fact, dropped.

The Bangladesh case study, conducted by Brack, reported that the micro-credit intervention allowed the child survival rate of participants in that program to approach the level of child survival in wealthy households. This particular intervention, which wasn't a health intervention *per se* but a micro-credit intervention, enhanced health equity by reducing the gap between rich and poor in terms of health outcomes. The Foundation is very interested in analyzing what was the particular pathway for these results. Was it the mother's empowerment? Was it knowledge gained? It is not clear what the specific link was and what it was that improved the child survival. What does this means for the Foundation's programming strategy? The challenge will be to shift to an outcome oriented approach to health care. The Foundation will focus on individuals who are unable to pay user fees and on those who are unable to pay but somehow still find the way to cover the costs.

Financing, particularly through taxes and financing arrangements in poor rural areas, will be a major line of inquiry for the Initiative's policy group. Further priority areas will include integrating equity oriented policies into the context of rapid health sector reform and developing user friendly tools to measure, monitor, and evaluate the parity dimensions of health equity. In addition to the Global Health Equity Initiative, interest in new initiatives related to health equity has mushroomed, which provides for an extremely favorable advance of the health equity agenda at the global level.

United Nations Development Program (UNDP)

UNDP's unit in charge of these issues is the Program and Policy Group, whose mandate is to collaborate with other UN agencies and other partners in the areas reviewed at this meeting, especially in poverty; equity; gender issues; education; and, more recently, children.

Pairing economic research with social research may provide information on attitudes and practices supported by some social research tools. We need to have better links between data from the models and current work and transmission to the policy makers.

UNDP's role has been to analyze the research's implications for policy, advice, and advocacy. The agency should aim at providing more support for comparative studies and for exchanges among researchers, and shift towards smaller meetings in which both decision-makers and the researchers can participate. This could be a first step in disseminating the results.

UNDP also would like to ensure that gender issues and the special needs of women are taken into account. We strive on being credible and we need to try to develop across the board norms and standards that will make our research results more user friendly. The importance of reviving past research in Latin America and the Caribbean, such as the Jamaica Poverty Report, also should be noted.

In terms of advocacy, UNDP works with parliamentarians, ensuring that health, equity, and gender figure prominently in our government's agenda.

Finally, UNDP is talking not only about poverty alleviation, but also about poverty eradication. We will continue the commitment to work with PAHO in the dissemination of research and publication in the area of gender, gender equity, and health, and will participate in the dialogue between our counterparts and ourselves. UNDP will support mechanisms that will further discussions and the sensitization of social research.

The World Bank

The World Bank is currently undergoing a period of introspection, realizing that the mission of the Bank, which is poverty reduction, will need to be more effective at reducing poverty than it had been in the past. Broadly defined, the new emphasis on poverty reduction means not just raising the incomes of the poor, but also improving human development outcomes. This would include, for example, improving health nutrition and population incomes of the poor.

Clearly, this is a shift away from thinking about processes, projects, and programs and toward outcomes, and showing clear linkages between what the Bank does and outcomes. In fact, many of the indicators that the Bank will be using in future documents to monitor its performance will be outcome indicators and project type indicators.

This inevitably means rethinking the support functions within the Bank. For example, the poverty reduction network has changed from devoting its time to operations to figuring out what the Bank should be doing in this new wave of thinking. Health nutrition and population features high in this new way of thinking. New documents will be published next Spring, including the document "The Poverty Reduction Strategy Paper", which will be a joint World Bank, International Monetary Fund work.

There also will be a summary document on poverty as part of the World Bank's web site, which will attempt to synthesize what is known about the determinants of poverty and health and poverty outcomes among the poorest. We hope that this will be useful to other agencies as well.

The Health, Nutrition, and Population (HPN) sector is producing fact sheets based on demographic and health survey data, which are presented by wealth quintile constructed through a principle component analysis of information on household characteristics and asset ownership, as well as information on a full range of health and poverty outcome indicators and usage indicators. Those will be accessible from outside the Bank through the Worldwide Web.

HPN has a research program that functions in tandem with the development of an economic research group that looks at various issues related to poverty and health. Health nutrition outcomes among the poor can be enhanced by improving access to an equalization of care and establishing the financial protection of households.

We look forward to an international conference that will boost this new way of thinking within the health nutrition population sector and the appearance of new sector strategy documents with stronger emphasis given to the poor.

World Health Organization (WHO)

A task force on health and poverty has been recently created in the Organization. The task force will coordinate and research on issues related to poverty reduction, health and economic growth, and policy development, among others.

In terms of the work of the Sustainable Development and Healthy Environment cluster and, especially, of the Department of Health and Sustainable Development, there already is work in that direction. A closer look may be taken at health sector practices that can benefit the poor, perhaps through the area of health care financing. Or, other sectors that influence poverty and poverty reduction, such as the environmental sector, may be examined.

WHO also needs to look at other sectors, such as education and international trade. In addition, the Organization intends to work on health matters as a part of the development process in particular initiatives, such as micro-credit schemes. What can they do for health? How can health be put to some of the regulations of micro-credit schemes?

There are several projects that relate more directly to the work that we have been discussing here. One project looks at the relationship between health and growth at the microeconomic level, using international panel data. Another looks at inequity in health and another, at equity in financing. Moreover, there are currently four pilot health, health state, and health status projects being undertaken, and they are improving the instruments that are currently being used for self reporting of health status. Finally, the *World Health Report 2000* focuses on health systems and addresses some of the issues that will interest the audience here, such as the interaction between public and private sectors and the role of the State.

Inter-American Development Bank (IDB)

The Inter-American Development Bank's main activities include lending money to governments from the 26 member countries in Latin America and the Caribbean. The lending level has increased dramatically in the last five years, from around US$ 5 billion a year to US$ 10 billion dollars a year. Health represents only about 3% of that portfolio. The Bank is basically a net consumer of research, not a net producer of research; but we want good quality information because we are trying to improve our programs.

IDB is undertaking little research, and we also have very little administrative budget allocated to do research. The Bank spends around US$ 250,000 a year on research and health in various topics, but the real money in IDB-financed research is through the loans. The governments, through IDB loans, have funds available for doing research related to the focus or the objectives of the loan, whether it is improving financing or delivery systems, or targeting the poor. One of the challenges for the Bank is to make sure that that money is directed to the areas of our priority for research, and that the research is of good quality.

IDB does not have a specific strategy in health, but there are two related activities in place. One is the work to improve health service systems, and the second involves health promotion activities. There is an increasing emphasis on those activities in Bank loans, but they tend to be within the context of projects.

In coordination with other institutions the Bank is trying to finance research on national health accounts. It has studies on hospital management, and there also are joint studies with PAHO and the World Bank on reproductive health. Now there are three new areas of research being developed, related to the best ways to deliver basic services to the poor, occupational health questions, and insurance regulations.

As international organizations, we must strive to do a better job at improving data collection, standardization of data, and availability of data. Demographic and health surveys are an excellent way to generate a great deal of data and making it available. Studies would emerge if data were available. If you look at studies on inequality—for example, studies on inequality done in the 1960s and 1970s—one finds a great deal of literature on Brazil and nothing on Mexico. This is basically because Brazil made its data available and Mexico did not. There are academic communities interested in doing this kind of work, if we make the data available.

IDB's Office of the Chief Economist has systematized a series of household labor surveys, and it is trying to make those available on the web. The same thing could be done with PAHO's epidemiological data, such as the health accounts data that it is being generated. If possible, real data on institutions and so forth could be made available. Advocacy for better research and evaluations is an important thing to be doing.

The Pan American Health Organization (PAHO)

PAHO's unit responsible for bringing about this meeting is the Division of Health and Human Development. The Organization is fully committed to the work discussed in this meeting, as well as to the development of methodologies, conceptual frameworks, and new measurement tools. It must be done and the best way to do it is through partnerships. PAHO has excellent working relationships with each and every partner that has spoken here, as well as with others.

Many issues that are crucial for this work have been addressed during this meeting. PAHO is engaged in identifying existing sources of data and information so they can be better utilized. The information has potential, but the health sector must have more say in how these tools are designed and deployed. This—helping the health sector become part of these systems and methods—is one of the greater challenges that that the Organization faces.

PAHO also needs to have a better and clearer conceptual framework of the relationships among health, economic growth, and poverty reduction and a framework that must rest on solid information and on data. Therefore, there is a great need to strengthen the resource capabilities within institutions and to conduct research those issues that have policy implications. We need to have a better dialogue with policy makers regarding how to utilize these research findings, and this dialogue must embrace both government policy makers and the emerging and ever-stronger civil society in the Region. This could become one of the main determinants in the changes that inevitably will have to come about.

In a year, the Organization will be able to show data from a multilevel analysis conducted in Bolivia, Nicaragua, Peru, Colombia and Brazil. PAHO also has begun to study the impact of health sector reform on gender equity, which clearly is another area of concern that needs to be better documented. There is empirical evidence that some health sector reform processes have been detrimental to women's access to health care and to the quality of care that they receive. In fact, women already pay more than men do for health care in our Region. This is another issue that the Organization wants to better document and to provide information about for those groups that can raise these issues and advocate for them at the proper level. PAHO's Division of Health Systems and Services Development also is coordinating an important effort to monitor equity and access to health care.

The Organization's work on national health accounts is helping to standardize the information that countries produce, and this information provides a baseline to analyze how the health sector expenditure is behaving. It is an extremely important input for understanding equity and distribution issues in the countries. PAHO also is working to understand how globalization and integration affect health and equity and health, particularly in terms of access to certain quotes and services at global or regional scales.

The dissemination of research results is one of the key areas that the Organization must focus on. Information can be disseminated at the country level through meetings, policy discussions, meetings with top level advisers or policy makers, as well as with civil-society organizations. Moreover, traditional and new ways of disseminating information, including electronic means, must be tapped. These are some of the challenges that lie ahead for all of us, so that our goals remain interesting, useful, and feasible.

We are pleased to see that every organization here has expressed an interest in this issue, and also to see that what we do in this Region can complement what is done at the global level. This meeting holds great promise, as it heralds our institution's future work together. We must guide our joint efforts by areas of mutual interest, specificity in our objectives, and joint programming. PAHO is prepared to harness some of its resources to see that these specific things get done. We look forward to cooperating with all of you.

List of Participants

Arnab Acharya
University of Sussex
Program Manager/Team Leader
Brighton, BN1 9RE
United Kingdom
Email: j.a.mcwilliam@ids.ac.uk
Fax: (44) 1273-621202
Telephone: (44) 1273-606261

Mrs. Danielle Benjamin
Senior Program Advisor for Gender and
Health
Regional Bureau for LAC
UNDP
New York, N.Y. 10017
Telephone: (212) 906-6303
Fax: (212) 906-5363
Email: Danielle.Benjamin@undp.org

Dennis Brown
The University of the West Indies
St. Autustine Campus, Trinidad and Tobago
Email: dav@africana.com
Fax: (868) 663-4948
Telephone: (868) 645-3232 (X-3053)

Guy Carrin
WHO/HSD
1211 Geneva 27, Switzerland
Email: carring@who.ch
Fax: (41 22) 791-4153

José Luis Estrada
UAM-Iztapalapa
Col. Purísima y Michoacán s/n
Iztapalapa
México, D.F., Mexico
Email: jlel@xanum.uam.mx
Fax: (52 5) 7243-6403
Telephone: (52 5) 724-4771

Julio Frenk
Evidence and Information for Policy
WHO
CH - 1211 Geneva 27, Switzerland
Email: frenkj@who.ch

Debra Jones
The Rockefeller Foundation
Health Sciences
420 Fifth Ave.
New York, N.Y. 10018-2702
Email: djones@rockfound.org
Fax: (212) 852-8279
Telephone: (212) 852-8321

Deon Filmer
The World Bank
1818 H St., N.W.
Room MC3 615
Washington, D.C. 20433
Fax: (202) 522-1153
Telephone: (202) 483-3510
Email: Dfilmer@workdbank.org

Davidson Gwatkin
The World Bank
1818 H St., N.W.
Room G7 - 091
Washington, D.C. 20433
Email: dgwatkin@workdbank.org
Fax: (202) 522-3235
Telephone: (202) 473-3223

David Mayer
CIDE
Carretera México-Toluca 3655
Lomas de Santa Fé
01210 México, D.F., Mexico
Email: mayerfou@dis1.cide.mx
Fax: (525) 727-9878
Telephone: (525) 727-9800

Carlos Montoya
Universidad de Chile
Condell 303
Providencia, Santiago, Chile
Email: cmontoya@machi.med.uchile.cl
Fax: (56 2) 204-7848, Anexo 754
Telephone: (56 2) 204-7848

Humberto Mora
FEDESARROLLO
Investigador Asociado
Calle 78 No. 9-91
Santafé de Bogotá, Colombia
Email: hmora@fedesarrollo.org.co
Fax: (571) 212-6073
Telephone: (571) 312-5300/3717 (X-310)

María Dolores Montoya Díaz
Universidad de São Paulo
Ribeirão Preto
Brasil
Email: madmdiaz@usp.br
Telephone: (55 11) 6959-5281

Brian Nolan
Economic and Social Research Institute
4 Burlington Road
Dublin 4, Ireland
Email: Brian.Nolan@esri.ie
Fax: (353 1) 668-6231
Telephone: (353 1) 667-1525

Margarita Petrera
OPS/OMS
Lima, Peru
Email: mpetrera@per.ops-oms.org
Fax: (511) 442-4634
Telephone: (511) 421-3030, ext. 272

Martín Valdivia
Grupo de Análisis para el Desarrollo -
GRADE
Av. Del Ejército
1870 Lima 27
Apartado 18-0572
Lima 18, Peru
Email: jvaldivi@grade.org.pe
Fax: (511) 264-1882

Adam Wagstaff
The World Bank
1818 H St., N.W., Room MC3-559
Washington, D.C. 20433
Email: awagstaff@worldbank.org
Telephone: (202) 473-0566
Fax: (202) 522-1153

Michael Ward
The World Bank
1818 H St., N.W., Room MC2-729
Washington, D.C. 204433
Email: mward@workdbank.org
Fax: (202) 522-364
Telephone: (202) 473-6318

José Vicente Zevallos
International Finance Corporation
2121 Pennsylvania Ave., R- 8K-120
Washington, D.C. 20433
Fax: (202) 974-4348
Telephone: (202) 458-9657
Email: Jvzevallos@worldnet.att.com/
josezevallos@ifc.org

PAHO/WHO Officers

George Alleyne
Director
PAHO/WHO
525 23rd Street, N.W.
Washington, D.C. 20037

Carol Dabbs
USAID
Team Leader, LAC/RSD-PHN
Room 5.09-103, RRB
1300 Pennsylvania Av., N.W.
Washington, D.C. 20523
Email: cdabbs@usaid.gov
Fax: (202) 216-3262
Telephone: (202) 712-0473

Sonia M. Draibe
University of Campinas
Rua São Vicente de Paula 526 Apt. 91
CEP 01229-010
Sao Paulo, Brasil
Email: smdraibe@uol.com.br

Telefax: (55 11) 3667-0289
Fax: (55 11) 3667-0631

Suzanne Dureya
Consultant
Inter-American Development Bank
1300 New York Av., OCE-W 0436
Washington, D.C. 20577

Bob Emrey
USAID
G- PHN- HN-HSPR
3.07-103
1300 Penn. Ave.
Washington, D.C. 20523
Email: bemrey@usaid.gov
Fax: (202) 216-3702
Telephone: (202) 712-4583

Ichiro Kawachi
Harvard School of Public Health
677 Huntington Ave.
Boston, MA 02115
Email: nhike@gauss.bwh.harvard.edu
Fax: (617) 432-3123
Telephone: (617) 432-0235

Felicia Knaul
WHO - AHE
Geneva, Switzerland
Email: knaulf@who.ch
Fax: (41 22) 791-4839

Gerald T. Keush
Director, Fogarty International Center
National Institutes of Health
Bethesda, MD 20892
Email: keushg@nih.gov
Fax: (301) 402-2173
Telephone: (301) 496-1491

Elsie Le Franc
The University of the West Indies
Cave Hill, Barbados
email: elefranc@uwichill.edu.bb
Fax: (246) 424-7291
Telephone: (246) 417-4478

Eduardo Lora
IADB
1300 New York Av., OCE-W 0436
Washington, D.C. 20577

Javier Martínez
DFID's Latin America Programs
C/Ausias March 6B
08810 Sant Pere de Ribes
Barcelona, Spain
Email: jmartinez@vvirtual.es
Fax: (34) 93 896-4806
Telephone: (34) 93 896-4803

William Savedoff
Inter-American Development Bank
Office of Chief Economist
1300 New York Av., OCE-W 0436
Washington, D.C. 20577
Fax: (202) 623-2481
Telephone: (202) 623-1932

Amala de Silva
c/o Mrs. Kei Kawabata, Team Coordinator
WHO
CH - 1211 Geneva 27, Switzerland
Email: kawabatak@who.ch
Fax: (41 22) 791-4828
Telephone: (41 22) 791-3160

Alfredo Solari
Senior Health Advisor IADB
1300 New York Av., OCE-W 0436
Washington, D.c. 20577

Rubén Suárez
6208 Leeke Forest Ct.
Bethesda, MD 20817
Email: Rubensu@email.msn.com

Karl Theodore
The University of the West Indies
Director
St. Augustine, Trinidad & Tobago
Email: karlt@tstt.net.tt
Telefax: (868) 662-9459

Duncan Thomas
RAND/UCLA
1700 Main St.
Santa Monica, CA 90401
Email: dthomas@rand.org
Fax: (310) 451-6935
Telephone: (310) 825-5304

Juan Antonio Casas
Director
Division of Health and Human Development
PAHO/WHO
Washington, D.C. 20037
Telephone: (202) 974-3210
Fax: (202) 974-3652
Email: casasjua@paho.org

Edward Greene
Public Policy and Health Program
Division of Health and Human Development
PAHO/WHO
Washington, D.C. 20037
Telephone: (202) 974-3122
Fax: (202) 974-3675
Email: greeneed@paho.org

Ana Mendoza
International Resident
Public Policy and Health Program
Division of Health and Human Development
PAHO/WHO
Washington, D.C. 20037
Telephone: (202) 974-3690

Raúl Molina
Public Policy and Health Program
Division of Health and Human Development
PAHO/WHO
Washington, D.C. 20037
Telephone: (202) 974-3142
Fax: (202) 974-3675
Email: molinara@paho.org

César Vieira
Coordinator
Public Policy and Health Program
Division of Health and Human Development
PAHO/WHO
Washington, D.C. 20037
Telephone: (202) 974-3235
Fax: (202) 974-3675
Email: veirace@paho.org